RADIOGRAPHIC TECHNIQUE IN SMALL ANIMAL PRACTICE

JAMES W. TICER, D.V.M., Ph.D.

Diplomate, American College of Veterinary Radiology,
Veterinary Radiologist, Berkeley Veterinary Medical Group

W. B. SAUNDERS COMPANY

Philadelphia • London • Toronto

W. B. Saunders Company: West Washington Square
Philadelphia, Pa.   19105

1 St. Anne's Road
Eastbourne, East Sussex BN21 3UN, England

833 Oxford Street
Toronto, M8Z 5T9, Canada

Library of Congress Cataloging in Publication Data

Ticer, James W

Radiographic technique in small animal practice.

Includes index.

1. Veterinary radiography.   I. Title. [DNLM: 1. Animals,
   Domestic.   2. Technology, Radiologic — Veterinary.
   SF757.8 T555r]

SF757.8.T52   636.089′607′572   74–24520

ISBN 0–7216–8860–8

Radiographic Technique in Small Animal Practice   ISBN 0-7216-8860-8

Last digit is the print number: 9   8   7   6   5   4   3   2

To my wife, Vivian

CONTRIBUTORS

JAMES K. BURT, D.V.M., M.S.
Diplomate, American College of Veterinary Radiology. Professor, Department of Veterinary Clinical Sciences, College of Veterinary Medicine, Ohio State University, Columbus. Senior Attending Clinician, Ohio State University Veterinary Teaching Hospital, Columbus, Ohio.
Contrast Pleurography

ROGER M. CLEMMONS, D.V.M.
Teaching Associate, School of Veterinary Medicine, Washington State University, Pullman, Washington.
Subtraction Radiography

CHARLES R. CONRAD, D.V.M.
Practitioner, Fort Plain Animal Hospital, Fort Plain, New York.
Cerebral Arteriography; Cerebral Ventriculography

LOUIS A. CORWIN, JR., D.V.M., Ph.D.
Diplomate, American College of Veterinary Radiology. Associate Professor, College of Veterinary Medicine; Assistant Professor, School of Medicine, University of Missouri, Columbia, Missouri.
Radiation Protection

STEPHEN J. ETTINGER, D.V.M.
Diplomate, American College of Veterinary Internal Medicine. Clinical Associate Professor of Medicine, School of Veterinary Medicine, University of California, Davis. Veterinary Cardiologist, Berkeley Veterinary Medical Group, Berkeley, California.
Angiocardiography; Pneumopericardiography

JACK C. GEARY, D.V.M.
Diplomate, American College of Veterinary Radiology. Professor and Director of Radiology, New York State College of Veterinary Medicine, Cornell University, Ithaca, New York.
Tomography

NEIL KOOYMAN, M.B.A.
Sales Manager, California X-Ray Company, Concord, California.
Equipping Radiology Department

J. E. OLIVER, JR., D.V.M., Ph.D.
Diplomate, American College of Veterinary Internal Medicine. Professor and Head, Department of Small Animal Clinics, School of Veterinary Medicine, Purdue University, West Lafayette, Indiana.
Cerebral Arteriography; Cerebral Ventriculography

EDWARD A. RHODE, D.V.M.

Diplomate, American College of Veterinary Internal Medicine. Professor of Medicine and Associate Dean of Instruction, School of Veterinary Medicine, University of California, Davis, California.

Angiocardiography

CHARLES R. ROOT, D.V.M., M.S.

Diplomate, American College of Veterinary Radiology. Associate Professor of Veterinary Radiology, Department of Veterinary Clinical Sciences, School of Veterinary Medicine, Louisiana State University, Baton Rouge, Louisiana.

Contrast Radiography of Abdomen

SAM SILVERMAN, D.V.M.

Diplomate, American College of Veterinary Radiology. Department of Radiological Sciences, School of Veterinary Medicine, University of California, Davis, California.

Avian Radiography

GARY L. WOOD, D.V.M.

Resident in Cardiology, Veterinary Medical Teaching Hospital. School of Veterinary Medicine, University of California, Davis, California.

Angiocardiography

WILLIAM J. ZONTINE, D.V.M., M.S.

Diplomate, American College of Veterinary Radiology. Lecturer, Department of Radiological Sciences, School of Veterinary Medicine, University of California, Davis, California.

Bronchography

PREFACE

Six years ago I left the rewards and frustrations of teaching and the shelter of academia to establish a consultative and referral practice in veterinary radiology. During these years I have had the privilege and probably the unique opportunity of working closely with many practicing veterinarians as a consultant in radiographic technique and radiologic diagnosis. Generally, I have found that the ability to render an accurate radiologic diagnosis is compromised by referral radiographic examinations that are technically deficient. Some of these are a result of improper exposure or darkroom techniques or of inadequate equipment, but by far the most common error encountered is improper patient preparation or positioning. From these observations, this book was conceived.

The purpose of this book is to provide a source of information on radiographic technique in small animal practice for use by veterinary students, by practitioners and by their technical assistants. The format presents the more theoretical aspects of radiographic technique in the first part of the book and an atlas on technique and positioning in the second part. I have tried to keep the theoretical concepts that are necessary for an understanding of radiographic technique in practical perspective in an effort to make their consumption more tolerable. The atlas on technique and positioning is arranged according to regional anatomy and, in most cases, pertinent radiographic anatomy is illustrated by line drawing overlays and labels. No attempt has been made to illustrate pathologic anatomy except where illustration of a particular technique is enhanced by its use.

I am very fortunate in having obtained contributions in specific areas from several experts in their fields. Without their efforts, this book would not have been possible and I am deeply indebted to them.

The errors and omissions that may be present in this book should be brought to my attention, since improvement can only be made with knowledge.

The effort necessary to produce this volume required the assistance of several individuals. In addition to my colleagues who gave so generously of their time and knowledge to provide contributions for the text, many other persons gave me encouragement and technical help. My partners at the Berkeley Veterinary Medical Group, Drs. S. Gary Brown and Steve Ettinger, have continually provided me with the necessary stimulation to remain abreast of the current trends in our profession. Without the editorial assistance of Ms. Barbara Warren, the original manuscript would have remained a clutter of extraneous verbiage.

The advice and direction provided by Mr. Carroll Cann has been outstanding. As veterinary editor for the W. B. Saunders Company, his encouragement and friendship were a vital stimulus in undertaking the task of producing this book. Miss Catherine Fix of the editorial department, Mr. Ray Kersey of the illustration department, and Ms. Lorraine Battista of the design department of the W. B. Saunders Company have been extremely helpful during the production of the book. Mrs. Laura Tarves, as production manager for veterinary titles, has made the flow from manuscript to printed page go smoothly.

There is nothing that I can write that would adequately express my gratitude for the efforts of my wife, Vivian, during the production of this book. She possesses the unique ability of translating my handwritten hieroglyphics into a typewritten page, which she did with great skill. Her encouragement and assistance have made my career and this book possible.

JAMES W. TICER

CONTENTS

SECTION I

PHYSICAL PRINCIPLES

X RAY GENERATION

INTRODUCTION

Fundamentally, an x-ray tube consists of a source of electrons and a target with which the electrons can interact after being accelerated across a given space. The resultant electron-target interaction generates X rays and heat. The electron source is usually a cathode that has been heated to a temperature required to impart escape velocities to the electrons. Electrons are thereby made available in a semifree state, as a cloud adjacent to the cathode surface.

By applying a positive potential to the target (anode) side of the tube through a voltage source that has its negative side attached to the cathode, the electron cloud can be accelerated across the vacuum and caused to collide and interact with the target material. By controlling the time for which the positive potential is applied to the anode, the number of generated X rays may be regulated. The three basic components of a functional x-ray generator are an electron source, a positive accelerating voltage and a timing mechanism.

TYPES OF ELECTRON-TARGET INTERACTIONS

Usually, an accelerated electron must undergo several interactions with target atoms before losing all its energy. Two types of energy losses occur—collisional losses and radiation losses. Stated simply, collisional losses involve the outer electrons of the target atom and generate heat, whereas radiation losses involve the nucleus of the target atom and are responsible for the x-radiation generated (Johns, 1961). The number of these individual interactions may be as high as many thousands for an accelerated electron used in diagnostic radiography.

Collisional Interactions

Two types of collisional interactions are illustrated diagrammatically in Figure 1–1. In the first type (Fig. 1–1 A), an incoming electron may excite an outer orbital electron of the target atom by passing in near proximity to its orbit, thus transferring energy. This allows the orbital electron to increase its distance from the nucleus, or raise its orbit. When the excited orbital electron returns to its original orbit, energy is irradiated as heat (Johns, 1961).

A second type of collisional interaction (Fig. 1–1 B) may occur if the incoming electron possesses sufficient energy to remove an outer orbital electron from a target atom. The target atom is then ionized. The ejected electron (if it possesses energies in excess of the order of 100 electron volts) and the incoming electron then undergo additional interactions with target atoms. The total energy loss is eventually dissipated as heat (Johns, 1961).

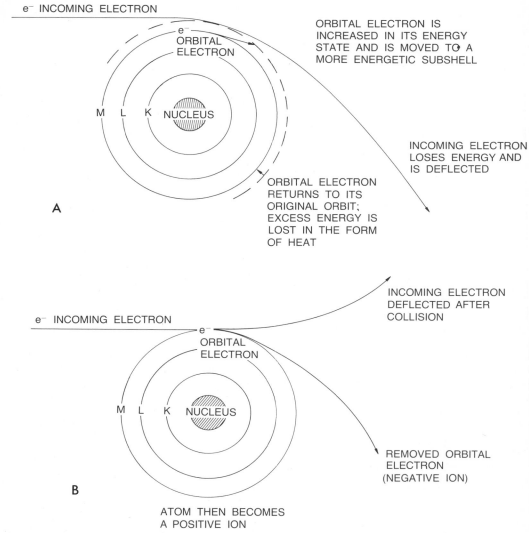

Figure 1–1. Collisional interactions. *A,* Collisional interaction produced when an incoming electron excites an outer orbital electron of the target atom by passing in near proximity to its orbit, thus transferring energy. This allows the orbital electron to increase its distance from the nucleus, or raise its orbit. When the excited orbital electron returns to its original orbit, energy is irradiated as heat. *B,* Collisional interaction produced when an incoming electron possesses sufficient energy to remove an outer orbital electron from a target atom. The target atom is then ionized. Energy lost by the incoming electron is irradiated as heat.

Heat Losses

When an accelerated electron beam interacts with a tungsten x-ray tube target, more than 99 per cent of the energy dissipated is in the form of heat from collisional interactions. The remaining energy is irradiated in the form of X rays.

Tungsten targets are used in diagnostic x-ray tubes because they possess a high melting point and have the ability to generate x-ray energies that are useful in diagnostic radiography. The tungsten target is usually embedded in copper, since this metal has the ability to conduct heat away from the target efficiently. Heat loss also occurs by direct radiation to surrounding material.

In order to appreciate the magnitude of the energy that must be dissipated as heat, one should review the principle of power distribution in an electrical circuit. Energy developed in the anode of an x-ray tube is given by:

$$P = VI$$

where P is the power expressed in joules[1] per second or watts, V is the potential difference in volts across the circuit, and I is the current in amperes flowing through the circuit. As an example, a diagnostic x-ray tube operating at 100 kilovolts (KV) (100,000 volts) and 300 milliamperes (ma) (0.3 amperes) has a rate of energy dissipation of $VI = 100,000 \times 0.3 = 30,000$ watts. This is approximately five times the rate of energy dissipation that is created by a large cooking element of an electric stove.

It is obvious that prolonged current flow (amperage) created by exposures that exceed the capabilities of an x-ray tube should not be permitted. Excessive heating of the target results in melting of the tungsten element, with its secondary effect of decreased x-ray output for a given number of electrons interacting with the tungsten element. Figure 1–2 illustrates damage caused by target overheating. Diagnostic x-ray tubes should, therefore, never be used for x-ray therapeutic purposes.

Generally, the larger the target, the more efficient will be the heat dissipation. For purposes of constructing a diagnostic x-ray tube, however, a small target size is desirable (Cahoon, 1965; Carlson, 1967; Fuchs, 1966).

Tube Rating Charts

Tube rating charts are provided for all x-ray tubes to assist the operator in determin-

[1]The joule is 10 million ergs. Power is the rate of doing work and is measured in joules per second (1 joule per second = 1 watt).

ing the maximum exposure characteristics that permit safe operation. By maintaining exposure factors below these factors, heat developed at the anode will not result in melting. Figure 1–3 illustrates a typical chart for anode size of 2.0 mm. An upper limit of exposure time may be determined by following the milliamperage value on the ordinate to the appropriate kilovoltage value curve. The maximum exposure time for safe operation is then determined by drawing a vertical line to the abscissa, on which the scale of time in seconds is recorded. For example, a tube operated at 300 ma and 80 KV would have an exposure time limit of approximately 1.5 seconds to remain within safe operating limits. Prolonged tube life may be assured by operating the x-ray equipment within safe limits.

Radiative Interactions

Radiative interaction occurs when the incoming electron possesses sufficient energy to remove an inner (K or L shell) orbital electron from the target atom (Johns, 1961). The ejected electron is replaced by an outer orbital electron and the difference in the binding energies of the ejected electron and the replacement electron is irradiated as characteristic x-ray radiation (Fig. 1–4 A). The term "characteristic" is derived from the fact that these radiations are characteristic for a given target atom, since the differences in orbital electron-binding energies are unique.

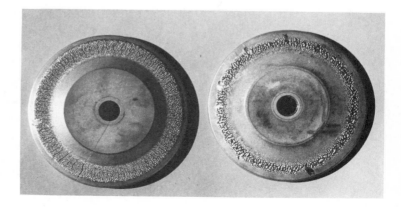

Figure 1–2. Damaged anodes. Heat damage (melting) to x-ray tube targets (rotating anodes) due to improper use.

RATING CHART FOR SINGLE-PHASE FULL-WAVE RECTIFICATION

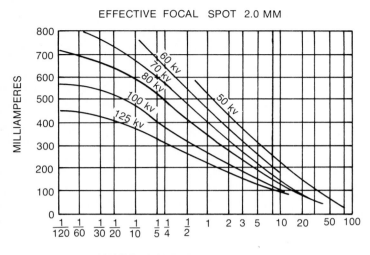

EFFECTIVE FOCAL SPOT 2.0 MM

MAXIMUM EXPOSURE TIME IN SECONDS

Figure 1–3. Tube rating chart for a tube operated with a single-phase, full-wave rectified generator. Maximum milliampere and exposure times for a given kilovoltage operation for safe x-ray tube operation may be calculated from this chart. Rating charts are characteristic for each tube type and are not interchangeable.

A second type of radiative interaction occurs when incoming electrons approach the nucleus of a target atom and are attracted toward the positive nucleus. The attraction of these two opposite charges causes the incoming electron to orbit partially around the nucleus. The change in electron direction results in reduced velocity.

The energy lost by decreasing the velocity is irradiated in the form of x-radiation (Fig. 1–4 *B*). The sudden deceleration, or "braking," of the incoming electron gives rise to the German term "bremsstrahlung" or braking radiation. This type of x-radiation is more probable with increased energies of incoming electrons.

The energy of the resulting bremsstrahlung radiations varies with the energy of the incoming electron and the angle of the interaction with the target atom. In contrast to characteristic radiations, bremsstrahlung radiations possess a spectrum of energies.

Spectrum of X-ray Energies Generated

With the energies used in diagnostic radiography (40 to 120 KV), the majority of the x-radiation generated is in the form of bremsstrahlung radiation. Bremsstrahlung radiation energies vary with the energies possessed by the accelerated electrons and are a function of the magnitude of the voltage applied between the anode and cathode of the x-ray tube as well as of the proximity to the nucleus where the reaction occurs. Thus, a wide range of x-ray energies is generated.

Figure 1–5 illustrates the spectrum of characteristic and bremsstrahlung radiations generated by a tungsten target for accelerating voltages of 65, 100, and 150 KV. Note that the energy of the peaks created by the characteristic radiations of tungsten does not vary with the voltage applied across the x-ray tube. Only the relative number increases with increased accelerating voltage.

The bremsstrahlung radiation spectrum, on the other hand, shows an increase in the maximum energy as the accelerating voltage is increased. This phenomenon accounts for the relative increase in x-ray beam energy as the kilovoltage (accelerating voltage) of the x-ray machine is increased.

The dashed lines in Figure 1–5 represent the theoretical distribution of bremsstrahlung radiation. In the low energy region, the curve decreases rapidly to zero

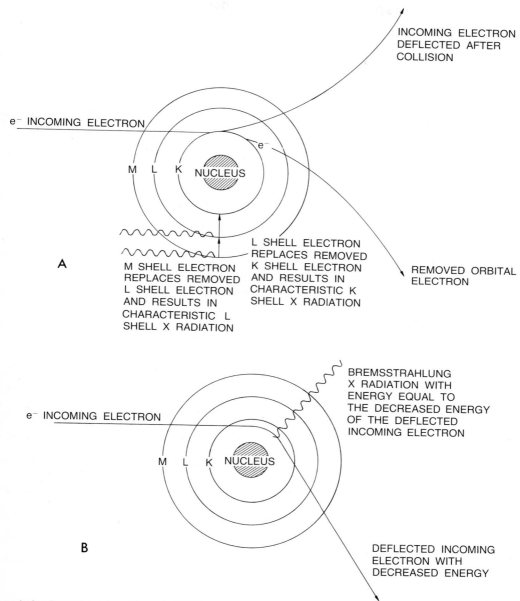

Figure 1–4. Radiative interactions. *A*, Radiative interaction produced when an incoming electron possesses sufficient energy to remove an inner orbital electron from the target atom. The ejected electron is replaced by an outer orbital electron and the difference in binding energies of the ejected electron and the replacement electron is irradiated as characteristic X radiation. *B*, Radiative interaction produced when incoming electrons approach the nucleus of a target atom and are attracted toward the positive field, resulting in the electron partially orbiting the nucleus. The change in direction reduces velocity and this loss is irradiated in the form of X radiation termed "bremsstrahlung" radiation.

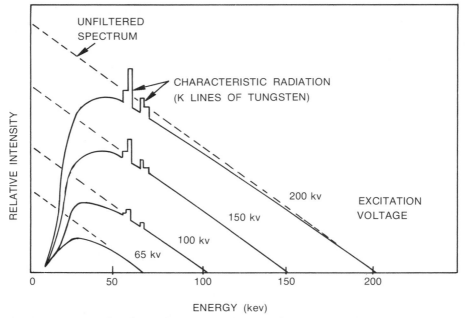

Figure 1–5. X-ray spectrum. Graphic representation of the variation of x-ray energies generated as a function of the energy of bombarding electrons interacting with a tungsten target. (From Johns, H. E., *The Physics of Radiology*, 2nd ed., 1961. Courtesy of Charles C Thomas, Publisher, Springfield, Illinois.)

at approximately 10 KV. This phenomenon occurs because the relatively decreased energy levels of bremsstrahlung radiations below 10 KV are not able to penetrate the target metal, vacuum tube wall and other filtering material placed in the x-ray beam.

The usefulness of the x-ray beam spectrum for diagnostic radiography decreases rapidly below approximately 40 KV, since penetration of the patient's body parts is not easily accomplished below this energy level. To prevent absorption of relatively nonpenetrating, low energy X rays by the superficial layers of a patient's body, they are removed from the primary x-ray beam by the addition of a thin layer (2 to 3 mm) of aluminum (added filtration).

It is important to recall that the distribution of the low energy X rays is not affected by increased operating voltages. Increasing the voltage applied across the tube only increases the maximum energy of the x-ray spectrum and does not increase the minimal energy. Filtration of the x-ray beam with aluminum to remove the less penetrating X rays, therefore, remains as important for high voltages as it is for low voltages.

Heel Effect

There is an unequal distribution of the x-ray beam intensity as it leaves the x-ray tube (Fig. 1–6). This variation has a definite relationship to the angle of the x-ray tube target. When the angle of the target is 20 degrees from the central ray, distribution of beam intensity decreases rapidly toward the anode (positive) side of the tube. This phenomenon is due to absorption of the x-ray beam by target and anode material. The x-ray beam on the cathode (negative) side of the tube is slightly more intense than the central ray. This is the so-called "heel effect."

This phenomenon may be used to good advantage when radiographing parts of unequal thickness. By placing the thickest part of the patient toward the cathode of the x-ray tube, a more uniform density of the radiograph may be obtained. The heel effect can be used most effectively when radiographing relatively long patients with marked differences in part thickness, such as the abdomen of a dog with a deep thorax. This method should always be considered when using a 14 × 17 inch cassette. The heel effect is not noticeable when radiographing parts that are less than 12 inches in length.

X-RAY TUBE CONSTRUCTION

An x-ray tube is essentially a large diode-type electronic tube. The heated cathode acts as a source of electrons and the anode acts as the positive plate that contains an embedded tungsten target (Fig. 1–7). These elements are placed within a glass envelope

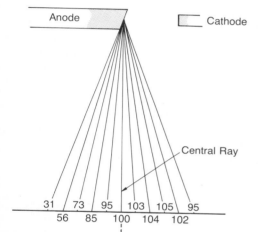

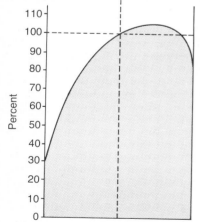

Figure 1–6. Heel effect. The unequal distribution of x-ray beam intensity is shown to decrease rapidly toward the anode of the x-ray tube, producing the so-called heel effect. This phenomenon is due to absorption of the x-ray beam by the target and the anode material.

which is then evacuated to form a vacuum. This vacuum will prevent rapid oxidation of the elements. A thin window area is formed in the glass envelope to act as an exit for the x-ray beam to decrease the x-ray-absorbing qualities of the glass. The entire tube is then enclosed in a metal container to control the escape of stray radiation and to protect the glass envelope from physical damage.

The cathode is usually placed in a shallow depression called a focusing cup. An electrical potential is applied to the focusing cup to control the electron beam diameter, thereby confining the electron beam to the target area. A decreased target area (focal spot) increases the detail of the resultant radiographic image and, therefore, the focal spot should remain as small as possible. The lower limit of focal spot size is governed by the ability of the anode to dissipate the heat of collisional electron interactions within the target material.

The effective focal spot size may be decreased by placing the face of the target at approximately 20 degrees to the cathode (Fig. 1–8). The effective focal spot size is made smaller than the actual focal spot size due to an artifact of geometric projection. Manufacturers of x-ray tubes designate the size of the effective focal spot. The so-called 1.0 mm focal spot tube, therefore, has a *projected* focal spot measuring 1 mm × 1 mm.

Dissipation of heat may also be enhanced by placing the tungsten target material in the form of a strip around the circumference of a high speed rotating disc (Fig. 1–9). This device prevents continuous bombardment of the same target surface and thus allows cooling of the target element. Rotating anode tubes may contain a focal spot of approximately one sixth the size required for stationary anode tubes. X-ray machines with high milliamperage capabilities require the use of rotating anode x-ray tubes to prevent excessive heat damage to the target surface. Rotating anode x-ray tubes, therefore, are a good investment despite their increased cost.

Some x-ray tubes have two cathodes and focusing cups, each producing a different electron beam diameter for use in differing exposure techniques. Thus, when decreased milliamperage is required, the smaller effective focal spot may be used to increase radiographic detail.

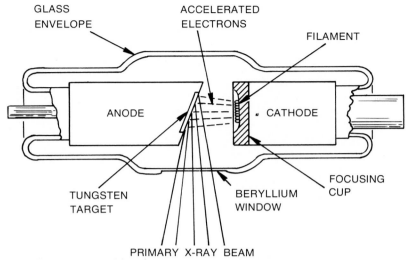

Figure 1–7. Diagram of simple x-ray tube.

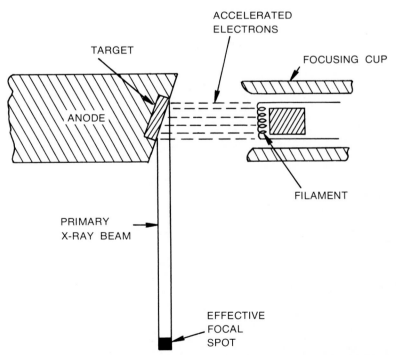

Figure 1–8. Effective focal spot. Effective focal spot is decreased by placing the target at 20 degrees to the cathode.

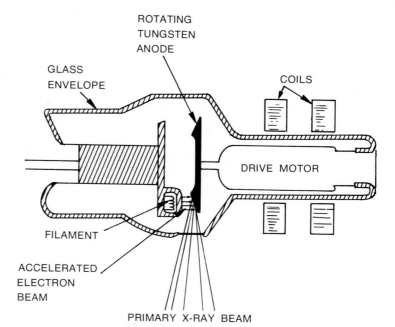

Figure 1–9. Rotating anode. Dissipation of heat is enhanced by placing the target material in the form of a strip around the circumference of a high speed rotating disc.

ELECTRICAL CIRCUITS FOR X-RAY TUBE CONTROL

High Voltage Circuit

Relatively simple electrical circuitry is necessary to provide the x-ray tube with a source of high voltage potential for accelerating electrons from the cathode to the anode. This circuitry is shown diagrammatically in Figure 1–10. High voltage is generated by a step-up transformer. By adding an appropriate number of windings to the transformer's secondary, the input of 60 cycles alternating voltage may be increased from 110 or 220 volts to the required 40 to 120 KV.

Variation of the voltage applied to the

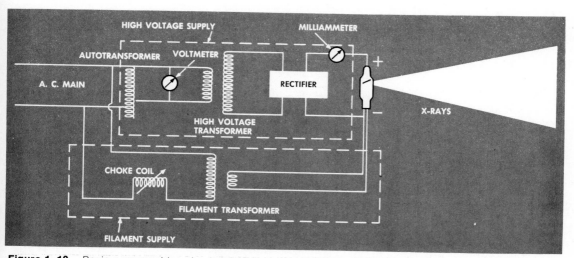

Figure 1–10. Basic x-ray machine circuitry. Diagrammatic illustration of the basic circuitry necessary to provide the x-ray tube with a source of high voltage potential for accelerating electrons from cathode to anode (target). (From Eastman Kodak Co., *The Fundamentals of Radiology*. Radiographic Markets Division, Eastman Kodak Co., Rochester, N.Y.)

primary winding of the high voltage transformer permits one to control the output voltage in the secondary winding, and thereby to control the voltage applied across the x-ray tube. This is accomplished by an autotransformer. An autotransformer differs from other transformer types by having both the primary and secondary windings contained in one winding. A switching device allows voltages to be obtained from various levels on the winding. The kilovoltage selection switch on the x-ray machine control panel is connected to this mechanism on the autotransformer.

Filament Circuit

A simple stepdown transformer (Fig. 1–10) is applied between the input voltage of the x-ray machine and the cathode filament, since the filament voltage supply must be relatively low, while the current flow or amperage must be high. The number of electrons available for flow to the target of the x-ray tube is a function of cathode heat.

Increased cathode heat results in increased electron availability and thus in an increased electron flow and an increased number of X rays generated.

Decreasing the amperage in the cathode filament results in decreased heat and, thereby, decreased availability of electrons. Control of the amperage in the cathode filament therefore accomplishes direct control over the number of X rays produced in a given time period.

Amperage control is accomplished by inserting a choke coil (Fig. 1–10) in the input side of the primary winding of the filament transformer. The impedancy (resistance in an alternating current circuit) may be varied by inserting or retracting the core of the coil. This mechanism is connected to the milliampere control of the x-ray control console.

Timer

Completion of a functional x-ray machine requires only the addition of an accurate timer switch in the primary windings of the high voltage transformer. This device will control the amount of time for which high voltage is applied across the x-ray tube and thereby control the duration of x-ray generation.

Various mechanical and electronic devices have been manufactured for this purpose. Electronic timing devices are necessary for the short exposure times required in diagnostic veterinary radiography. Though these are more expensive, the increased expense must be accepted as a necessary investment.

Rectification Circuits

Rectification of the alternating voltage applied to the x-ray tube increases the efficiency of the unit. Basically, "self-rectification" is a term used to describe the limitation of current flow across the x-ray tube in one direction, that is, from the cathode to the anode. The inefficiency of a self-rectified x-ray machine can only be tolerated in portable equipment.

When an alternating 60-cycle voltage is applied to the x-ray tube, electrons flow from the cathode to the anode only when a positive voltage is applied to the anode. During one half of every cycle, a negative potential is applied to the anode, resulting in no electron flow and no x-ray generation. The result is 60 pulses of X rays generated every second.

By placing a valve tube (diode) in the high voltage supply, the anode of the x-ray tube can be protected from the extremely high negative voltages (Fig. 1–11), and the cathode from high positive potentials. This protection becomes important practically when high milliamperage generators are used, because increased current (electron) flow results in anode heating sufficient to make some electrons available in the form of an electron cloud, similar to the phenomenon occurring at the heated cathode. If a high positive voltage is applied to the cathode, an electron beam will be accelerated toward the filament of the cathode, causing severe damage due to electron bombardment.

Prolongation of x-ray tube life is accomplished by the addition of valve tube rectification. The efficiency of a valve-rectified x-ray generator is, however, not appreciably increased over the self-rectified system,

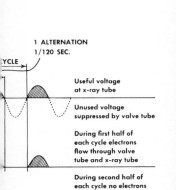

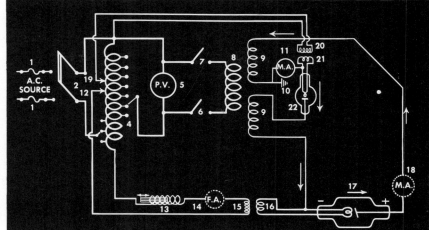

LEGEND FOR CIRCUIT DIAGRAMS

1. Fuses
2. Switch
3. Autotransformer
3A. Autotransformer line-voltage compensator
4. Autotransformer control
5. Prereading voltmeter
6. Circuit breaker
7. Automatic timer
8. Primary of high-voltage transformer
9. Secondary of high-voltage transformer
10. Ground
11. Milliammeter
12. Circuit connector for cathode filament

13. Voltage control for cathode filament with adjustable iron core
14. Ammeter for cathode filament
15. Primary of cathode filament transformer
16. Secondary of cathode filament transformer
17. X-ray tube
18. Milliammeter in high-voltage circuit
19. Circuit connector for valve-tube filament
20. Primary of valve-tube filament transformer
21. Secondary of valve-tube filament transformer
22. Valve tube

Figure 1–11. Half-wave rectification circuit. Circuit for half-wave rectification by means of a single valve tube. (Arrows indicate electron flow.) The resulting voltage wave form is shown on the left. (From Eastman Kodak Co., *The Fundamentals of Radiography*. Radiographic Markets Division, Eastman Kodak Co., Rochester N.Y.)

since one half of the voltage input cycle is wasted. The resultant x-ray generation is similarly pulsed at a rate of 60 per second.

By adding four valve tubes to the high voltage supply in such a manner that positive voltage is always applied to the anode of the x-ray tube, the efficiency of operation is increased by 100 per cent (Fig. 1–12). A pulsing positive voltage is then applied to the x-ray tube anode at the rate of 120 times per second. This results in twice the x-ray output than is achieved with the half-wave rectified units. The advantage of the full-wave rectified generator becomes obvious when one considers that exposures can be made in half the time—a consideration that is extremely important in veterinary radiography, where patient movement is always a problem.

Condenser Discharge Units

An alternate method of generating the extremely high voltages necessary to produce diagnostic radiographs is by the use of a condenser discharge generator. High voltage is generated by charging a relatively large condenser with a low-power circuit taken from the input voltage available. This voltage input may be from a standard 110 volt supply. A charge is allowed to build up to the desired kilovoltage.

The voltage is then switched to the x-ray tube, where it discharges in a fraction of a second. The resulting electron flow generates X rays in a similar manner to when an alternating voltage source is used. The condenser discharge generator has the advantage of giving high voltage performance

LEGEND FOR CIRCUIT DIAGRAMS

1. Fuses
2. Switch
3. Autotransformer
3A. Autotransformer line-voltage compensator
4. Autotransformer control
5. Prereading voltmeter
6. Circuit breaker
7. Automatic timer
8. Primary of high-voltage transformer
9. Secondary of high-voltage transformer
10. Ground
11. Milliammeter
12. Circuit connector for cathode filament

13. Voltage control for cathode filament with adjustable iron core
14. Ammeter for cathode filament
15. Primary of cathode filament transformer
16. Secondary of cathode filament transformer
17. X-ray tube
18. Milliammeter in high-voltage circuit
19. Circuit connector for valve-tube filament
20. Primary of valve-tube filament transformer
21. Secondary of valve-tube filament transformer
22. Valve tube

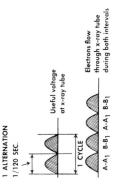

1 ALTERNATION
1/120 SEC.

Useful voltage at x-ray tube

1 CYCLE

A-A₁ B-B₁ A-A₁ B-B₁

Electrons flow through x-ray tube during both intervals

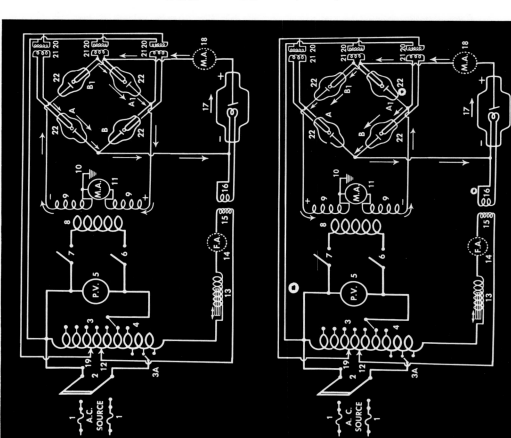

Figure 1–12. Full-wave rectification circuit. Circuit for full-wave rectification in which four tubes are used. The resulting wave form is shown on the right. (From Eastern Kodak Co., *The Fundamentals of Radiography*. Radiographic Markets Division, Eastman Kodak Co., Rochester, N.Y.)

from low voltage supplies. This is an obvious advantage in mobile equipment and should find a use in veterinary radiography, where mobility and high voltage performance often are needed.

REFERENCES

Cahoon, J. B.: Formulating X-ray Techniques. 6th ed. Durham, North Carolina, Duke University Press, 1965.

Carlson, W. D.: Veterinary Radiology. 2nd ed. Philadelphia, Lea and Febiger, 1967.

Eastman Kodak Company: The Fundamentals of Radiography. 11th ed. Rochester, N. Y., 1968.

Fuchs, A. W.: Principles of Radiographic Exposure and Processing. 2nd ed. Springfield, Ill., Charles C Thomas, Publisher, 1966.

Glasser, O., Quimby, E. H., Taylor, L. S., Weatherwax, J. L., and Morgan, R. H.: Physical Foundations of Radiology. 3rd ed. New York, P. B. Hoeber, Inc., 1961.

Johns, H. E.: The Physics of Radiology. 2nd ed. Springfield, Ill., Charles C Thomas, Publisher, 1961.

Lapp, R. E., and Andrews, H. L.: Nuclear Radiation Physics. 3rd ed. Englewood Cliffs, N. J., Prentice-Hall, Inc., 1963.

Ticer, J. W.: Production of diagnostic radiographs in veterinary medicine. I. Machine factors. Calif. Vet., 23:18–21, 1969.

2

IMAGE FORMATION AND RECORDING

INTRODUCTION

The usefulness of a radiographic examination is necessarily limited by the quality of the image recording process. Distortion caused by faulty geometric projection of the part examined is frequently a cause of poor quality radiographs. The vast majority of unsatisfactory radiographic examinations are, however, caused by poor radiographic density, contrast or detail. Multiple factors relating to the patient type, radiographic technique and darkroom methods affect the production of high quality radiographic examinations.

GEOMETRY OF IMAGE FORMATION

An accurate recording of patient shape is necessary in order to obtain quality radiographs. Distortion of the projected image may result in inaccurate interpretation. It is therefore important to understand the effect of geometric projection of the subject onto the recording surface.

To preserve accurate geometric projection, the subject to be examined and the recording surface must be parallel. Figure 2–1 A illustrates this effect. Note that, when relatively large areas are radiographed, it is not necessary for the x-ray source to be di-

rectly above the part examined if the part and the recording surface are parallel (Eastman Kodak Co., 1968). If the part being examined is not parallel to the recording surface, geometric distortion results (Fig. 2–1 B). This fact becomes important in veterinary radiography when the long bones of the appendicular skeleton are examined. An example of the artifactual shortening of the femur that may occur if the bone is not parallel to the recording surface is illustrated in Figure 2–2 A and B.

Although geometric shape is preserved by a parallel positioning of subject and recording surface, a significant enlargement in the recorded image occurs when the distance between the subject and the recording surface is increased (Fig. 2–3 A and B) (Carlson, 1967; Eastman Kodak Co., 1968). Figure 2–4 illustrates this magnifying effect when a lateral recumbent radiographic view of both scapulo-humeral articulations are produced simultaneously. Note that the humerus lying farther from the recording surface is artifactually enlarged.

The geometric relationships between areas of radiolucency and radiodensity are important to consider, especially when the vertebral column is radiographed. Figure 2–5 A and B illustrates these relationships in the radiographic examination of the caudal cervical vertebrae in a ventrodorsal projec-

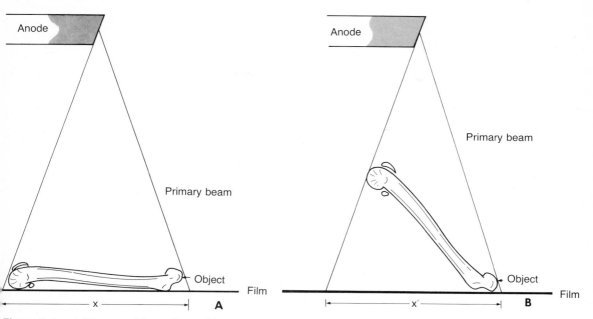

Figure 2–1. *A,* Diagram of the radiographic projection when a long bone such as a femur is placed parallel to a recording surface such as a film. Note that there is only a minor artifactual recorded length increase, especially when the part is placed close to the film. *B,* Diagram of the radiographic projection when a femur is placed at an angle to the film. Note that there is an artifactual shortening when projected onto the recording surface.

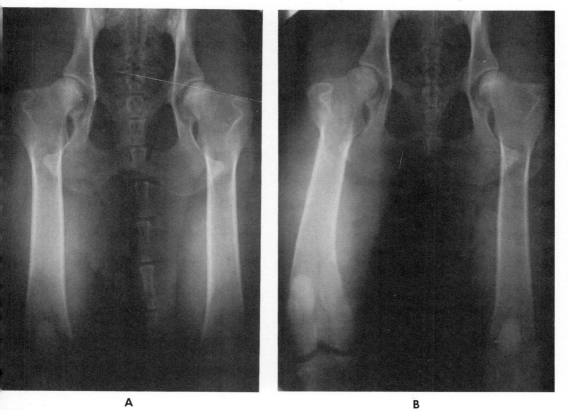

Figure 2–2. *A,* A radiograph produced with both femurs placed parallel to the film. *B,* A radiograph produced with the left femur placed parallel to the film and the right femur placed at an increased angle by allowing the hip to flex. This is the same dog as in *A.*

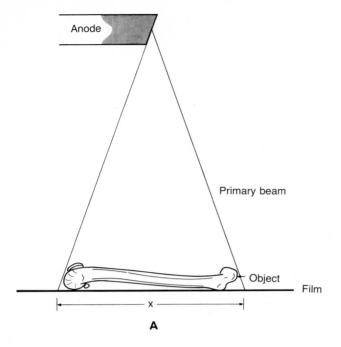

A

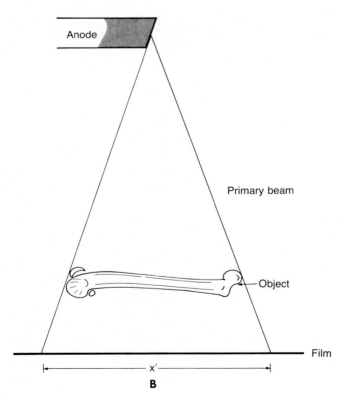

B

Figure 2–3. *A,* Diagram of the effect of placing the patient in close proximity to the film. Note that very little magnification occurs. Increasing the distance between the x-ray source and the film (FFD) would decrease the magnitude of this artifact. *B,* Diagram of the magnification effect produced by increasing the distance between the patient and film.

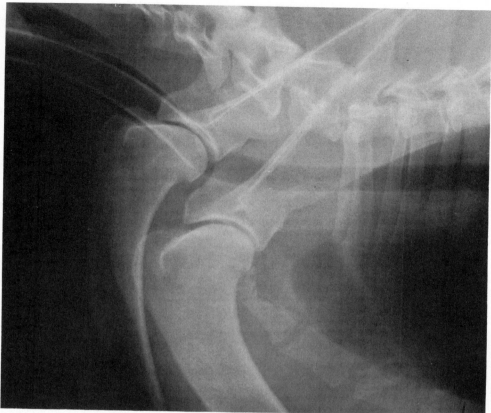

Figure 2–4. A lateral radiographic projection illustrates the principle shown in Figure 2–3. Note that the humerus and ribs that are farthest from the film are magnified. Radiographic detail is also decreased by increasing the distance between the patient part and the film, which is also illustrated in this study.

tion. Note that either elevating the caudal cervical vertebrae or shifting the angle of the x-ray tube caudally results in an improved projection of the intervertebral spaces, as shown in Figure 2–6 *A* and *B*.

Accurate projection of interfaces between a series of radiolucent and radiodense objects, such as vertebrae, requires that these parts be parallel to the recording surface. Figure 2–7 *A* shows the inaccurate projection of cervical vertebrae in a lateral recumbent view when these parts are allowed to sag toward the recording surface, thus producing artifactually narrowed intervertebral spaces (Bartels and Hoerlein, 1971; Carlson, 1967). If the midcervical region is elevated, a more accurate projection is obtained (Fig. 2–7 *B*). Note that the intervertebral spaces are now nearly the same width.

A further example of the geometric projection of radiolucent-radiodense planes is found in the artifactual narrowing of intervertebral disc spaces that occurs as the distance from the central ray of the x-ray beam is increased (Bartels and Hoerlein, 1971). Figure 2–8 illustrates this principle in a lateral recumbent radiography of a lumbar vertebral column. Note that the intervertebral spaces appear to decrease caudal to the L-1, L-2 interspace, where the central ray of the x-ray beam was placed. This fact becomes particularly important when evaluating radiographs for possible intervertebral disc herniations. Multiple lateral recumbent views of the vertebral column, with the central ray of the x-ray beam placed at several different levels, are necessary for accurate evaluation of a series of intervertebral spaces.

(*Text continued on page 23.*)

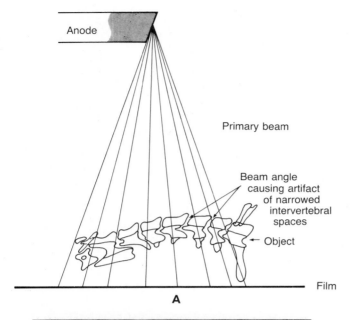

Anode

Primary beam

Beam angle
causing artifact
of narrowed
intervertebral
spaces

Object

Film

A

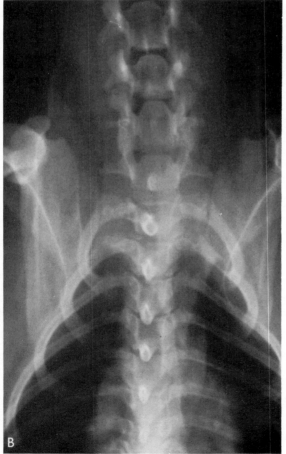

B

Figure 2–5. *A,* Diagram of the radiographic projection produced when the patient is placed in a ventro-dorsal position and the x-ray beam is placed perpendicular to the film. *B,* A radiograph produced under these conditions. Note the artifactually narrowed intervertebral spaces in the caudal cervical and cranial thoracic region.

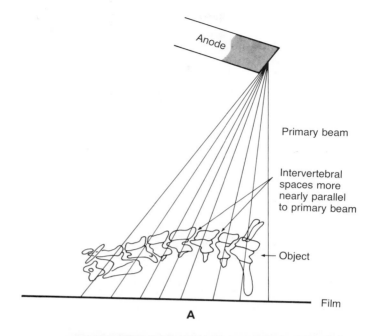

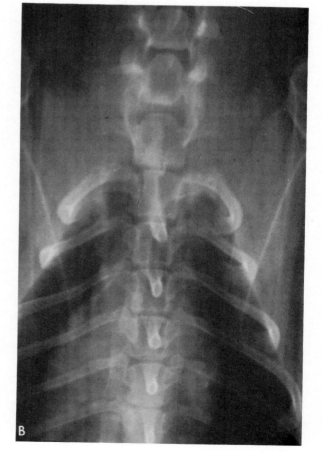

Figure 2–6. *A,* Diagram of the radiographic projection produced when the patient is placed in a ventro-dorsal position and the x-ray beam is directed approximately 15 degrees caudal from the perpendicular. *B,* A radiograph produced under these conditions. Note the nearly accurate projection of the intervertebral spaces.

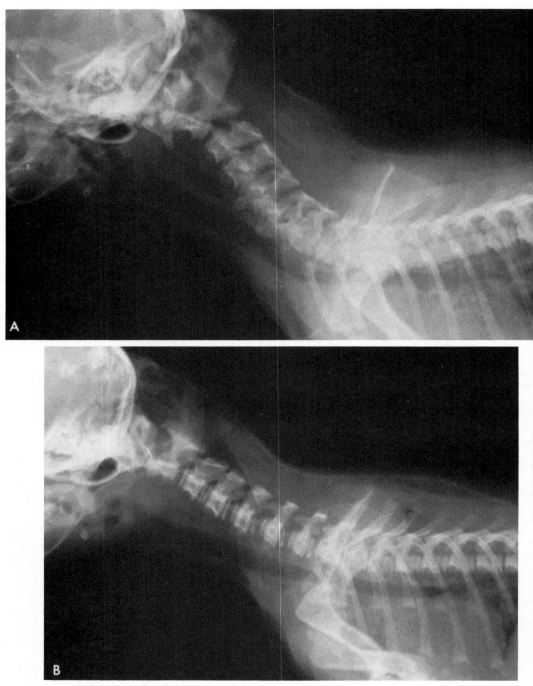

Figure 2–7. *A*, A lateral radiograph of the cervical region of a 7 week old Dachshund produced by allowing the central cervical vertebrae to sag toward the film. Note that this position artifactually produces a bizarre appearance of the central and caudal vertebral bodies and intervertebral spaces which does not allow for adequate radiographic interpretation. *B*, A lateral radiograph of the cervical vertebrae in the same position as in *A* produced by maintaining a parallel relationship between the film and the vertebral bodies of the entire cervical and thoracic region. Note the normal appearance of the epiphyseal lines and the narrowed intervertebral space between C-3 and C-4.

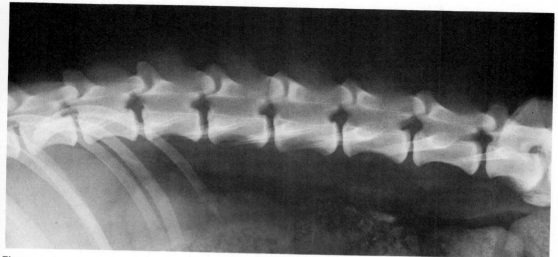

Figure 2–8. A lateral radiograph of the lumbar vertebrae produced with the central x-ray beam centered at L-2. Note the artifactually narrowed intervertebral spaces both cranial and caudal to this body, produced by the increased angle of incidence.

RADIOGRAPHIC CONTRAST

The differences in the densities of the various subjects on a finished radiograph are termed radiographic contrast (Carlson, 1967; Eastman Kodak Co., 1968). These differences are a function of both film contrast and subject or patient contrast. Generally, film contrast is constant and, for practical purposes, need not be considered as a variable in veterinary radiography.

Modern medical x-ray film usually exaggerates the differences in x-ray image contrast by a factor of two (Eastman Kodak Co., 1968). This means that for a given density difference between two tissues, such as bone and muscle, approximately twice this difference will be recorded on a finished radiograph, compared to the original image displayed on a fluoroscopic screen. Proper developing technique must also be maintained to preserve this contrast created by film type.

Differences in density found on a finished radiograph are, in part, a function of the differences in x-ray absorption by the tissues of the patient and also of the average atomic number of the components of the various tissues (Johns, 1950). This is true only for x-ray absorption in the energy range used in medical radiography, where the principal mode of x-ray absorption is by the photoelectric effect (Johns, 1961). This mechanism of electromagnetic energy absorption varies with the number of electrons per gram of absorbing material, which in turn varies with atomic number (Johns, 1961). An increased average atomic number of the absorbing material will, therefore, result in increased x-ray absorption. (Recall that a higher atomic number represents an increase in the proton number and, therefore, an increase in the number of orbital electrons, since the proton or atomic number is equal to the orbital electron number in electrically neutral substances.) It is easy to see that calcium- and phosphorus-containing bone will absorb a greater number of x-rays than muscle, which contains relatively more atoms of low atomic numbers, such as nitrogen, oxygen, and hydrogen. These differences in absorption rate for x-ray energies used in medical radiography make possible the recording of contrast on a finished radiograph.

Increased x-ray energies (produced by increased accelerating voltage applied across the x-ray tube) result in both increased penetrability of the x-ray beam and decreased difference in contrast at subject interfaces, such as bone and muscle (Glasser et al., 1961). Figure 2–9 shows graphically that the number of electrons per gram of absorbing material becomes less im-

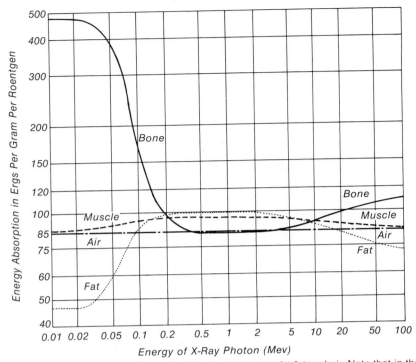

Figure 2–9. A graph of the absorption of x-ray photons by bone, muscle, fat and air. Note that in the range below 0.2 Mev (200 Kev) the difference in absorption ability between these media increases rapidly with decreasing electromagnetic energy. This is due to the photoelectric absorption effect and accounts for the selection of this energy range for use in medical radiography, since the resultant radiographic image depends on the different absorption rates of various tissues. (After Johns, H. E.: Radiation therapy: depth dose. *In* Glasser, O. (Ed.), *Medical Physics,* Vol. II. Chicago, Year Book Publishers, Inc., 1950.)

portant to the differential absorption of X rays as the energy of the x-ray beam increases. This phenomenon is caused by a relative decrease in the photoelectric mode of electromagnetic energy absorption (which is a function of the number of electrons per gram of absorbing material) as x-ray energy is increased. In the upper range of x-ray energies used in medical radiography, the Compton absorption mechanism becomes increasingly important (Johns, 1950). This absorption mechanism is independent of the number of electrons per gram of absorbing material and therefore produces decreasing density differences at subject interfaces recorded on a finished radiograph (Johns, 1961).

Increased x-ray energies result in a finished radiograph of lower contrast but with an increased scale of contrast (Cahoon, 1965; Fuchs, 1966), which means that there are relatively more shades of grey and fewer

contrasting black and white surfaces. This effect is best illustrated by radiographing a series of aluminum blocks of increasing thickness with x-ray beams of increasing energies (Fig. 2–10). Note that as the voltage used to generate the x-ray beam is increased from 40 to 100 KV, the ability to determine differences in the aluminum block thickness is improved. The relatively low energy x-ray beam generated with 40 KV produces fewer tones of grey on the finished radiograph, whereas increased x-ray energies produce more tones of grey and possess an increased scale of contrast (Cahoon, 1965; Eastman Kodak Co., 1968; Fuchs, 1966). The decreasing differential absorption effect on increasing kilovoltage becomes particularly important when an increased scale of contrast is desired for the radiographic examination of subjects possessing subtle differences in density, such as fascial planes of muscle and the serosal surface—peritoneal fat interfaces of the abdomen. Generally, the examination of bone structures require low kilovoltage (low scale of contrast) in order to differentiate the interfaces of bone and soft tissue. Soft tissue structures should be examined with a relatively higher KV x-ray beam, which produces the increased scale of contrast necessary to differentiate subtle density differences.

RADIOGRAPHIC DENSITY

Radiographic density is defined as the degree of blackness possessed by a finished radiograph. Dark areas on a finished radiograph are produced by deposits of metallic silver in the film emulsion. These areas appear dark when light is transmitted through a radiograph.

In a finished radiograph, increased silver retention occurs in areas where increased x-ray beam penetration has occurred. It follows that such body parts as air-containing lungs will produce a radiographic image that is blacker than the bones of the thoracic cage.

Increased radiographic density may be produced by increasing the number of X rays penetrating the patient or by increasing developing time or temperature. The number of penetrating X rays may be increased by increasing the milliamperage (electron flow from the x-ray tube cathode to the anode), or by increasing the time of exposure. Both techniques result in increased total x-ray production per exposure.

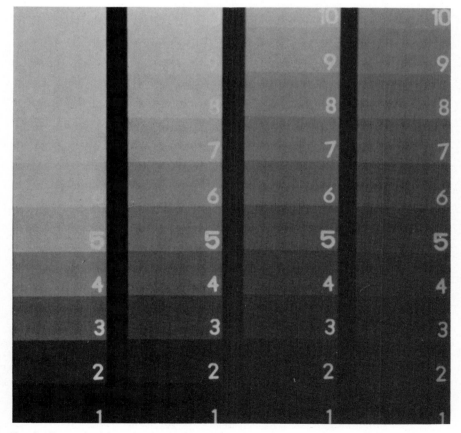

Figure 2–10. Radiograph of four aluminum step wedges produced with increasing kilovoltage from left to right. Kilovolt values of 40, 60, 80 and 100 were used. Milliampere second (mas) values were lowered simultaneously to ensure constant density. Note the increasing penetrability of the more energetic beams, illustrated by number 10 step visualization. There is also better differentiation between the steps as KV is increased, resulting in the production of more shades of grey.

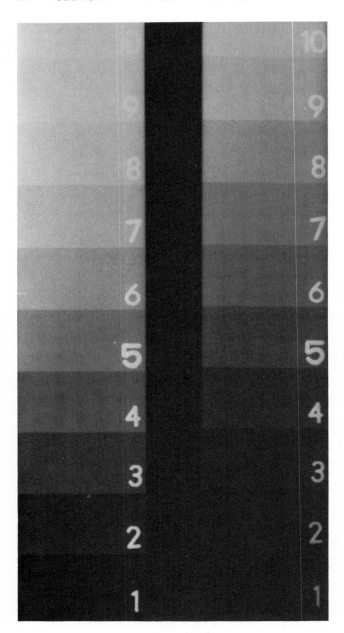

Figure 2–11. Radiograph of two aluminum step wedges produced by 6.7 and 13.3 mas at 60 KV. Note that with a constant KV setting, the number of shades of grey (steps penetrated) does not change with increasing mas values. Only the overall radiographic density has increased as a result of an increase in the total number of X rays available to expose the film.

Figure 2–11 illustrates the effect of doubling the milliamperage during a given exposure time. Note that the overall blackness or density has increased, but the scale of contrast is not affected—i.e., the number of shades of grey has not changed. The same effect could be produced by doubling the time of exposure, thereby producing twice the number of X rays. Increasing the milliamperage or the time of exposure therefore determines the quantity of X rays available to penetrate the patient and expose x-ray film but does not affect the quality of the resultant image (Cahoon, 1965; Eastman Kodak Co., 1968; Fuchs, 1966).

Increased accelerating voltages applied across the x-ray tube affect both the image quality and the quantity of X rays available. Increasing the kilovoltage results in increased penetrability of the x-ray beam and increases the overall density of the finished radiograph, since more X rays are made available to be recorded on the film. This effect, unlike the increases in milliamperage or time, is accompanied by an increase in the scale of contrast (Fig. 2–10).

RADIOGRAPHIC DETAIL

Radiographic detail is essentially a visual quality (DuPont de Nemours Co.). Radiographs possess good detail when the tissue interfaces, such as the juncture of bone and soft tissue, are sharp (clearly delineated) and possess good contrast (Cahoon, 1965; Ticer, 1969).

The production of good detail in radiographs depends upon many factors. Sharpness of definition may be increased by using an x-ray tube with an effective focal spot that is as small as is practical, consistent with heat tolerance of the x-ray tube target (Eastman Kodak Co., 1968; Fuchs, 1966). This principle is illustrated diagrammatically in Figure 2–12 A and B. Note that

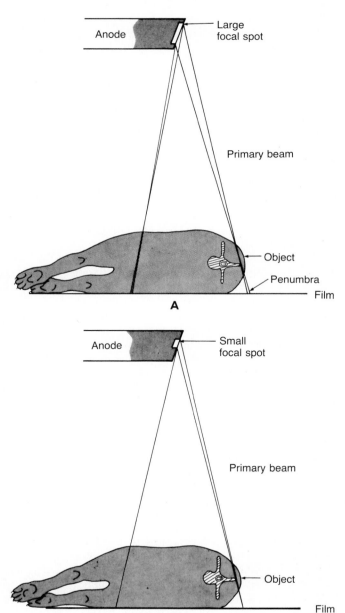

Figure 2–12. A, Diagram of the effect of increased x-ray tube focal spot (target) size on the production of a penumbra, which results in blurring of the edges of the various radiographic densities. B, Decreasing the x-ray tube focal spot size produces less penumbra effect, with the result that there is decreased blurring at the edges of various radiographic densities. This yields increased radiographic detail.

the larger the effective focal spot, the more pronounced will be the penumbra effect, which produces a blurred tissue interface.

The magnitude of the penumbra effect may also be decreased by increasing the focal-film distance (FFD) (Cahoon, 1965; Fuchs, 1966). The FFD is the distance from the x-ray tube target to the recording surface, or film. There is, however, an upper practical limit to the FFD, which is governed by the marked decrease in the x-ray beam intensity at the recording surface as the FFD is increased. This intensity decrease occurs at a rate inversely to the square of the distance, so that by doubling the distance, the x-ray beam intensity will be decreased by a factor of four and will possess one fourth the original intensity (see Chap. 4). In practice, this means that the exposure must be increased four times if the FFD is doubled to maintain equal density. This factor becomes very important in veterinary radiography, where short exposure times are needed to decrease detail loss caused by recording imperceptible patient motion on the finished radiograph. A practical FFD is 36 to 40 inches (Ticer, 1969); this distance seems to be sufficient to avoid noticeable detail loss due to the penumbra effect.

The penumbra effect may also be diminished by decreasing the distance between the subject and the recording surface (Fuchs, 1966). This factor is of practical importance when producing lateral oblique views of the mandible or temporomandibular articulation or lateral views of limbs, where a minimal distance between the subject and the film may be maintained by placing the part being examined closest to the film.

High detail x-ray film and intensifying screens also increase the sharpness of the recorded image, thereby improving radiographic detail. Good film-intensifying screen contact is also a necessary item for the preservation of sharpness. The use of nonscreen x-ray film will eliminate the two variables of intensifying screen detail loss and poor screen-film contact. However, the increased exposure time required to produce radiographs with nonscreen technique renders this method of increasing radiographic detail impractical for general veterinary radiographic technique, since longer exposure times increase the chances that patient

motion will cause loss of detail. For this reason, nonscreen technique should be reserved for high detail radiography of the peripheral appendicular skeleton, skull and in some cases, spinal examinations.

The detail and usefulness of veterinary radiographic examinations is often limited by imperceptible patient motion during exposure (Carlson, 1967; Ticer, 1969). This is particularly true when examining the thorax or cranial abdomen, where diaphragmatic movement often causes blurring of tissue interfaces. Therefore, the fastest exposure times should be used in veterinary radiography, where control of patient motion is less than ideal.

Subject contrast also affects radiographic detail (Eastman Kodak Co., 1968). Skeletal structures may be examined using a relatively low KV technique which produces a shortened scale of contrast that improves radiographic detail. Some loss of detail must be accepted when high KV technique is used for examining soft tissue structures, for which subtle differences in density require radiographs with a longer scale of contrast.

Subject contrast and, subsequently, radiographic detail may also be improved by decreasing the scatter radiation, which reduces the contrast of finished radiographs (Cahoon, 1965; Carlson, 1967). Cones or diaphragms and grids are used to control stray radiation.

Cones and Diaphragms. Controlling the volume of the patient's body irradiated during a diagnostic procedure not only increases the safety factor by preventing unnecessary patient exposure, but also decreases scatter radiation to which the operator may be exposed unnecessarily. Limiting the area of the primary x-ray beam also has the effect of reducing fog-producing scatter radiation from reaching the recording surface (Carlson, 1967). An unrestricted, primary x-ray beam irradiates a large volume of patient tissue, which, in turn, causes an excessive amount of scatter radiation to reach the recording surface (Fig. 2–13 A).

Control of the patient volume being irradiated during a given exposure is accomplished by placing either a cone or a collimator containing a diaphragm in the primary beam (Fig. 2–13 B and C). The major disadvantage of the use of cones to restrict the primary beam is that they are available in fixed sizes and must be changed when a different area of the patient is radiographed. The chance of error or misuse is inherent in the mechanical maneuver required to change the cones.

By far the most satisfactory method of controlling the primary x-ray beam is the use of a collimator (Fig. 2–13 C), which contains movable lead leaves that may be adjusted to conform precisely to the area being examined. The collimator has the added advantage of usually having a localized light incorporated within its structure. This light beams upon the area to be examined and has dimensions similar to the controlled x-ray beam. This mechanism has the obvious advantage of aiding in accurate patient positioning within the area of the primary x-ray beam.

Filters. A thin sheet of aluminum called a filter may be placed over the window of the x-ray tube for the purpose of removing the less energetic, less penetrating X rays from the primary beam. The resultant filtered x-ray beam is thereby rendered void of this useless, stray portion of the generated x-ray spectrum. Filtered, primary x-ray beams decrease the amount of undesirable exposure to patient skin, thereby reducing the relative radiation hazard (see Chapter 6). Filtered x-ray beams also have the advantage of reducing fog-producing scatter radia-

tion, thus increasing both radiographic contrast and detail.

Grids. As thickness of the part of the patient's body being examined increases, there is an increase in the amount of secondary, scatter radiation produced (Carlson, 1967; Fuchs, 1966). Generally, subjects greater than 9 cm thick produce sufficient secondary scatter radiation to cause contrast and detail loss on the finished radiograph, even when proper beam restriction and filtration have been accomplished. This necessitates the use of devices that will limit exposure of the x-ray film to the primary beam by removing those scattered X rays that cause loss of detail. This is accomplished by the addition of a grid between the patient and the film.

A grid is a series of thin, linear strips of alternating radiodense and radiolucent materials, which are encased in a rectangular wafer (Fig. 2–14). Generally, the radiodense strips are made of lead, and the radiolucent strips are made of plastic. The placement of the strips, their height, and the number of strips per linear inch of grid width are variables that are adjusted to the specific requirements of the examination being performed.

PARALLEL GRIDS. Parallel grids are those grids composed of strips that are placed perpendicular to the grid surface

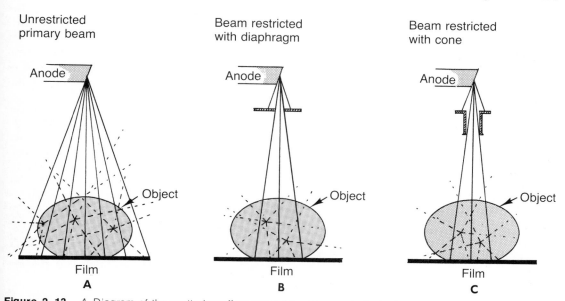

Unrestricted primary beam	Beam restricted with diaphragm	Beam restricted with cone
A	B	C

Figure 2–13. *A,* Diagram of the scattering effect caused by an uncontrolled primary x-ray beam. The increased volume of tissue irradiated results in increased scatter radiation. *B,* Decreased scatter radiation obtained when the area of exposure is controlled by means of a diaphragm. *C,* Decreased scatter radiation produced when the area of exposure is controlled by means of a cone.

Figure 2–14. A 17 × 17 inch grid encased in a rectangular wafer of aluminum.

(Fig. 2–15). These parallel lead strips absorb oblique, scattered radiation, while the radiolucent strips allow the X rays traveling perpendicular to the grid surface to pass through and expose the film (Johns, 1961). Grid efficiency is governed by the grid ratio. Grid ratio is defined as the ratio of the height of the strips to the width between the opaque strips (Johns, 1961). For example, a grid with lead strips that are 2.5 mm high and 0.5 mm apart would have a 5:1 ratio. Increased efficiency of scatter radiation clean-up occurs with increased ratio. A grid with a 5:1 ratio is, therefore, less efficient than a 10:1 ratio grid.

Increased grid ratios necessitate increased exposure requirements, since the percentage of radiographic density caused by scattered radiation decreases. Therefore, to obtain the same radiographic density, a greater number of primary X rays is needed for a 10:1 ratio grid compared to a grid with a 5:1 ratio (see Chap. 4).

Parallel grids have a distinct disadvantage in that an x-ray beam emanating from a small source (such as a tube target) interacts with the periphery of the grid at an increasing angle, thus reducing the number of primary X rays reaching the film near the periphery. This disadvantage increases with increased grid ratio, thus limiting the use of parallel grids to those with small ratios (5:1 or 6:1).

FOCUSED GRIDS. To compensate for the decreasing peripheral radiographic density produced with parallel grids, the so-called focused grid was designed (Fig. 2–16). This grid is constructed so that the lead strips are placed parallel to the primary x-ray beam and at increasing angles to the grid surface near the periphery of the grid. This design allows the primary beam to expose the periphery of the film with nearly the same intensity as the central ray.

Placing a series of lead strips in the primary beam causes the recording of an image of the grid on the radiograph. This image appears as a series of thin white lines. Decreasing the width of these lines may be accomplished by increasing the number of

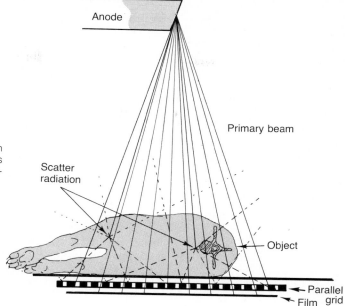

Figure 2–15. Diagram of a cross section of a parallel grid. Note that all lead strips are placed perpendicular to the grid surface.

lines per linear inch of grid width. A grid of 80 to 100 lines per inch provides radiographic images that are so fine that they generally do not produce interference with the diagnostic quality of the radiograph. Increasing the number of lines per inch obviously increases the cost of these fine-lined grids. An increased number of lines per inch also increases the ratio of the grid, since the space between the lead strips is decreased. Hence, increased exposure is required. Since increased exposure requirements generally dictate increased exposure time, high ratio, fine-lined grids have a distinct disad-

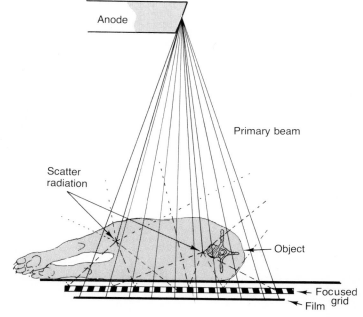

Figure 2–16. Diagram of a cross section of a focused grid. The lead strips are placed at decreasing angles to the grid surface as the distance from the center is increased. This serves to maintain the parallel relationship between the x-ray beam and the grid strips for the entire distance across the grid.

vantage in veterinary radiography, where patient movement is sometimes difficult to control. However, with high milliamperage x-ray machines, short exposure times may be maintained, thus eliminating this disadvantage (see Chap. 4).

BUCKY DIAPHRAGM. By moving the grid at right angles to the grid strips during exposure, the white line images of the lead strips may be blurred and thereby made indistinguishable. This is accomplished by a Potter-Bucky diaphragm, sometimes called a Bucky. This mechanism is usually suspended in a cabinet beneath the x-ray tabletop. A tray is placed in this cabinet for holding a cassette or film.

Movement of the grid may be produced by several methods. Older equipment utilize a spring-loaded slide. After compressing the spring device, release must be coordinated with exposure so that the grid is in motion during the time of the exposure. Travel time for the grid must therefore be longer than the exposure time. On the other hand, the speed of travel must be sufficient to cause blurring of the lines. Mechanical, or, preferably, electrical release that is coordinated with exposure within the x-ray equipment is obviously preferred. Motor-driven Bucky mechanisms are also preferred, since they require no manual loading of a spring-drive mechanism. Some modern drive mechanisms provide constant motion of the grid. This type of device is called a reciprocating Bucky.

By rendering grid lines indistinguishable, Bucky mechanisms allow the use of grids with fewer lines per inch, with decreased exposure requirements. This factor is very important in veterinary radiographic equipment, especially in those x-ray machines with intermediate milliamperage capabilities.

A drawback to the use of Bucky diaphragms in veterinary radiography is the noise produced by certain mechanisms. Motor-driven mechanisms (particularly reciprocating devices) are quieter and tend not to frighten the nonsedated patient.

X-RAY FILM

X-ray film is formed by layering a silver halide-containing emulsion on each side of a supporting polyester sheet (Fig. 2–17). When exposed to radiant energy, silver halide (mostly silver bromide) crystals become more susceptible to chemical change. These chemically susceptible crystals form the so-called latent image. Reduction of the sensitized silver halide crystals to metallic silver is accomplished by a developer solution in a darkroom. Removal of the unreduced silver halide crystals is accomplished by a separate fixer solution. The remaining metallic silver appears as black particles, which compose the negative image of a finished radiograph.

The sensitivity of x-ray film allows latent image formation when the film is exposed to all forms of radiant energy, including X rays, gamma rays, particulate radiations (alpha and beta particles), heat and light. Latent image formation can also occur in the presence of excessive pressure. Handling and storage of film to avoid exposure to these elements obviously becomes a primary factor in the production of diagnostic radiographs.

X-ray film used in medical radiography is available in various sensitivity ranges, depending upon the requirements of the examination. X-ray film that can be used with intensifying screens is designed to be most sensitive to ultraviolet and visual light in the blue-violet range. Light radiated from the fluorescing calcium tungstate crystals of intensifying screens is within this range. Film used with intensifying screens requires less exposure and is preferred in general veterinary radiographic examinations because decreased exposure times are possible. X-ray film designed to be used without intensifying screens is more sensitive to x-ray energies than to light. This nonscreen film is used when increased detail is needed, such as in examinations of the peripheral appendicular skeleton.

The sensitivity rating of an x-ray film is

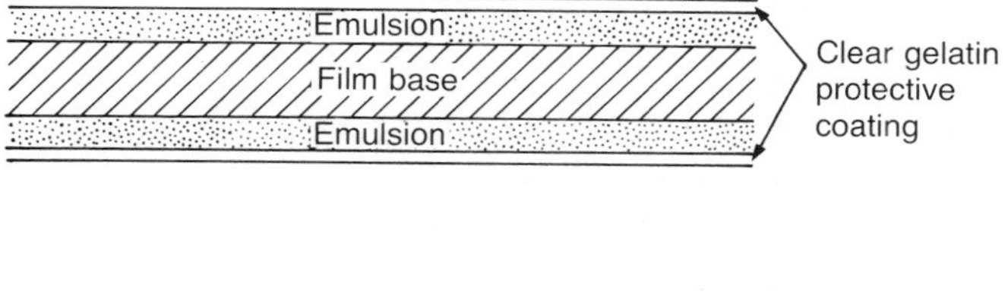

Clear gelatin protective coating

Figure 2–17. Diagram of a cross section of x-ray film.

determined by the exposure required to produce a radiograph of a given density (degree of blackness). Film that is very sensitive is referred to as being fast or high-speed. High-speed films are therefore those films that require less total exposure to produce a given density than film of average (par) speed.

Increased film speed is generally accomplished by increasing the size of the silver halide crystals. Although larger black particles of reduced silver impart more density per unit of exposure, they also result in a radiograph with a more granular appearance because these particles are within the range of easy visibility. This increased granularity decreases radiographic detail considerably. The use of high-speed film should therefore be reserved for situations where low milliamperage x-ray equipment is necessary. For most other examinations, par speed film or nonscreen film should be used.

INTENSIFYING SCREENS AND CASSETTES

X-ray intensifying screens are sheets of luminescent chemical applied to a supporting base. These screens fluoresce when irradiated and emit foci of light in areas in which X rays have penetrated a patient being examined. By placing film in direct contact with the surface of these screens, an accurate recording of the resulting image may be made. Approximately 95 per cent of the film's silver halide crystal exposure occurs from the light of fluorescing crystals in the screens. Approximately 5 per cent of the total film exposure is accomplished by direct x-ray interactions. The use of intensifying screens allows the total exposure to be decreased to a small fraction of that which would be required if screens were not used (Fuchs, 1966). Intensifying screens also increase the contrast of the resultant radiograph and thereby improve radiographic detail.

Intensifying screens are mounted in pairs in a cassette (Fig. 2–18). The cassette is a light-tight metal case designed to support a pair of intensifying screens and x-ray film, and to apply moderate pressure to insure good screen-film contact. The front of the cassette is made of plastic or a low atomic number metal such as magnesium, and the back of the cassette is a hinged metal lid. A pad of oil-free felt, glass fiber, or isocyanate foam is placed between the lid and the back screen. This pad forms a light seal around the edges and serves as a means of evenly distributing moderate pressure on the screens and film. A second screen is mounted on the inside of the cassette front in such a way that when film is placed in the cassette, a screen is in direct contact with the emulsion on each side of the x-ray film. The lid is equipped with springs or other types of latches that are designed to insure against light leaks and to exert uniform pressure to preserve good screen-film contact. Figure 2–19 diagrammatically illustrates a cross section of a loaded cassette.

Film exposure is accomplished by passing an x-ray beam through the patient, the front of the cassette, the front screen, the film and the back screen. Since X rays are absorbed by the front screen, this screen is thinner than the back screen. The X rays interact with screen crystals (usually calcium tungstate), which fluoresce ultraviolet and visible blue-violet light, which then exposes the silver halide crystals of the x-ray film, thus forming the latent image. The use of par (average) speed screens allows the production of radiographs with as much as 25 times less exposure than those made without intensifying screens (DuPont de Nemours Co.).

Cardboard cassettes for holding nonscreen x-ray film are designed to provide a light-tight envelope and support. A sheet of lead on the back side increases radiographic detail by preventing back-scatter X rays from exposing the film. Medical nonscreen film is available in ready-to-use, light-tight envelopes and does not require the use of cardboard cassettes. These ready-to-use packs are recommended for low volume radiology departments. Nonscreen film is extremely pressure sensitive and should be protected with a cardboard sheet if used without cardboard cassettes. This protection is essential when radiographing the peripheral limbs of dogs and cats, where toenail pressure may cause artifacts, which will appear as white lines, on the radiograph.

Intensifying screens are available in various speeds and are designed for specific purposes. The primary factor affecting speed and radiographic detail is the thickness of the chemical layer of lumines-

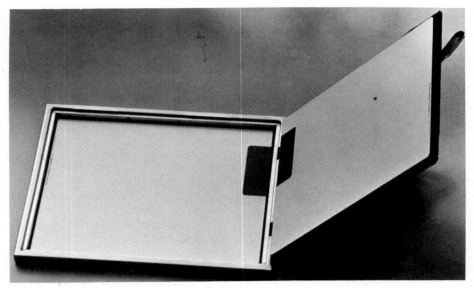

Figure 2–18. Film cassette with lid open to show the intensifying screens on both the front and the lid. The lead blockers are seen on the screens. These prevent film exposure in the regions covered both by physically blocking x-ray exposure and through the lack of fluorescing crystals in the underlying areas. This unexposed area may then be used to imprint identification material with a light flasher.

cent calcium tungstate (Johns, 1961). X radiation interacts with the luminescent crystals both on the surface and within the depth of the screen. Fluorescence from the underlying crystals is reflected and refracted toward the surface, thereby causing a diffusion of light from the point of x-ray interaction, which results in the recording of an unsharp image with consequent loss of radiographic detail. With increasing screen thickness, less exposure is required to produce a given radiographic density, since there will be a greater number of fluorescing cyrstals for each x-ray interaction. The speed of the intensifying screen is then increased at the expense of radiographic detail. It is evident, therefore, that a compromise is necessary between screen speed and radiographic detail.

Crystal size also is a factor in determining screen speed, just as it is with film speed. However, this factor is of less importance than screen thickness. Within certain limits, the larger the luminescent crystal, the greater will be the fluorescent emission, since x-radiation impinging upon any part of a crystal causes the entire crystal to fluoresce (Johns, 1961). Increased crystal size therefore results in both greater granularity of the finished radiograph and increased speed of the intensifying screen. High-speed screens usually have increased luminescent crystal size with consequent sacrifice of radiographic detail. Conversely, slow or detail screens use smaller crystals and produce greater radiographic detail.

A dye may be added to the luminescent layer in order to absorb refracted and re-

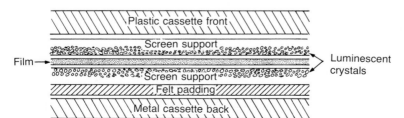

Figure 2–19. Diagram of a cross section of a loaded cassette, showing the relationship of the film to the intensifying screens.

flected light from the deeper underlying screen crystals, thereby improving radiographic detail. These dyes tend to absorb the deeper, less direct light rays, while those rays emitted from the surface tend to expose the x-ray film. The use of a dye results in a decreased light emission for a given x-ray interaction, and this decreases the speed of the screen. Dyes are therefore generally used for slow-speed detail screens.

By combining in various ways the factors of layer thickness, dyes, and crystal size and type, a correct balance of speed and detail may be produced. Various screen speeds, generally designated as detail, fast detail, par (average) and high, are available commercially. Exposure requirements to produce a given radiographic density usually double between the various speed screens. For example, twice as much exposure is required for the use of par speed screens compared to high-speed screens.

FLUOROSCOPIC METHODS OF RECORDING MOTION STUDIES

Fluoroscopy. A fluorescent screen may be used to record an x-ray image instead of film. Recording an image on a fluorescent screen has the obvious advantages of instant display and the ability to record dynamic events. Many special radiographic procedures require the use of such equipment.

A conventional fluoroscope screen consists of a fluorescent material mounted on a plastic sheet approximately 3 mm thick, which is covered (on the operator side) by a layer of glass containing lead salts of sufficient quantity to stop X rays, thereby preventing exposure of the operator to the primary x-ray beam (Johns, 1961). The fluoroscope screen is placed immediately adjacent to the patient while the x-ray beam is directed through the patient onto the screen. The resultant image is thereby displayed on the screen (Fig. 2–20). Spot film devices may be used to insert an x-ray cassette into the beam, allowing the production of a permanent record when desired for certain phases of a dynamic study.

Fluoroscope screens are essentially the same as intensifying screens. The fluorescent crystals generally used are of zinc cadmium sulfide, since these crystals show maximum sensitivity at about 5300 Angstrom units (one Angstrom unit equals 10^{-8} cm), which is very near the peak sensitivity of the rods of the retina (Johns, 1961). Crystals exposed to the x-ray beam fluoresce with an intensity that is directly proportional to the number of X rays interacting with the fluorescent screen. It is obvious that increased patient thickness requires increased primary exposure to the patient and secondary exposure to the operator. Patient exposure rates of 3 to 300 milliroentgens per minute (mr/min) are needed to produce screen images in the visible range in a darkened room with properly adapted eyes (Chamberlain, 1942). This exposure level produces an image approximately 1/30,000 of the brightness of this page being read under normal conditions (Johns, 1961).

It is obvious that special conditions must be met to allow adequate visualization of the fluoroscopic image. The decreased illumination of the fluoroscopic image requires maximum use of rod vision, which necessitates adapting the eyes to dark prior to viewing. Most frequently, dark adaptation is accomplished by wearing red goggles for approximately 15 minutes prior to fluoroscopic viewing. Adaptation is rapid (between 10 and 20 minutes) after excluding all but

Figure 2–20. Diagram of the relationships of the x-ray tube, patient and viewing screen using a conventional fluoroscopic table.

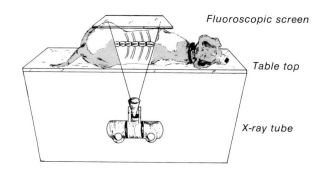

Fluoroscopic screen

Table top

X-ray tube

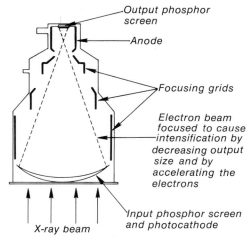

Output phosphor screen

Anode

Focusing grids

Electron beam focused to cause intensification by decreasing output size and by accelerating the electrons

Input phosphor screen and photocathode

X-ray beam

Figure 2–21. Diagram of an image intensifier which is used to replace the conventional fluoroscopic screen.

red wavelengths from the retina. The room must also remain dark during the examination, which produces further disadvantages for the conventional fluoroscopic equipment. Attempts to increase the image brightness to a level of intensity that would allow the use of cone vision have been made, but the amount of patient exposure became prohibitive.

Image Amplifiers. To eliminate the many inherent disadvantages of the conventional low output fluoroscope screen, an electronic device for image amplification was developed. These devices, called image amplifiers, consist of a fluorescent screen which is bonded to a light-sensitive photocathode, incorporated into a suitable vacuum envelope (Fig. 2–21). The light patterns produced by the fluorescent screen are converted into low energy photoelectrons, which are then accelerated toward a fluorescent anode or output viewing screen which is smaller in diameter than the original input screen. Focusing electrodes are used to maintain image sharpness, thus preserving detail. Increased image brightness is accomplished by decreasing (concentrating) the size of the image at the smaller output screen and by accelerating the photoelectrons, which

causes them to interact with the output phosphor at markedly increased velocities. In addition, the photoemissive cathode which is applied to the input screen is more sensitive than the human eye to the light radiated from the x-ray sensitive fluorescent screen.

Image amplification by this method may be viewed directly or after a mirror and lens apparatus angulates the image toward the operator; or the image may be viewed indirectly by a closed circuit television system, consisting of a camera and a monitor. Permanent records of the motion studies may be produced on videotape, or by using a 16 mm or 35 mm cine film, as well as 70 mm or 90 mm spot films. Various combinations of these capabilities may be obtained to meet the requirements of the particular radiology department (see Chap. 5).

REFERENCES

Bartels, J. E., and Hoerlein, B. F.: Radiographic examination. *In* Hoerlein, B. F., Canine Neurology: Diagnosis and Treatment. 2nd ed. Philadelphia, W. B. Saunders Co., 1971.

Cahoon, J. B.: Formulating X-Ray Techniques. 6th ed. Durham, N.C., Duke University Press, 1965.

Carlson, W. D.: Veterinary Radiology. 2nd ed. Philadelphia, Lea and Febiger, 1967.

Chamberlain, W. E.: Fluoroscopes and fluoroscopy. Radiology, *38*:382, 1942.

DuPont De Nemours and Company: Split-Second Exposure. Wilmington, Delaware.

Eastman Kodak Company: The Fundamentals of Radiography. 11th ed. Rochester, N.Y., 1968.

Fuchs, A. W.: Principles of Radiographic Exposure and Processing. 2nd ed. Springfield, Ill., Charles C Thomas, Publisher, 1966.

Glasser, E., Quimby, E. H., Taylor, L. S., Weatherwax, J. L., and Morgan, R. H.: Physical Foundations of Radiology. 3rd ed. New York, P. B. Hoeber, Inc., 1961.

Hagar, R. A.: Machlett Dynascope X-Ray Image Intensifier Tubes. Part II. Qualitative Theory and Construction. Cathode Press. Springdale, Conn., The Machlett Laboratories, Inc., Vol. 22, No. 3, 1965.

Johns, H. E.: Radiation therapy: depth dose. *In* Glasser, O. (Ed.), Medical Physics, Vol. II. Chicago, Ill., The Year Book Publishers, Inc., 1950.

Johns, H. E.: The Physics of Radiology. 2nd ed. Springfield, Ill., Charles C Thomas, Publisher, 1961.

Ticer, J. W.: Production of diagnostic radiographs in veterinary medicine. II. Recording factors. Calif. Vet., *23*:30–32, 1969.

3
DARKROOM THEORY AND TECHNIQUE

FILM PROCESSING TECHNIQUE

Film processing is an extremely important part of quality radiography. Many correctly positioned and exposed radiographic examinations are spoiled by improper processing methods. Proper processing can only be accomplished routinely in an environment that is conducive to careful film and cassette handling. Knowledge of processing technique alone will not insure against poor results if adequate facilities and equipment are not provided.

DARKROOM AND DARKROOM EQUIPMENT

Darkroom facilities need not be large or elaborate for the average veterinary practice (see Chap. 5) but must be efficiently designed to allow a "dry bench" area for load- and unloading cassettes, an area for proper film storage, and an area for wet tanks or automatic processor. Additional features such as a cassette transfer box from the x-ray room to the darkroom and a film dryer are desirable but not absolutely necessary (Ticer, 1969). A list of darkroom equipment appears in Table 3–1.

The processing tanks should be placed at a remote position from the dry bench. This separation prevents solutions from being splashed on dry films or intensifying screens. An added precaution against accidental contamination of film and screens by solutions or water is the placement of a towel rack and towel next to the dry bench so that hands may be dried after placing a film in the tanks.

TABLE 3–1
DARKROOM EQUIPMENT

Tanks for developer, fixer and wash water*
Film storage bin
Film dryer
Cassette transfer box
Safelight illuminators
Film hangers*
Timer*
Flash labeler
Labeling cards
Radiographic view box*
Corner cutter*
Thermometer*
Solution stirring paddles*
Exhaust fan

*This equipment is unnecessary with automatic processing.

It is desirable to provide a hard-surfaced wall behind the dry bench, rising approximately 20 inches above the bench surface. The hard surface will prevent the wall from being damaged by opened cassette lids.

Multiple electrical outlets should be placed above the hard-surfaced wall in order to provide easily accessible electrical power for the operation of dry bench equipment, such as the flash printer, safelights, view box and timer. By keeping the electric cord lengths short, the bench top may remain clutter-free.

Processor Tanks

The processor tanks should be large enough to accept a 14 × 17 inch film hanger. Developer solution capacity is determined by the caseload in the radiology department, which affects the rate of solution depletion. Generally, the five gallon insert tank is adequate for the average clinic practice (Eastman Kodak Co., 1968). Increased tank size should be obtained for higher caseload practices. The fixer tank should be larger than the developer tank since the fixer solution tends to deplete at a faster rate than the developer solution owing to volatilization of active ingredients.

Covers should be provided for both the developer and fixer tanks. This will decrease the rate of volatilization and evaporation of the solutions. The wash tank need not be covered.

Stainless steel tanks provide corrosion-free, low maintenance service. In addition, the heat conduction efficiency of these tanks allows more rapid heating and cooling of the solutions by the surrounding wash water (Eastman Kodak Co., 1968).

Stainless steel or rubberized stirring rods are necessary to mix the developer and fixer solutions. A floating thermometer should be provided in the developer tank to monitor solution temperature.

A mixer valve on the hot and cold water lines supplying the wash tank compartment will aid in the maintenance of a standard temperature for the entire tank, including the developer and fixer tanks. A modern shower-bath mixer control may be installed with relatively little expense and allows easy control of the temperature of the water in the wash tank and solution insert tanks (Ticer, 1969). A refrigerated developer tank may be desirable in areas where summer temperatures cause the cold water temperature to exceed 75° F. Flow rate for the wash tank water should be sufficient to allow a complete change of water at least 10 times per hour. This rate allows complete washing of films in approximately 20 minutes.

Periodic cleaning of tank surfaces must be a routine procedure in darkroom maintenance. If spilled solutions are not wiped up at once, they evaporate, leaving a chemical dust that may contaminate and damage film and screens.

Automatic Processors

The interior of the darkroom should contain the input tray for the large automatic processor. The processor may be installed in the wall in such a manner that the output film bin is outside the darkroom.

Small, low capacity processors may be installed on a bench top. Bench top installation allows both the input and output trays of the unit to be inside the darkroom. The room must therefore be large enough to allow easy operation and servicing of the unit. It may be necessary to build a special bench for the processor in order to avoid crowding the dry bench area.

Film Storage

X-ray film is a delicate, sensitive product and must be handled and stored properly to insure maximum usefulness. The product must be protected from light, electromagnetic radiation (X rays and gamma rays), various gases, heat, moisture and pressure (Eastman Kodak Co., 1968). The film storage area must be designed to mimimize the exposure of stored x-ray film to these elements.

Purchasing x-ray film in small amounts decreases the possibility of prolonged exposure to most of the damaging elements (even when the storage method consists of closing the top of the box in which the film was purchased). Additional protection may be provided by storing opened film boxes in a darkened cabinet. This cabinet should be located at a maximum distance from the x-ray machine in order to avoid exposure to scattered radiation.

Ideally, unexposed film should be stored in a room with a temperature between 50 and 70° F, and opened film boxes kept at a relative humidity of 30 to 50 per cent (Eastman Kodak Co., 1968). Film should never be stored in a drug room or next to sources of formalin, hydrogen sulfide, hydrogen peroxide, or ammonia vapors (Eastman Kodak Co., 1968). Films should be placed on end since stacking tends to produce pressure artifacts after exposure and development. The oldest film should always be used first.

Film storage bins that can be installed under the dry bench for easy access are available commercially (see Chap. 5). The increased accessibility of film for cassette loading makes these bins a highly desirable accessory to the darkroom equipment; they should always be considered when new darkrooms are being built or when an old darkroom is being remodeled.

Cassette Transfer Box

For increased efficiency of cassette handling, one may add a cassette transfer box between the darkroom and the x-ray room (Ticer, 1969). This container is installed in the wall and is accessible from either side. An interlock mechanism prevents inadvertent opening of the box on the light side (x-ray room) while the darkroom is in use. This box provides a convenient and readily accessible storage area for loaded cassettes (Fig. 3–1).

Darkroom Illumination

Either direct or indirect lighting is satisfactory for illuminating darkrooms. White light illumination is necessary to visualize maintenance procedures adequately. Control of these lights should be within the darkroom.

Safelights. Safelight lamps are an indispensable item since they provide light of a quality that is safe for x-ray film handling and processing. Excessive exposure of film to safelight lamps will, however, result in fog due to activation of silver halide crystals and will cause an overall grey quality to the developed radiograph. Careful arrangement of these lamps is therefore an important item to consider when planning a darkroom.

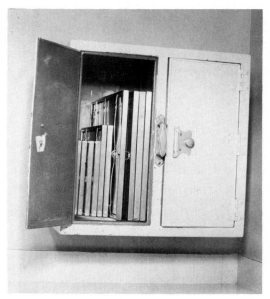

Figure 3–1. Cassette transfer box is installed in the wall between the x-ray room and the darkroom. This box provides a convenient storage place for loaded cassettes that are readily accessible from either room.

Three zones of safelight intensity are desirable: the brightest zone where the films are washed and put in the dryer; a medium zone where the films are developed and fixed; and a dim zone over the dry bench where the cassettes are loaded and unloaded and the film is placed on hangers (Eastman Kodak Co., 1968).

Indirect lighting is suggested for general darkroom illumination (Eastman Kodak Co., 1968). In addition, one or two direct lamps may be located over the processing areas. Proper light color and intensity are essential for high quality radiography. The proper color is provided by filtration on the face of the lamp. Most medical x-ray film has maximum sensitivity to the blue light emitted by the intensifying screen and may be safely handled when this wavelength is filtered from the light source. This is generally accomplished by a Wratten Series 6B filter (Selman, 1972). A red or ruby bulb should never be used as a safelight. The dim illumination emitted from these bulbs is not safe since the blue light spectrum has not been filtered. Filters should be inspected periodically for cracks that leak unfiltered light.

The intensity of the safelight illumination should be low but not so dim that lack of illumination interferes with efficient operation. A white frosted $6\frac{1}{2}$ to 10 watt bulb is adequate for most lamp fixtures. These fixtures should be placed 48 inches (122 cm) above the working surface.

Light Leaks. White light leaks around darkroom doors and ventilators and through wall cracks make quality radiography impossible since film exposed to unfiltered light, even of very low intensity, results in a finished radiograph with an overall grey appearance, thus markedly decreasing radiographic contrast. Light seals at the darkroom door margins should fit properly. Closure of the door should not require unnecessary effort, yet the seal should fit tightly enough to eliminate light leaks. Visual examination for light leaks should be made after the eyes are properly adapted to the dark, which usually requires approximately five minutes in the darkroom. A guillotine-type seal at the bottom of the door is efficient and decreases wear that results from opening and closing the door.

The darkroom walls should be a color that will reflect the safelight illumination, thus increasing lighting efficiency. Black or dark walls are not necessary or desirable. They only increase the need for light intensity.

Safety Test. Testing safelight illumination is accomplished by first subjecting film in a cassette to a moderate x-ray exposure. This exposure will increase the sensitivity of the film to fog-producing light (Selman, 1972). Density should be in the grey range, which will allow identification of increased exposure that is produced by light. The proper density can usually be achieved with 1 to 2 mas and 40 to 50 KV exposure.

The test is performed by (1) unloading the film in the darkroom and placing it on the loading bench; (2) covering half of the film with cardboard or black paper and exposing the other half to safelight conditions for slightly longer than is usually required to handle a routinely exposed film; (3) developing the film as usual and examining it for increased density in the light-exposed area. Increased density indicates unsafe conditions. The source of light leak must then be determined.

Radiographic Illumination. A fluorescent radiographic viewing illuminator should be mounted over the washing compartment so that wet films may be examined without contaminating processing solutions. This viewer is not necessary when automatic processing is used.

Ventilation

Adequate darkroom ventilation provides an environment that is free from volatile chemicals. Proper air circulation also helps control temperature and humidity. A light-tight exhaust fan installed in the ceiling, when accompanied by a light-tight air-intake louver, usually permits sufficient air circulation. Heater exhausts from film dryers and automatic processors should be vented to the exterior of the darkroom.

Hanger Storage and Care

Film hangers should be stored in a readily accessible area above or below the processing bench. They should be segregated by size. Periodic adjustment of film hanger tension will result in bulge-free film placement during processing. Excessive film bulge may allow film-to-film contact and thereby decrease the quality of the developing or fixing process. Proper spring tension is obtained when the distance between the upper clips and the lower clips is approximately $\frac{1}{2}$ inch greater than the length of the film they accommodate (Eastman Kodak Co., 1968). The springs may be bent to provide this distance.

Corner clips should be inspected and cleaned periodically. Gelatin from film emulsion adheres to clip surfaces and provides a medium for solution absorption, thereby increasing the possibility of transporting excessive chemicals from one solution to another. Solution contamination may result in streaks on the corners of a finished radiograph. Excessive gelatin build-up may also result in inefficient gripping of film corners. A solution of trypsin and sodium bicarbonate will dissolve or loosen these contaminants so that they can be brushed away in a water rinse.

A corner cutter should be provided to remove the rough projections on the corners of dried films that have been processed on hangers (Fig. 3–2). These protrusions pre-

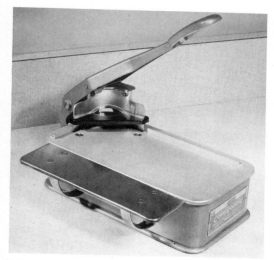

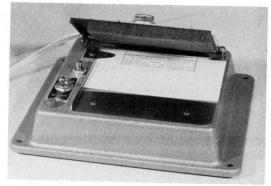

Figure 3–3. Light flasher for labeling radiographs before development.

Figure 3–2. Corner cutter used to trim the corners of dried radiographs for the purpose of removing the sharp projections caused by hanger clips.

vent sliding the films into an evelope with ease. Damage to film surface also occurs when these projections are sharp. Corner cutting is not necessary when film is processed automatically.

Film Labeling

Many methods of film labeling are available. Lead numbers and letters placed on the cassette at the time of exposure are reproduced in white on the finished radiograph. However, the inefficiency of handling such letters and numbers renders this method unsatisfactory.

Another method of labeling consists of writing the identifying information on a piece of graphite-impregnated tape and placing this on the cassette at the time of exposure. Since various exposures are required for the various radiographic examinations performed, back-up x-ray absorbing materials are necessary to insure a readable density for the resultant label. This requirement decreases the efficiency of this labeling system, making it less than desirable.

By far, the most satisfactory darkroom labeling method utilizes a light flasher to imprint the desired information on the exposed film (Fig. 3–3). Use of this system requires a small, leaded blocker in the upper left-hand corner of the intensifying screens

to prevent exposure of the film in that region to either x-rays or intensifying screen light (Fig. 3–4). Information is imprinted on this unexposed region by placing a card containing the desired information (Fig. 3–5) and the film in the light flasher, where light is passed through the card and onto the film. The printed material is thereby placed on the film in the form of a latent image and is developed when the radiograph is processed (Fig. 3–6).

The cards used in light-flasher labeling should be of high quality material since poor quality paper tends to produce a mottled background. These cards, with the desired printed information, may be obtained from

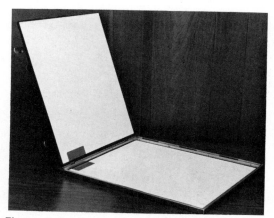

Figure 3–4. An open cassette showing the lead blockers in the upper left-hand corner of the intensifying screens. The lead blockers serve to eliminate both the x-ray and intensifying screen light exposure of the film in the region that they cover. This area is then available to be labeled by a printed card in the light flasher.

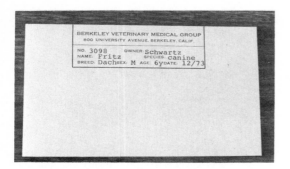

Figure 3–5. A sample label card that is used to imprint identification on an undeveloped radiograph.

any film supplier. The cost of the light flasher is minimal. The lead blockers for the intensifying screens are readily available commercially.

In addition to identification labels, left and right markers and timing indicators for contrast studies should be provided in the form of leaded indicators placed on the cassette at the time of exposure.

Timers

Since the rate of the chemical reaction involved in developing radiographs is dependent upon temperature, some type of timing apparatus is necessary for accurate, reproducible results. The time of development must be determined by the temperature of the developing solution.

Timers vary in both cost and ease of operation. Although small, wind-up egg timers may be adequate for the radiology department with a light work load (Ticer, 1969), an electrical, pre-set timer is more functional for the busy facility (Fig. 3–7).

HANDLING FILM AND CASSETTES

Film Handling

X-ray film is a delicate product that is sensitive to damage and alteration by many physical factors, including electromagnetic energy (X rays, gamma rays, light), pressure, heat, moisture and various gases and fumes. Handling and storage methods must, therefore, take these factors into consideration.

When handling a sheet of film, pressure, creasing, buckling and friction must be avoided. Care must be exercised when removing a film from a carton or a cassette in order to avoid rapid film movement across a surface. This action tends to cause static electrical discharge, which produces a tree-like black artifact on the finished radiograph (Fig. 3–8). Excessively low humidity will also predispose film to static discharge artifacts. In extremely dry climates, clothing articles of artificial materials such as nylon and dacron should not be worn by darkroom workers, since these materials tend to in-

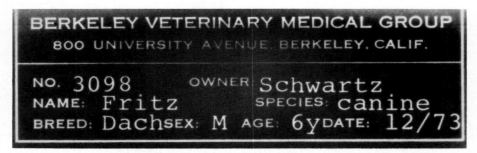

Figure 3–6. The resultant image of the label card imprinted on the edge of a finished radiograph.

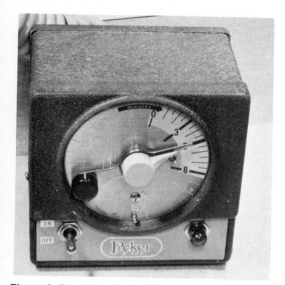

Figure 3–7. A timer is used for accurate timing of the x-ray development process. This model has an automatic reset feature.

crease the likelihood of static electrical build-up and discharge.

Lifting film from a box or cassette should be done with the thumb and one finger. Film without interleaving paper should be handled by the corners. Film shipped in containers with paper interleaving wrappers on the individual films has much less likelihood of having fingerprints on the film surface. These films should, nevertheless, be handled with care, since bending and folding can cause artifacts on the finished radiographs.

After exposure, the film is removed from the film container (envelope or cassette) and placed on a processing hanger. The hanger is inverted and the film, being held by the thumb and finger at the corner, is attached first to the left clip and then to the right clip. The hanger is inverted and the upper left and right clips are attached in such a manner that the springs on the upper clips pro-

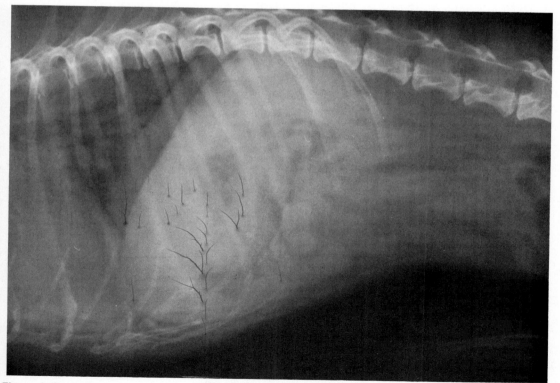

Figure 3–8. Radiograph of an abdomen with superimposition of the black, tree-like artifacts caused by static electrical discharge.

vide a taut film that will not bulge during processing.

Care of Screens and Cassettes

Loading and unloading cassettes must be done with extreme care, since physical wear and tear are responsible for shortening the useful life of these rather delicate instruments. To prevent excessive wear on screen surfaces, manufacturers coat the surface areas with a protective layer of thin transparent material. Since close screen-film contact is necessary for the production of high detail radiographs, this protective layer must be very thin. Care should be taken to avoid contact with abrasive materials. When loading a cassette, the film should be dropped into position and not allowed to slide across the screen surface (Fig. 3–9). This is particularly important when using film with square corners. Rounded corners are obviously preferred.

When removing a film from a cassette, rock the cassette on its hinged end with the lid open. The film will fall free against the fingers and can then be removed. The cassette should not remain open while films are being developed. Close the lid and reopen when ready to reload.

Always load and unload cassettes on the dry side of the darkroom, away from solutions that may contaminate screen surfaces (Ticer, 1969). The dry bench surface should be wiped clean daily.

Since there is a momentary vacuum in the inside of a cassette when it is opened, particles such as dust, lint and hair will be drawn into the cassette. Hair or any similar object caught between intensifying screens and film prevents the fluorescent light of the screen from exposing the silver halide crystals of the film. A white artifact of the size and shape of the contaminant will appear on the finished radiograph. White artifacts are also produced by splashes of fixer or developer and by fingerprints on intensifying screens (Fig. 3–10). As a general rule, well-circumscribed white artifacts on a finished radiograph are produced by screen contaminants. Similar artifacts can obviously be produced by defects that remove fluorescent crystals from a screen surface.

Other common screen and cassette defects that result in poor quality radiographs are poor film-screen contact, worn lid felt and loose, broken or bent hinges. Poor screen-film contact results in an excessive divergence of fluorescent light emitted by the screen. This will produce an area of decreased detail, manifested by a fuzzy, poorly defined image. Poor screen-film contact can be caused by a warped cassette front, a sprung or cracked cassette frame, warped screens, a foreign body beneath the

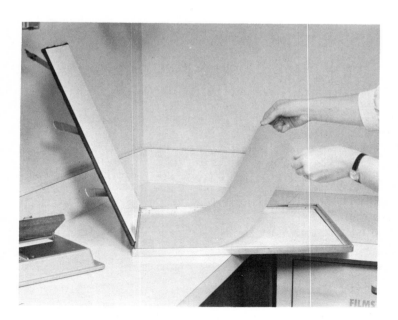

Figure 3–9. Proper cassette loading. The film is held by the edge and dropped into place.

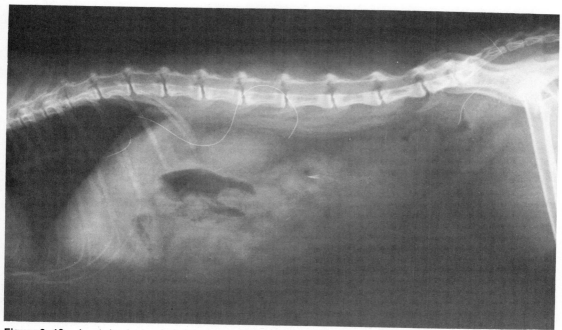

Figure 3–10. An abdominal radiograph showing the imprints of hair and other debris that were present between an intensifying screen and the film.

surface of a screen, or worn, bent or broken latches.

A simple test of poor screen-film contact may be made by radiographing a wire mesh screen. A copper or brass screen of uniform one-eighth inch mesh is laid over a loaded cassette and exposed at approximately 40 KV and 2 mas, at a 40 inch FFD (see Chap. 4). If the developed radiograph shows areas of dark, fuzzy or blurred outlines, there is poor contact between the screens and the film in that area (Fig. 3–11). A close examination of these areas will show a lack of sharpness or detail of the wire images. It is helpful to stand back a few steps when inspecting the film on a illuminator. The viewing angle should be about 45 degrees.

Trying to determine the cause of the poor screen-film contact without the aid of a qualified representative of the company that produced the cassette is not advisable. When the cause is not obvious, seek help, since these instruments are expensive. Repair of faulty cassettes should be the job of a factory representative.

Routine inspection and cleaning of intensifying screens and cassettes are necessary for the production of diagnostic radiographs and should be done at least once a month — more often in departments with a high caseload or in an area such as an inner city where soot and other air contaminants are likely to settle on screen surfaces.

Screen cleaning should be done with a commercially available cleaning solution and a soft, lint-free cloth. Cassettes should not be left open longer than is required for the cleaning solution to dry.

Occasionally, screen (white) artifacts may be detected on finished radiographs between regular cleaning intervals. In this case, it is extremely helpful to be able to find the contaminated cassette so that unloading and cleaning of all cassettes of that particular size may be avoided. A simple method of identification is to record the serial number that appears on the edge of most screens on the outside of the cassette lid. Because this black number is opaque to fluorescent light, it is recorded on each film exposed in the cassette. An alternative method is to write a number (1, 2, 3, etc.) on the edge of the screen with a black ink pen (Magic Marker) and then to record this number on the cassette lid. This number will also be recorded on each film exposed in the cassette.

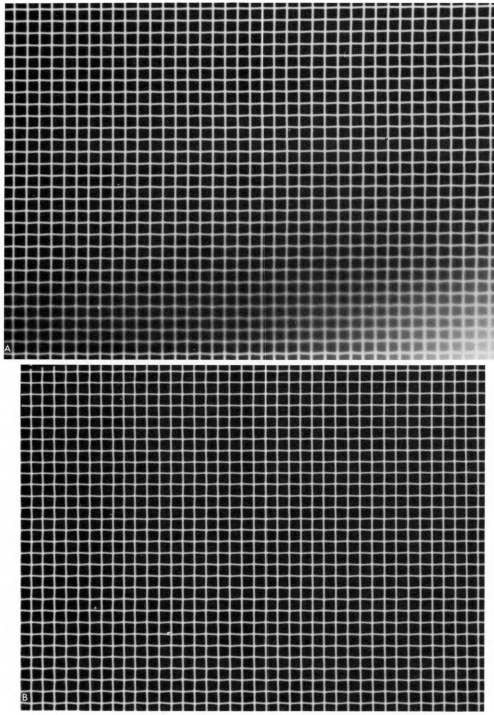

Figure 3–11. *A,* Radiograph of a wire mesh screen showing the loss of detail produced by poor intensifying screen-film contact. *B,* Radiograph of a wire mesh screen showing the increased detail produced by close intensifying screen-film contact.

PRINCIPLES OF PROCESSING

Radiographic Photography

X-ray film consists of a layer of silver bromide-containing emulsion on each side of a supporting base (see Chap. 2). Each silver bromide crystal contains a small impurity of silver sulfide, which serves as a sensitive speck or development center (Selman, 1972). When photons of light or X rays interact with the silver bromide crystals, the valance (outer) electron of the bromide ion is liberated and drifts to the sensitive speck (silver sulfide), to which it imparts a negative charge. The positive silver ion is then attracted to the negatively charged sensitive speck, where it is reduced to a silver atom. This process may be repeated often in a short time interval. The number of susceptible crystals that are affected depends upon the number of photons interacting with a given area of the film.

Crystals in which the sensitive specks have acquired silver atoms during exposure are invisible and constitute the *latent image* (Selman, 1972).

When the latent image is exposed to reducing agents in the developer solution, the process initiated by the photon interaction is continued. The sensitive speck acts as a development center for the entire crystal. Electrons are made available from reducing agents, allowing an increase in the number of reduced silver atoms (metallic silver), which appear as black foci on the finished radiograph. The finished radiograph, therefore, consists of dark areas of metallic silver in a very fine state of subdivision. The amount of metallic silver deposited in a given area is directly proportional to the intensity of the initial x-ray exposure received by a given area.

During development, the bromide ions diffuse out of the developed crystals and into the surrounding solution. This process and the gradual exhaustion of the electron supply in the reducing agents result in deterioration of the developer.

The development process is governed by the kinetics of chemistry and therefore proceeds at a greater rate with increasing temperatures. The process is also time-dependent and is subject to increasing intensity with increased time. From these relationships, the so-called time-temperature development process was evolved. This relationship dictates decreased development time when solution temperature is increased and, conversely, increased development time when solution temperature is decreased. Standard manual developing requires from three to five minutes at 68° F to obtain optimum film density, depending on the products used. With manual processing, the chemistry of the film and reducing agents in the developer solution provides maximum latitude at 68° F. Increasing the developing temperature decreases the latitude, which has the practical result of decreasing the magnitude of allowable error in developing time; hence, the films must be removed from the developer with more exact timing. Decreasing developing temperature and increasing developing time have the practical disadvantage of decreasing darkroom efficiency.

Fixer solutions remove the unexposed and unreduced silver salts from the film emulsion. Sodium thiosulfate (hypo) is the chemical used to accomplish this action in powder fixers, whereas ammonium thiosulfate is used in liquid fixers (Eastman Kodak Co., 1968). These chemicals "clear" the film so that the black metallic silver image formed by the reduced silver salts may be visualized. Improperly cleared film contains unexposed silver salt crystals, which darken when reduced by the action of light and tend to obscure the radiographic image. The magnitude of this artifact tends to increase with storage time.

Fixer solutions also contain a hardener (usually salts of aluminum) that is used to prevent excessive swelling and softening of the emulsion during washing, which serves to prevent slippage of the emulsion on the film base. Film hardening also reduces drying time.

Acetic acid or another acidic medium is used for the clearing agent and to neutralize any alkaline developer that may be residual in the film (Selman, 1972). The volatility of acetic acid makes it necessary to provide a cover for the fixer tank to insure long life for the solution.

A finished radiograph is essentially a negative of the structures being examined, since the regions of increased silver reduction are those where increased patient penetration by the x-ray beam occurred—i.e., the soft tissues and air-containing structures. In areas where penetration is decreased (such as under bony structures), there is a decreased degree of silver reduction, and the resultant image is relatively clearer after the fixation process. This image mimics that of a negative in ordinary photography.

Preparation of Solutions

Tank Cleaning. Preparation and maintenance of processing solutions is a very important aspect of high quality diagnostic radiography. Replacement of old solutions should always be preceded by a thorough cleaning of the processing tanks. The cleaning of these tanks may be simplified by using a commercially prepared stainless steel tank cleaner. Generally, a thorough washing with a good detergent followed by rinsing with fresh water is sufficient. Wipe the tank dry with a clean cloth or cellulose sponge. Avoid abrasive cleaning products.

Algae build-up on the walls of the water compartment is a problem in some areas. Filtration of the incoming water supply is an effective method of controlling this problem. Filters with a mean pore opening of not more than 35 micrometers are recommended. A water flow capacity of at least five gallons per minute should be available after filtration.

Algae may be removed from the tank walls by several methods. Commercially available algicides may be used. A dilute solution of laundry bleach may also be used effectively. Thorough rinsing with water should precede reuse. In severe problem areas, the water compartment may be allowed to dry over the weekend as an aid to algae control. Ultraviolet irradiation of the drained tank has been suggested; however, in most cases, the developer and fixer solution inserts provide a shield for a large number of algae.

Mixing Solutions. Developer and fixer chemicals may be purchased in concentrated liquid form or as a dry powder. Regardless of the type used, the manufacturer's directions should be followed carefully. Mixing and storage containers should be made of corrosion-resistant materials such as enamel, glazed earthenware, polyethylene or polypropylene plastic, glass, hard rubber, or stainless steel with 2 to 3 per cent molybdenum (Eastman Kodak Co.,

1968). Never use reactive metals such as tin, copper, zinc, aluminum, or galvanized iron. Tanks or containers that have soldered joints should not be used since chemical reaction between solder and processing solutions may cause chemical fog on film.

Proper dilution of concentrated solutions or dry chemicals depends on knowledge of processing tank capacity. This may be measured by actually filling these tanks with water, using a gallon container, or by calculation, using a constant (231 cubic inches per gallon) to convert cubic inches to gallons:

$$\frac{\text{Width} \times \text{Length} \times \text{Depth (Solution Level)}}{231}$$

$$= \text{Capacity (gal.)}$$

If significant bulge of the tank sides occurs when the tank is filled, it is preferable to actually measure the capacity.

Solution level should be approximately one inch below the height of the tank so that solutions will cover the film hangers.

Preparation of liquid chemicals is a simple matter of diluting the concentrated solution in the processing tanks. It is good practice to partially fill the tank with water, add the concentrated solution and then fill the tank to the desired level. This will prevent inadvertently filling the tank with too much water, leaving insufficient room for the concentrated solution.

Preparation of dry chemicals requires much more attention to detail. Since powdered chemicals are extremely reactive, dust control must be maintained throughout the mixing procedure. In fact, these chemicals are best prepared in a concentrated solution form in a room other than the darkroom. If solutions are prepared from dry chemicals directly in the processing tank, certain precautions must be taken to control chemical dust. Close and store all cassettes, close all windows and doors and turn off fans. Immediately after mixing the solution, all benches should be wiped with a damp cloth and the floor mopped.

The actual mixing of dry chemicals for processing solutions is accomplished by filling the tank half full with water at approximately 80° F (27° C). Add chemicals slowly while stirring. After the chemicals are in solution, bring the water level to desired height using cold water. Adding cold water will bring the solution toward a desirable processing temperature of about 68° F. Any scum, lint or dust should be removed prior to processing films. This may be accomplished by drawing an absorbent paper towel across the solution surface.

Replenisher Technique

Developer Solution. The chemical activity of the developer solution diminishes as the reducing agents become exhausted. In addition, a volume loss occurs as the developer solution is physically carried out of the tank on the surface of developed films. Evaporation accounts for minimal losses if the tanks are kept properly covered.

Depletion of the reducing agent concentration and volume loss must be compensated for by a systematic replenisher plan if uniform radiographic quality is to be maintained. Replenisher systems are designed to maintain both the volume and the activity of the developer solution. The most satisfactory method seems to be merely adding a concentrated developer solution to the original solution as volume is needed. By using a concentrated replenisher solution, replacement of the depleted developing chemical may be accomplished while adding minimally to the volume. When properly calculated, the replenisher solution concentration may be made to approximate the depleted chemicals and volume simultaneously. These calculations are made on the assumption that approximately $2^3/_4$ ounces of solution are carried out of the tank with every 14 × 17 inch film (Eastman Kodak Co., 1968). This means that approximately one gallon of replenisher solution will be used for every fifty 14 × 17 inch films developed. A proportionately smaller amount of solution is carried out on smaller films, and these films deplete the reducing agent at a proportionately decreased rate. Commercially available replenisher solution should be used, thus making it unnecessary to compute the concentration of replenisher needed.

In practice, small amounts of the replenisher solution are added at frequent intervals so that the volume of developer solution is kept nearly constant. The solution should be stirred vigorously after each solution addition.

Replenishment to maintain volume and concentration should not continue indefinitely, since aerial oxidation and the accumulation of gelatin, sludge and mechanical impurities eventually make it necessary to replace the entire developer solution with new materials. This replacement should be done every two to three months with average usage, more often with heavy usage (Eastman Kodak Co., 1968; Selman, 1972).

Fixer Solution. Fixer solution also diminishes in chemical activity with usage, and increased fixing time is then required to adequately fix and harden films. Maintenance of the fixer solution concentration increases the efficiency of the film processing operation. A simplified method of maintaining fixer concentration is to remove a small amount of old fixer solution and add a like amount of fresh, normally concentrated fixer solution. Removal of some old solution is necessary since water is carried into the fixer tank on each film processed. The volume of fixer solution to be discarded can be calculated based on the number of films processed, but the variables of acetic acid volatilization and water evaporation make this calculation unnecessarily complex. In practice, discarding old solution and adding fresh solution in a volume equal to the developer volume being replenished maintains adequate fixation and hardening activity.

Manual Method of Time-Temperature Processing

X-ray processing solutions interact with film at rates governed by the kinetics of chemistry. Thus, increased processing temperature results in faster reaction rates which, in turn, reach the same end point in a shorter period of time. The end point of the developing process is consistent, reproducible radiographic density and contrast. It follows that for a given radiographic density, increased developer temperature requires removal of the film from the developer solution after a shorter period of time than would be necessary with solutions of lower temperatures. This concept has resulted in the so-called "time-temperature" method of processing x-ray films.

In practice, processing solution temperatures below 60° F result in inadequate development and fixation due to the sluggish activity of the chemical reactions, and temperatures above 75° F result in excessive development speeds that are not practical for manual control. In addition, temperatures above 75° F may soften film emulsion and may cause excessive chemical fog. A temperature of 68° F produces optimum radiographic quality while providing a maximal latitude of error. That is, noticeable differences in radiographic quality will not exist if moderate over- or under-developing time has occurred inadvertently. By keeping processing temperature constant, standardized processing time may be maintained for the developing and fixing reactions.

When it is necessary to process film at temperatures other than 68° F, adjustment in the processing time must be made. Higher temperatures require shorter processing times and lower temperatures require longer processing times. Variations from the optimal 68° F, five minute development time are given in Table 3–2. Standardization of three minute development time may be desired to decrease darkroom time; however, the five minute procedure is preferable since maximum radiographic contrast is obtained (Selman, 1972).

Developing Procedure. Solutions should be thoroughly stirred before processing film. This should be done if an interval of 3 to 4 hours has elapsed since the last film was processed. Preferably, different stirring paddles or plungers should be used for the developer and fixer. If these are not available, the stirrer should be thoroughly rinsed prior to stirring a different solution, in order to minimize cross contamination.

The solution temperature must be noted and the timer pre-set. The film or films are placed on hangers and then immersed in the developer solution. Agitate the hangers vertically several times to remove all air bubbles that may be in contact with the film surfaces.

Air bubbles cause underdevelopment of the film since contact with solution is not obtained. These artifacts appear as small, round, clear spots on the finished radiograph because the unreduced silver granules in these regions are dissolved and washed away during the fixation process (Eastman Kodak Co., 1968).

Film hangers should be separated by approximately 1 inch in the processing tanks.

TABLE 3–2

TIME-TEMPERATURE GUIDE FOR DEVELOPING X-RAY FILMS

Solution Temperature (°F)	Development Time (minutes)
75	3¼
70	4½
68	5
65	6
60	8½

Care should be taken to prevent the film from touching the tank wall since such contact will also cause localized underdevelopment.

The timer must be set for the predetermined amount of time dictated by solution temperature. At the end of development time, remove the hangers and allow drainage back into the tank for a maximum of 2 seconds. The final drippings contain badly oxidized developer and tend only to weaken and contaminate the remaining solution. Excessive drainage may also result in streaks or chemical fog.

Rinse the films by immersing in clean, fresh water, with vigorous agitation for 15 to 45 seconds (Eastman Kodak Co., 1968). Minimal rinsing time is required if the temperature is at 68° F and the films are agitated vigorously. Without thorough rinsing, fixation may occur unevenly and cause streaking of the finished radiograph (Selman, 1972). Be sure the tops of the hangers are rinsed well to avoid contamination of the fixer solution by the alkaline developer. Lift the hangers from the rinse water and allow to drain completely before placing films in the fixer solution. This will prevent dilution of the fixer solution.

Films should be placed in the fixer solution and agitated in the same manner used in the developing procedure. Agitation insures that fresh, nonstagnated solution will come in contact with the film surface. Fixing time should generally be twice the clearing time. During clearing, the milky appearance of the film disappears as the unreduced silver salts are dissolved. After clearing, time must be allowed for these salts to diffuse from the film. Hardening of the film also occurs during this time. Adequate emulsion hardening decreases drying time and insures preservation of the finished radiograph. Generally, his total time is five minutes for solutions of dry chemicals. Approximately twice this time is required to properly fix and harden nonscreen films because of the increased emulsion thickness (Eastman Kodak Co., 1968).

Films should never be viewed with white light until fixation has occurred for at least one minute. Films should not be allowed to dry during preliminary viewing and should be agitated well upon return to the fixer solution for the completion of fixation.

Removal of film from the fixer solution should be done in a manner similar to that used with the developer solution in order to decrease contamination of the fixer solution in the tank with the used solution that is in close contact with the film surface. These films may then be immediately immersed in the wash water.

Washing films requires approximately 20 minutes in fresh, running water. There should be a flow rate that results in a complete change of water at least 10 times per hour. Hanger tops should be below the surface of the water to insure removal of all solutions, thus preventing contamination of the developer solution when the hangers are used again. Nonscreen films require approximately 40 minutes to wash adequately (Eastman Kodak Co., 1968; Selman, 1972). Exact timing is not necessary; however, care should be taken to avoid lengthy wash-

ing since prolonged exposure to water tends to cause excessive emulsion swelling and increases the drying time required.

Drying of washed radiographs may be accomplished by suspending the hangers at room temperature. This method is to be discouraged in all but departments with very low caseloads since the hangers are not available for reuse until drying is complete, and a shortage of hangers usually results.

Film dryers using temperatures below 120° F enhance the drying process markedly and make the operation of the radiology department more efficient. After drying is completed, films should be removed promptly since prolonged exposure to high temperatures may result in brittle, cracked finished radiographs.

After removal of the radiographs from the hangers, sharp corners should be removed so that handling and storage may be accomplished with minimum danger of scratching the finished surface. Sorting and filing of the radiographs in properly labeled storage envelopes should be performed immediately to avoid misplacement of valuable diagnostic information. Figure 3–12 shows an adequate storage envelope which provides easy identification of the radiograph and a summary of important facts that may be needed in radiographic interpretation. A summary of manual processing technique is given in Table 3–3.

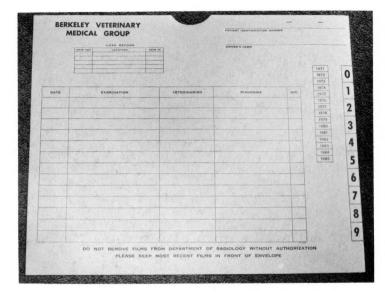

Figure 3–12. A usable radiographic storage envelope.

TABLE 3–3

SUMMARY OF MANUAL PROCESSING
TECHNIQUE

Stir solutions.
  Use separate paddles for developer and fixer
  solutions.

Check developer temperature.
  Adjust to 68° F if possible.

Load film on hanger.

Set timer.
  Time is determined by time-temperature relationship (see Table 3–2).

Immerse film in developer.
  Agitate vertically several times.

Rinse hands, dry and reload cassettes.

Remove film from developer after proper time
interval.
  Do not allow drainage back into developer
  solution for more than 2 seconds.

Rinse 15 seconds.
  Agitate film vertically. Drain well.

Immerse in fixer solution.
  Agitate vertically several times. Leave in fixer
  for 5 minutes (10 minutes for nonscreen film).

Remove film from fixer.
  Do not allow drainage back into fixer solution.

Immerse in running wash water for 20 minutes
(40 minutes for nonscreen film).

Remove from wash water and drain.

Dry on racks or in warm air dryer.
  Keep films separated.

Remove from hanger and trim corners to remove
sharp clip marks.

Store in well-identified envelopes.

Warm Weather Processing. The most satisfactory method of compensating for over-
warming of the cold water supply during
warm weather is to provide a refrigerated
developer solution insert for the processor
tanks. When this is not possible and the
temperature of the cold water supply exceeds 75° F, a restrainer should be added to
the developer. The addition of 2.5 ounces of
sodium bicarbonate per gallon of diluted developer has been used satisfactorily.

With increasing temperatures, warm developer solutions tend to be absorbed on the
film at a greater rate and the film therefore
needs to be rinsed for a longer period of

time before being placed in the fixer solution.

Acetic acid may be added to the fixer
solution periodically during warm weather
to insure proper hardening action. This addition may be necessary to replace losses
from volatilization or from neutralization by
developer alkali carried over in excessively
swollen emulsion.

Warm wash water tends to wash more
rapidly than does cold wash water. Since
prolonged immersion of film tends to cause
emulsion frill, wash time should be decreased.

When relatively small (3 to 5 gallon) solution inserts are used, overnight cooling of
solutions may be aided by removal of a
gallon of both the developer and fixer solution into separate glass containers for
storage in a refrigerator overnight. Replac-
ing the cooled solutions each morning will
aid in reducing the solution temperatures.

A summary of common darkroom causes
of unsatisfactory radiographs is given in
Table 3–4.

Automatic Processing

Automatic x-ray film processing has minimized the traditional bottleneck created by
the time and effort that is required for manual processing in many radiology departments. The savings in labor and time
required to produce a finished radiograph
and the consistent radiographic quality produced by an automatic processor make it a
highly desirable instrument for all but the
small radiology department.

Basically, an automatic processor mechanically transports a film through the developer, fixer, wash and dryer at a uniform
rate, which results in a finished (dry) radiograph within as little as 90 seconds (Fig. 3–
13). Specially formulated chemicals and film
are necessary to accomplish this high-speed,
high-temperature process.

Replenisher rates are governed by the
length of the films being processed. Generally, these devices are adjusted to correspond to the short side of the film; hence,
films should be placed in the processor side-
ways to avoid overreplenishment.

Automatic processors are complex mechanical devices and should be maintained
by professional service personnel where
(*Text continued on page 57.*)

TABLE 3–4

COMMON DARKROOM CAUSES OF UNSATISFACTORY RADIOGRAPHS

Low Density

I. UNDERDEVELOPMENT
  A. Improper development
    1. Time too short
    2. Temperature too low
    3. Combination of both
    4. Inaccurate thermometer
  B. Exhausted developer
    1. Chemical activity depleted
    2. Activity destroyed by contamination
  C. Diluted developer
    1. Water added to raise level instead of adding fresh developer
    2. Melted ice from cooling attempt
    3. Water overflow from wash tank
    4. Insufficient chemicals mixed originally (tank actually larger than judged)
    5. Improper developer additions
  D. Incorrectly mixed developer
    1. Exact capacity of tank unknown
    2. Mixing ingredients in wrong sequence
    3. Omission of ingredients
    4. Unbalanced formula composition

High Density

I. IMPROPER DEVELOPMENT
  A. Time too long
  B. Temperature too high
  C. Combination of both
  D. Inaccurate thermometer
  E. Insufficient dilution of concentrated developer
  F. Omission of bromide when mixing

Fog

I. UNSAFE LIGHT
  A. Light leaks into the processing room
    1. Leaks through doors, windows, etc.
    2. Poorly designed labyrinth entrance
      a. Bright light at outer entrance
      b. Reflection from white uniforms of persons passing through
    3. Sparking of motors
      a. Ventilating fans
      b. Dryer fans

    4. Light leaks from cassette transfer box
  B. Safelights
    1. Bulb too bright
    2. Improper filter
      a. Not dense enough
      b. Cracked
      c. Bleached
      d. Shrunken
  C. Turning on light before fixation is complete
  D. Luminous clock and watch faces
  E. Lighting matches in darkroom

II. RADIATION
  A. Insufficient protection
    1. During delivery or transportation
    2. Film storage bin
    3. Loaded cassette racks
    4. Not enough protection for loading darkroom
  B. Improper storage
    1. Radium or other isotopes nearby with improper shielding
    2. X-ray machine

III. CHEMICAL
  A. Prolonged development
  B. Developer contaminated
    1. Foreign matter of any kind (metals, etc.)

IV. DETERIORATION OF FILM
  A. Age (use oldest film first)
  B. Storage conditions
    1. Too high temperatures
      a. Hot room
      b. Cool room but near radiator or hot pipe
    2. Too high humidity
      a. Damp room
      b. Moist air
    3. Ammonia or other fumes present in darkroom or other working areas
  C. Delivery conditions
    1. Moisture precipitation when cold box of film is opened in hot, humid room
    2. Fresh boxes should be stored overnight at room temperature before opening

Table 3–4 continued on the following page.

TABLE 3–4

COMMON DARKROOM CAUSES OF UNSATISFACTORY RADIOGRAPHS (Continued)

V. EXCESSIVE PRESSURE ON EMULSIONS OF UN-PROCESSED FILM
   A. During storage
   B. During manipulation in darkroom

VI. LOADED CASSETTES STORED NEAR HEAT, SUNLIGHT OR RADIATION

Strains on Radiographs
  I. YELLOW
    A. Exhausted, oxidized developer
      1. Old developer
      2. Covers left off
      3. Scum on developer surface
        a. Oil from pipelines
        b. Impure water used when mixing
        c. Dust
    B. Prolonged development
    C. Insufficient rinsing
    D. Exhausted fixing bath

  II. DICHROIC (doubly refracting crystals exhibiting different colors when viewed in different directions)
    A. Old, exhausted developer
      1. Colloidal metallic silver
    B. Nearly exhausted fixer
    C. Developer containing small amounts of fixer
    D. Films partially fixed in weak fixer, exposed to light and refixed
    E. Prolonged intermediate rinse in contaminated rinse water

  III. GREEN TINTED
    A. Insufficient washing

Deposits on Radiographs
  I. METALLIC
    A. Oxidized products from developer
    B. Silver salts reacting with hydrogen sulfide in air to form silver sulfide
    C. Improper solder used in repair of hinges
    D. Silver loaded fixer

  II. WHITE OR CRYSTALLINE
    A. Milky fixer
      1. Acid portion added too fast while mixing
      2. Acid portion added when too hot

      3. Excessive acidity
      4. Glacial acetic acid mistaken for 28 per cent acetic acid
      5. Developer splashed into fixer
      6. Insufficient rinsing
    B. Prolonged washing

  III. GRIT

Marks on Emulsion Surfaces
  I. RUNS
    A. Insufficient fixing
      1. Weakened fixer
      2. Unbalanced formula
      3. Exhausted ingredients
      4. Low acid content
        a. Deficient when fresh
        b. Diluted from rinse water
        c. Neutralized by developer because of insufficient or no rinsing
    B. Drying temperature too high
    C. Contact with hot viewing box

  II. BLISTERS
    A. Formation of gas bubbles in gelatin
      1. Carbonate of developer reacting with acid of fixer
      2. Unbalanced processing temperatures
        a. Combination of hot fixer and cool developer
        b. Combination of cool fixer and hot developer
      3. Excessive acidity of fixer
      4. No agitation of film when first placed in fixer

  III. RETICULATION
    A. Nonuniform processing temperatures
      1. Developer (hot)
      2. Rinse
      3. Fixer (cool)
      4. Wash
    B. Weakened fixer with little hardening action

  IV. FRILLING
    A. Weakened fixer with little hardening action
    B. Hot processing solutions
      1. Developer
      2. Rinse

Table 3–4 continued on the opposite page

TABLE 3-4

COMMON DARKROOM CAUSES OF UNSATISFACTORY RADIOGRAPHS (Continued)

3. Fixer
4. Wash
C. Prolonged washing

V. AIR BELLS
A. Air bubbles trapped on film surfaces preventing development
B. Dropping film into developer without agitation as soon as immersed

VI. DRYING MARKS FROM UNEVEN DRYING OF GELATIN
A. Excessive drying temperatures
B. Extremely low humidity
C. Puddles (buckshot marks)
1. Drops of water striking semi-dried emulsion surface
D. Streaks
1. Drops of water running down semi-dried emulsion surface
a. Water trapped on hanger frames
b. Water splashes
c. Dirty hangers
d. Drying air flow too rapid

VII. WHITE SPOTS
A. Screens pitted
B. Grit or dust present on film or screens, or other contaminants
C. Chemical dust settling on film or screens (particles of certain chemical dusts will also cause black spots)

VIII. ARTIFACTS
A. Crescents—rough handling
B. Smudge marks—fingerprints or fingernail abrasions
C. Bands in marginal areas— usually due to screen mounting medium

Slow Drying
I. WATERLOGGED FILMS
A. Insufficient hardening in fixer
1. Too short fixing period
2. Weakened fixer from splashing wash water
3. Exhausted fixer
4. Insufficient acidity in fixer
B. Prolonged washing
C. Wash water too warm

II. AIR TOO HUMID

III. AIR TOO COLD

IV. DRYER AIR VELOCITY TOO LOW

Brittleness of Finished Radiographs
I. EXCESSIVE DRYING TEMPERATURE

II. EXCESSIVE DRYING TIME

III. EXCESSIVE HARDENING IN FIXER
A. Excessive fixation
B. Excessive acidity

Streaks on Radiographs
I. INSUFFICIENT AGITATION WHILE PROCESSING

II. FOG (RADIATION, CHEMICAL OR PRESSURE)

III. CHEMICALLY ACTIVE DEPOSITS (DRIED CHEMICALS ON HANGERS)

IV. SCRATCHES
A. Careless handling
B. Grit present in air, in cassettes, or on illuminator

VI. EXPOSURE TO WHITE LIGHT BEFORE COMPLETE FIXING

VII. UNEVEN DRYING DUE TO HIGH TEMPERATURE AND LOW HUMIDITY

Static
I. LOW HUMIDITY

II. IMPROPER HANDLING IN:
A. Removal from box
B. Removal from interleaving paper
C. Loading cassette
D. Unloading cassette
E. Loading hanger
F. Films stacked before processing

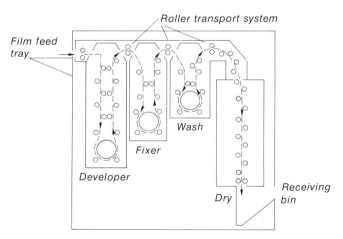

Figure 3–13. Diagram of the essential features of an automatic x-ray film processor. The roller assembly is designed to transport the film through the developer fixer and wash tanks, and finally to the dryer at a fixed rate, to ensure constant, predictable radiographic quality.

TABLE 3–5

COMMON CAUSES OF UNSATISFACTORY PROCESSING TECHNIQUE WITH AUTOMATIC PROCESSORS

Decreased Density
Under-replenishment
Developer temperature low
Exhausted developer. Drain and clean tanks every six months or after processing 50,000 films, whichever occurs first
Developer improperly mixed

Increased Density
Over-replenishment
Developer temperature high
Contamination of developer with fixer
Developer improperly mixed
Light leaks in processor cover or darkroom door

Failure of Film to Transport
Chemicals improperly mixed
Chemicals contaminated or diluted
Chemical temperature too high
Incorrect replenishment rates
Dirty racks, turnarounds, or crossovers
Racks or crossovers not seated properly or warped
Dirty wash water
Overlapped films
Tacky films in dryer section
Incorrect dryer temperature
Dryer air tubes incorrectly located or seated
Hesitation in drive assembly which causes film to pause in transit
Film not tracking through the processor on a straight course

Scratches
Guide shoe out of line or dirty
Dryer air tubes not seated properly

Processing Streaks
Rollers and crossovers encrusted with chemical deposits
Dirty wash water
Film not hardened properly by chemicals

Drying Streaks
Dirty air tubes
Film not hardened properly by chemicals

"Pi-Lines"*
Deposits on rollers in the developer tank

Insufficient Drying
Temperature too low
Thermostatic control or heater inoperative
High humidity in dryer section indicating one of the following:
1. Insufficient air venting resulting in back pressure
2. Damper in exhaust line not open far enough
3. Exhausting into an existing line carrying a higher pressure than that coming from the processor
4. Lack of or insufficient air conditioning
Film not hardened properly by chemicals

*"Pi-lines" are thin black longitudinal lines running across the film. They are most often seen in new machines, and will usually disappear after about 500 films have been processed.

such service is available. Only in rare instances should a veterinarian depend on his staff to perform this function.

A summary of common causes of unsatisfactory processing technique with automatic processing is given in Table 3–5.

REFERENCES

Carlson, W. D.: Veterinary Radiology. 2nd ed. Philadelphia, Lea and Febiger, 1967.

Carlson, W. D., and Corley, E. A.: Radiographic equipment and supplies. *In* Felson, B., Ed., Roentgen Techniques in Laboratory Animals. Philadelphia, W. B. Saunders Co., 1968.

Eastman Kodak Company: The Fundamentals of Radiography. 11th ed. Rochester, N.Y., 1968.

Fuchs, A. W.: Principles of Radiographic Exposure and Processing. 2nd ed. Springfield, Ill., Charles C Thomas, Publisher, 1961.

Johns, H. E.: The Physics of Radiology. 2nd ed. Springfield, Ill., Charles C Thomas, Publisher, 1961.

Selman, J.: The Fundamentals of X-ray and Radium Physics. 5th ed. Springfield, Ill., Charles C Thomas, Publisher, 1972.

Ticer, J. W.: Production of diagnostic radiographs in veterinary practice. III. Processing factors. Calif. Vet., *23*:19–21, 1969.

4

EXPOSURE FACTORS

Milliamperage, length of exposure, kilo-voltage, focal-film distance, grid ratio, and film and intensifying screen type are readily adjustable variables that affect the number and quality of X rays interacting with the image recording surface (film or fluoroscopic screen). Proper selection of these variable factors results in radiographs of diagnostic quality. After their initial selection, focal-film distance, film type, intensifying screen type and grid ratio generally become fixed; variations of milliamperage, length of exposure, and kilovoltage are then used as variables to produce adequate exposure. An understanding of these factors is necessary for the production of high quality diagnostic radiographs.

Milliamperage

The number of electrons moving from cathode to anode (current flow) within the x-ray tube is the principal factor controlling the number of X rays generated. Decreasing the electron flow results in a decreased x-ray output, and conversely, increasing the electron flow results in an increased x-ray output.

The measure of electron or current flow is the ampere (1 coulomb/sec or 6.3×10^{18} electrons/sec) (Harris and Hemmerling, 1955). Since the current flow through an x-ray tube is small, the standard measure is the milliampere (0.001 ampere). Most diagnostic x-ray tubes used in small animal radiography are operated with current flows of 25 to 300 milliamperes (ma). Some high capacity units may utilize up to 1000 ma current flow for certain specialized procedures.

Adjustment of the milliamperage control on an x-ray machine permits selection of the number of X rays desired per unit time. Increased radiographic density may be obtained by increasing the milliamperage, and decreased radiographic density may be obtained by decreasing the milliamperage (Carlson, 1967; Selman, 1972).

Length of Exposure

By varying the time for which the current is allowed to flow from cathode to anode, the total number of X rays generated in each exposure may be controlled. The total number of X rays reaching the recording surface ultimately determines the density of the resultant radiograph (Selman, 1972).

Milliampere-second Concept

Variation of both the milliamperage (controlling the number of X rays generated per unit time) and the time of exposure results in a variation of the radiographic density. An increase in milliamperage allows shortening of the exposure time, and conversely, a decreased milliamperage requires lengthening of the exposure time to maintain adequate radiographic density.

These relationships between milliamperage and exposure time have resulted in the concept of the milliampere-second (mas), which is the product of the milliamperes of current flow and the time (in seconds) for which the current is allowed to flow. Thus, an exposure made with 100 ma for 1/10 sec has a mas factor of 10. Likewise, an exposure made at 200 ma for 1/20 sec has a mas factor of 10. Both exposures generate the same number of X rays needed to produce radiographic density.

The radiograph produced at 1/20 sec is preferable in veterinary radiography, in which patient motion is likely to cause a loss of detail due to blurring of the radiographic image. Consequently, x-ray equipment with high milliamperage capabilities is needed for small animal radiography.

Kilovoltage

Voltage applied between the cathode and anode of the x-ray tube is used to accelerate electrons toward a collision interaction with the x-ray tube target. Higher voltages cause increased electron speed, thereby increasing the collision force. This results in a higher mean energy of the x-ray beam and ultimately causes increased penetrability of the X rays.

Voltages commonly used in small animal radiography range from 40,000 to 110,000 volts (40 to 110 kilovolts [KV]). Increasing kilovoltage increases radiographic density because a greater number of the total X rays generated penetrate the patient and expose the film. Generally, increased kilovolt values are used for thicker body parts since greater penetration is necessary to produce adequate radiographic density.

Higher kilovoltage and greater patient penetration increases the scale of contrast on the radiograph, which will possess more tones of grey that represent subtle density differences in tissue. For this reason, high kilovoltage radiographic technique is used for soft tissue examination where the small differences in tissue densities need to be illustrated radiographically. Conversely, bone examinations require the recording of relatively fewer tissue density differences, and a lower kilovoltage technique may be used.

The KV variation necessary to increase or decrease radiographic density varies with the original kilovoltage. Adequate radiographic density may be maintained by adding 2 KV for each centimeter increase in patient thickness when the original KV value is below 80. In the range from 80 to 100 KV, the addition of 3 KV for each centimeter increase in patient thickness is necessary. Above 100 KV, the addition of 4 KV per cm is necessary. Decreasing kilovoltage values may also be used to compensate for decreasing patient thickness.

Relatively large increases or decreases in radiographic density may also be accomplished by altering the KV value. The amount of kilovoltage change necessary to effectively double or halve the technique also varies with the original KV value (Table 4–1). These kilovoltage alterations are used to change radiographic density approximately the same as would be obtained by doubling or halving the mas.

Large alterations in kilovoltage may be used to increase or decrease the scale of radiographic contrast. For example, when soft tissue examinations require a long scale of contrast, the kilovoltage may be increased by an amount indicated in Table 4–1. Approximately the same radiographic density may be maintained by simultaneously halving the mas value.

High KV technique has the additional advantage of increasing the lattitude of the exposure. Latitude is a measure of allowable error in technique that will result in a diagnostic radiograph. In the range of 46 to 55

TABLE 4–1

CHANGES IN KV VALUES THAT RESULT IN RADIOGRAPHIC DENSITY CHANGE EQUIVALENT TO HALVING OR DOUBLING MAS

KV Range	KV Value[1]
41–50	8
51–60	10
61–70	12
71–80	14
81–90	16
91–100	18
101–110	20

[1]Amount to be subtracted for density change equal to halving mas or to be added for density change equal to doubling mas.

KV, an error in the x-ray machine setting of plus or minus 2 KV will result in an adequate radiographic density, whereas in the range of 86 to 95 KV, an error of 10 KV is allowable (Carlson, 1967).

Focal-Film Distance

The focal-film distance (FFD) is the distance from the x-ray tube target to the recording surface. Increasing the FFD decreases the total number of X rays available to penetrate the patient and expose the film.

This relationship follows the inverse square law, according to which the intensity of the x-ray beam at a point is inversely proportional to the square of the distance from the x-ray source (Matthews and Barnhard, 1968). Simply expressed, this relationship means that doubling the distance between x-ray tube target and the film will result in one-fourth the number of X rays being available to produce radiographic density, because, when the distance is doubled, the same radiation field is spread over an area four times as great.

The following simple calculations may be made to determine new mas requirements for maintaining proper radiographic density when the FFD is changed:

$$\text{old mas} \times \frac{[\text{new FFD}]^2}{[\text{old FFD}]^2} = \text{new mas requirement}$$

For example, if a satisfactory radiograph were produced with 10 mas at 20 inches FFD and the new FFD were 40 inches:

$$10 \text{ mas} \times \frac{40^2}{20^2} = \frac{16000}{400} = 40 \text{ mas}$$

The new value to maintain radiographic density would be 40 mas.

Grids

A grid improves radiographic contrast by preventing scattered radiation from exposing film (see Chap. 2). The efficiency of scatter radiation removal depends mainly on grid ratio and the number of lead strips per linear inch (Selman, 1972). Grids with increased ratio are more efficient at removing scatter radiation. Increasing the number of lead strips per inch decreases the efficiency since these strips must be thinner and consequently will absorb less angular (scattered) radiation, especially during high KV operation. With grids of equal ratio, the one with fewer strips per inch possesses the greater efficiency. Therefore, as the number of lead strips per inch increases, the grid ratio must also be increased to maintain the same efficiency of scatter radiation removal (Selman, 1972). Visibility of grid lines on the finished radiograph makes the use of grids with relatively fewer lines per inch objectionable except when moving grids are used.

Grids with increased ratio require increased exposure to maintain adequate radiographic density (Carlson, 1967; Selman, 1972). It is obvious, then, that there must be a compromise between the need for scatter radiation removal and the magnitude of exposure required. The need for scatter radiation removal in small animal radiography varies with the thickness and average density of the part being examined. Radiography of structures that have a high percentage of bone (such as the skull) requires the use of a grid for parts of relatively less thickness compared to less dense structures such as the thorax (Ticer and Evans, 1969).

Generally, patient parts with a thickness of 10 cm or more require the use of a grid to remove scatter radiation (Carlson, 1967). Non-obese patients that have relatively non-pathological thoracic cavities (up to 15 cm in thickness) may be radiographed without the use of a grid. Relatively dense skulls (less than 10 cm thick) of brachycephalic dogs may require the use of a grid.

Choice of grid ratios depends, in large part, upon the requirements for scatter removal and on the capabilities of the x-ray machine. Practices that radiograph a large number of relatively large dogs require the use of grids with ratios of at least 8:1, preferably 12:1. Since increased grid ratios require increased exposure, the choice of a grid must be tempered by the ability of the x-ray machine to generate sufficient mas with relatively short exposure times to produce adequate radiographic density.

X-ray machines with a 100 ma maximum output dictate the use of grids with an 8:1 ratio or less. These grids require two or three times the exposure needed for the non-grid technique. In practice, this means that exposure time must be doubled or tripled to maintain radiographic density. Grids should not be used that require increased exposure of such a magnitude that radiographic detail will be lost as a result patient motion, which may be perceptible with increased exposure times.

X-ray machines that have capabilities of generating 300 or 400 ma allow the use of grids with ratios of 12:1. Requirements for grids with ratios of greater than 12:1 are not found in small animal radiography because techniques using a kilovoltage above 100 KV are not often used. Efficiency requirements for grids with 16:1 ratios are needed only with high KV technique, where the production of scatter radiation is increased (Selman, 1972).

Increased exposure requirements vary with the grid ratio. The magnitude of the increased exposure should be determined by trial since other factors (such as the type of body part being radiographed) affect the proportion of primary to secondary (scatter) radiation emerging from the patient. Table 4–2 provides a guide for the start of a trial exposure technique.

For example, if a radiograph of a Boston Terrier skull 9 cm thick possesses adequate density when exposed at 100 ma, $1/20$ sec (5 mas) and 70 KV, but lacks detail because of scatter radiation, the use of a grid is indicated. If a grid with a 5:1 ratio is used, the exposure must be increased by a factor of 2. This is accomplished by increasing either mas or KV. Increases in milliampere-second usually provide the practical method of increasing exposure. Since most techniques utilize the maximum x-ray machine milliamperage, increased exposure time is used to increase mas. In practice, increasing the exposure by a factor of 2 is accomplished by doubling the time of exposure to $1/10$ sec. This effectively increases the mas to 10 (100 ma × $1/10$ sec).

Moving grids (grids mounted in a Bucky mechanism) are used to blur the visibility of the lead strips on the finished radiograph. Original mechanisms for moving the grid during exposure were known as the single-stroke type (Selman, 1972). The grid was caused to move by a spring-driven slide which was mechanically compressed by hand prior to the exposure. The spring-driven slide was released by a string or electromagnetic tripping device, allowing the spring to move the grid.

Reciprocating Bucky mechanisms are driven by a solenoid that works against a spring tension on the opposite end of the slide. This mechanism oscillates continuously without manual loading. Minimum exposure times with use of these mechanisms is $1/20$ sec, since faster exposure times tend to produce visualization of grid lines due to a relatively slow grid travel speed (Selman, 1972).

Recipromatic Bucky mechanisms are driven by an electric motor, and exposure times as short as $1/60$ sec are possible without grid line visualization (Selman, 1972).

There are several causes for the appearance of grid lines on radiographs made with moving grids. If exposures are made before or after grid movement occurs, grid lines will appear. Similarly, grid lines will appear if exposures are made before the grid reaches full speed. In all but the very old equipment, this problem has been eliminated by an electric contractor that prevents exposure until the grid is moving at full speed. Uneven or irregular movement of the grid may produce grid lines. Grid lines may also be visualized if the x-ray tube is not centered above the grid (particularly with a high ratio grid). Grid lines may appear if there is inadvertent synchronization of the peak x-ray output pulses and grid travel speed—i.e., a lead grid strip is present over the same point on the x-ray film during each maximum x-ray output (maximum x-ray output occurs in pulses of 120 times per second in full-wave rectified generators).

TABLE 4–2

SUGGESTED EXPOSURE INCREASES
WHEN USING GRIDS

Grid Ratio	Increase Exposure by a Factor of
5:1	2
8:1	3
12:1	4
16:1	4.5

Film Type

Several film types are available to the medical radiographer. The choice of film type is governed by the speed and detail requirements. High-speed film requires approximately one half the exposure needed by par speed film to produce a given radiographic density (Eastman Kodak Co., 1968). High-speed film, on the other hand, produces radiographs with a granular appearance that results in a loss of detail. For this reason, high speed film is only recommended for use with x-ray machines that have maximum capabilities of less than 60 ma.

Par speed film usually produces radiographic detail that is satisfactory for the average small animal diagnostic use. Detail or slow speed film may be desirable for certain specialized uses where fine structure is being examined. This film requires approximately twice as much exposure as par speed film.

Most high detail radiography should be performed with nonscreen film. This film type possesses approximately one fifth the speed of par speed film and therefore requires five times the exposure to produce the same radiographic density (Carlson and Corley, 1968; Matthews and Barnhard, 1968). This film should be used when examining peripheral skeletal structures or feline skulls of 5 cm or less in thickness. In certain specialized procedures (such as detailed examination of spinal disease), nonscreen film may be used with a grid (see Chap. 8). Exposure requirements for such uses must be further increased to compensate for increased exposure requirements of the grid. This nonscreen film/grid technique can, therefore, be used only with high milliamperage equipment.

Intensifying Screen Type

Intensifying screen speed, like film speed, varies the exposure requirements. Increasing the screen speed decreases the exposure requirements needed to produce similar radiographic density. Par speed screens require approximately twice the exposure to produce the same density as high-speed screens. The difference in radiographic detail is not as marked between par and high-speed screens as it is between par and high-speed film. The use of high-speed intensifying screens is therefore recommended for most small animal radiology departments because of the decreased exposure requirements (one half the exposure time).

Certain specialized examinations may require fast detail or detail screens which require two and four times the exposure, respectively, that is required for par speed screens. Due to the expense involved in purchasing these items, nonscreen film is usually recommended for high detail examination where the moderate decreased contrast of the nonscreen film does not present a problem.

TECHNIQUE CHARTS

A usable radiographic technique chart provides a convenient and reliable source of information about exposure factors that are needed for the production of diagnostic radiographs. Such a chart should be formulated for each x-ray machine. Even x-ray machines of the same make and model vary in both quantity and quality of output due to variations in input voltage, calibration, and condition of component parts. A chart constructed for one x-ray machine should not be used on another machine since these variables are often unique.

Although the art of quality radiography can only be achieved after extensive training and experience, an adequate compromise between poor quality and excellent quality can be obtained if a good technique chart is constructed and followed.

Variable KV Technique Chart

A basic variable KV technique chart may be constructed from data obtained during a series of trial exposures. A normal, non-obese, mature dog with a lateral abdominal measurement of 8 to 9 cm should be used as a test subject. Three test radiographs are made of the lateral abdominal projection. These test exposures may be made using one 14 × 17 inch film that is blocked off by lead sheets or by a folded lead apron over the areas not being exposed (Fig. 4–1). X-ray machine settings for the trial exposures vary with the film and intensifying screen type and with the capabilities of the x-ray machine. The following list of exposure factors are presented as a starting point:

1. Focal-Film Distance (FFD) = 36 inches.
2. Par (average) speed film. High speed film requires half the mas requirements

and should be used for x-ray machines with less than 60 ma capabilities.

3. High-speed intensifying screens. Par speed screens require twice the mas and should be used only with x-ray machines having 300 ma or greater capabilities.
4. Kilovoltage = 65 KV.
5. Milliampere-seconds = 1.66 mas for the first exposure, 2.5 mas for the second, and 5 mas for the third in a series of trial exposures. The other variables are not changed.
6. Standard film processing (developed at 68° F for 5 min.)

When determining the milliamperage and time settings to obtain the desired mas factors of 1.66, 2.5, and 5, the highest ma and the shortest time should be chosen. For example, if the maximum ma output of a machine is 100, the exposure time to be used may be calculated by rearranging the following mas formula:

$$mas = ma \times t \text{ in seconds}$$
$$t = \frac{mas}{ma}$$

The desired time then becomes:

$$t = \frac{1.66}{100} = \frac{1}{60} \text{ sec}$$

Solving the time requirement for 2.5 and 5 mas, the values of $\frac{1}{40}$ and $\frac{1}{20}$ sec, respectively, are obtained.

The fastest exposure time available is always used when determining x-ray machine settings for a given mas requirement. If the fastest time available, in combination with the highest ma, exceeds the desired mas, the milliamperage should be decreased. For example, if the x-ray machine has a 300 ma capability with a minimum of $\frac{1}{60}$ second timing, mas values of less than 5 may be calculated. The formula for mas (mas = ma $\times t$ in seconds) may be rearranged as:

$$ma = \frac{mas}{t}$$

The desired mas (in this case, 1.66) and minimal time factors are then substituted, and the milliamperage to be used is determined as follows:

$$ma = \frac{1.66}{1/60} = 100 \text{ ma}$$

Solving the ma requirement for 2.5 mas, the value of 150 ma is obtained.

After development of the trial exposures using standard processing (68° F for five minutes), the most "diagnostic" radiograph is selected. Variations of radiographic density should be observed on the three radiographs. If inadequate density is obtained on the 5 mas radiographs, make another exposure at 10 mas. On the other hand, if the 1.66 mas radiograph has excessive density, another exposure should be made using 0.83 mas.

For the purpose of illustration, assume that adequate radiographic density was obtained on the trial radiograph of an 8 cm canine abdomen using 5.0 mas. Insert those factors into a variable KV technique chart as illustrated in Table 4–3.

For this example, an x-ray machine of 100 ma, 100 KV, and $\frac{1}{60}$ sec timing capabilities will be used. The same calculation principle exists with any x-ray machine. Only the variables of milliamperage and time need to be adjusted to arrive at the proper mas value and the shortest time possible should be used in order to decrease the probability of recording imperceptible patient motion.

The variable KV chart is then completed by subtracting 2 KV for each decreased centimeter of thickness and adding 2 KV for each increased centimeter of thickness. After 80 KV is reached (at 16 cm on this chart), 3 KV are added for each centimeter increase in thickness up to the limits of the machine (100 KV).

Patient parts in excess of 9 cm should be radiographed with the aid of a grid in order to control fog-producing scatter radiation. In this example, a 5:1 ratio grid was added. Increased exposure is then required to maintain adequate radiographic density. Addition of a 5:1 ratio grid usually requires doubling the exposure (Table 4–1), which, in this case, was accomplished by doubling the mas from 5 to 10. Since the 100 ma used for the chart represents the maximum value for the machine, mas was doubled by doubling the exposure time from $\frac{1}{20}$ to $\frac{1}{10}$ sec.

At the 23 cm thickness line on the chart, the required kilovoltage is 102, which exceeds the limits of this x-ray machine. By subtracting 20 KV (Table 4–1) from the

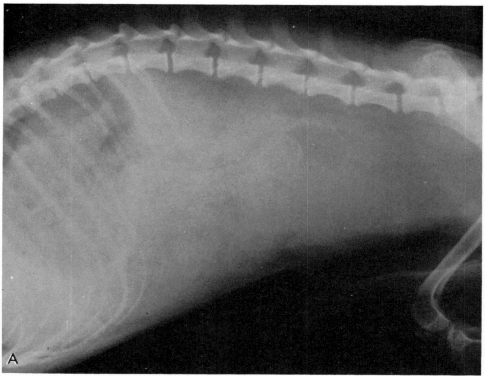

Figure 4–1. Three test radiographs of the lateral projection of the abdomen of an 8 cm thick poodle. The exposure factors of par speed film, high speed screens, 36 in. FFD and 65 KV were constant. *A* was produced at 1.66 mas, *B* at 2.5 mas, and *C* at 5 mas. The most desirable radiographic density was produced at 2.5 mas. In this case, the 2.5 mas factor would be used as the starting point for constructing a technique chart.

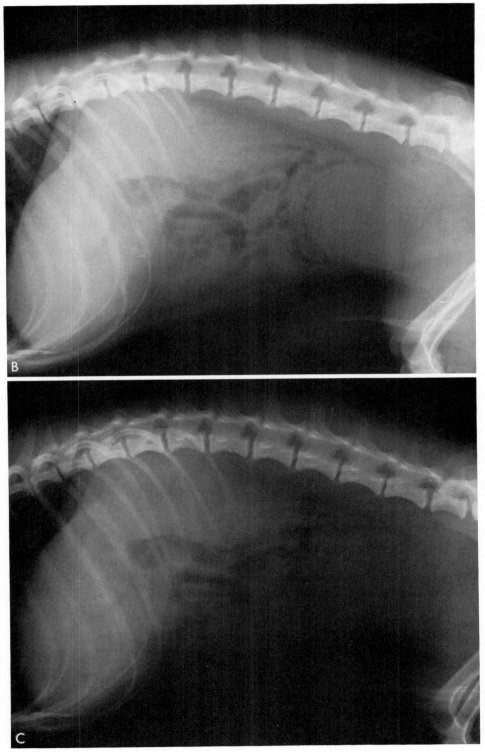

Figure 4–1 *Legend on opposite page.*

TABLE 4–3

VARIABLE KV TECHNIQUE CHART FOR AN X-RAY MACHINE WITH
100 MA, 100 KV, $1/60$ SEC CAPABILITIES

Thickness (cm)	KV	ma	Time (Seconds)	mas	FFD (Inches)	Grid (5:1 ratio)
1	51	100	1/20	5	36	No
2	53	100	1/20	5	36	No
3	55	100	1/20	5	36	No
4	57	100	1/20	5	36	No
5	59	100	1/20	5	36	No
6	61	100	1/20	5	36	No
7	63	100	1/20	5	36	No
8[1]	65	100	1/20	5	36	No
9	67	100	1/20	5	36	No
10[2]	69	100	1/10	10	36	Yes
11	71	100	1/10	10	36	Yes
12	73	100	1/10	10	36	Yes
13	75	100	1/10	10	36	Yes
14	77	100	1/10	10	36	Yes
15	79	100	1/10	10	36	Yes
16	81	100	1/10	10	36	Yes
17[3]	84	100	1/10	10	36	Yes
18	87	100	1/10	10	36	Yes
19	90	100	1/10	10	36	Yes
20	93	100	1/10	10	36	Yes
21	96	100	1/10	10	36	Yes
22	99	100	1/10	10	36	Yes
23[4]	82	100	1/5	20	36	Yes
24	85	100	1/5	20	36	Yes
25	88	100	1/5	20	36	Yes

[1] Trial radiograph with adequate density using these exposure factors.

[2] Grid added for thickness of 10 cm or greater. A 5:1 ratio grid requires twice the exposure (double mas by exposing at $1/10$ sec) to maintain adequate radiographic density (Table 4–2).

[3] 3 KV per cm of increased thickness is added above 80 KV.

[4] The kilovoltage requirements for 23 cm thickness would have been 102 KV, which is not within this x-ray machine's capabilities. Subtracting 20 KV resulted in halving the exposure, thereby bringing the KV setting down to 82. To compensate for this decrease, the mas was doubled, thereby maintaining radiographic density.

needed 102 KV value, the exposure may be effectively halved. The new value of 82 KV is then inserted on the 23 cm thickness line. To compensate for the decreased radiographic density that would occur, the mas value is then doubled from 10 to 20 by doubling the exposure time from $1/10$ to $1/5$ sec. The variable technique chart is then completed by adding 3 KV per cm thickness to the remaining lines.

Table 4–4 is a variable KV technique chart constructed for a 300 ma, 125 KV, $1/60$ sec capability x-ray machine, using the same starting point as was used for Table 4–3 (8 cm thick abdomen, 65 KV, 5 mas). The chart was constructed using the same

method of increasing and decreasing kilovoltage. Calculation of the exposure time using 300 ma yielded $1/60$ sec ($t = \dfrac{5 \text{ mas}}{300 \text{ ma}}$ $= 1/60$ sec).

An 8:1 ratio grid was used to increase the radiographic detail for parts greater than 9 cm thick, which required three times the exposure (Table 4–2). This was accomplished by tripling the exposure time.

Since the upper kilovoltage limit of this x-ray machine is 125 KV, the KV-mas alteration was not necessary at the 23 cm thickness line. Note that 4 KV per cm of increased thickness was added above 100 KV.

Thorax Technique Chart

The thorax possesses less x-ray absorbing tissues than other parts of the anatomy and therefore requires fewer X rays to produce a given radiographic density on the film. As a rule, thoracic radiography has 50 to 75 per cent the mas requirements of other body parts of similar thickness. A considerable amount of experience is necessary to be able to estimate the variation in thoracic tissue that must be penetrated by the x-ray beam.

Generally, thorax examinations for normal small animal patients require 50 per cent of the mas needed for other body parts (Carlson, 1967). Patients that are somewhat obese or those that have pathological states such as pleural effusion, pulmonary edema, or massive cardiomegaly require approximately 75 per cent of the mas needed for other body parts.

A usable technique chart for thoracic radiography (Table 4–5) may be constructed by modifying the variable KV chart shown in Table 4–3. This modification is accomplished by decreasing the mas factor by halving the exposure time. In thoracic radiography, a grid is needed only for thicknesses of 15 cm or more.

When radiographing patients that possess an increased ratio of soft tissue (fat or fluid) to air-filled lungs, the KV or mas values of the chart should be increased. Increasing the KV value is the method of choice for increasing the exposure factors in these cases, since short exposure times may be maintained. Increased kilovoltage values of 5 to 10 KV, depending on the patient type and

TABLE 4–4

VARIABLE KV TECHNIQUE CHART FOR AN X-RAY MACHINE
WITH 300 MA, 125 KV, $1/60$ SEC CAPABILITIES

Thickness (cm)	KV	ma	Time (Seconds)	mas	FFD (Inches)	Grid (5:1 ratio)
1	51	300	1/60	5	36	No
2	53	300	1/60	5	36	No
3	55	300	1/60	5	36	No
4	57	300	1/60	5	36	No
5	59	300	1/60	5	36	No
6	61	300	1/60	5	36	No
7	63	300	1/60	5	36	No
8	65	300	1/60	5	36	No
9	67	300	1/60	5	36	No
10[1]	69	300	1/20	15	36	Yes
11	71	300	1/20	15	36	Yes
12	73	300	1/20	15	36	Yes
13	75	300	1/20	15	36	Yes
14	77	300	1/20	15	36	Yes
15	79	300	1/20	15	36	Yes
16	81	300	1/20	15	36	Yes
17[2]	84	300	1/20	15	36	Yes
18	87	300	1/20	15	36	Yes
19	90	300	1/20	15	36	Yes
20	93	300	1/20	15	36	Yes
21	96	300	1/20	15	36	Yes
22	99	300	1/20	15	36	Yes
23	102	300	1/20	15	36	Yes
24[3]	106	300	1/20	15	36	Yes
25	110	300	1/20	15	36	Yes

[1]Grid added for thickness of 10 cm or greater. An 8:1 ratio grid requires three times the exposure (triple the mas by exposing at $1/20$ sec) to maintain adequate radiographic density (Table 4–2).

[2]3 KV per cm thickness increase is added above 80 KV.

[3]4 KV per cm thickness increase is added above 100 KV.

TABLE 4–5

VARIABLE KV TECHNIQUE CHART FOR THE THORAX
(MODIFIED FROM TABLE 4–3)

Thickness (cm)	KV	ma	Time (Seconds)	mas	FFD (Inches)	Grid (5:1 ratio)
5[1]	59	100	1/40	2.5	36	No
6	61	100	1/40	2.5	36	No
7	63	100	1/40	2.5	36	No
8	65	100	1/40	2.5	36	No
9	67	100	1/40	2.5	36	No
10	69	100	1/40	2.5	36	No
11	71	100	1/40	2.5	36	No
12	73	100	1/40	2.5	36	No
13	75	100	1/40	2.5	36	No
14	77	100	1/40	2.5	36	No
15[2]	79	100	1/20	5	36	Yes
16	81	100	1/20	5	36	Yes
17	84	100	1/20	5	36	Yes
18	87	100	1/20	5	36	Yes
19	90	100	1/20	5	36	Yes
20	93	100	1/20	5	36	Yes
21	96	100	1/20	5	36	Yes
22	99	100	1/20	5	36	Yes
23	82	100	1/10	10	36	Yes
24	85	100	1/10	10	36	Yes
25	88	100	1/10	10	36	Yes

[1] Started at 5 cm thickness because thorax measurements are usually greater than 5 cm.

[2] Grid added for thickness of 15 cm or greater. A 5:1 ratio grid requires twice the exposure (double mas by exposing at 1/20 sec) to maintain adequate radiographic density.

pathological state, will usually produce adequate radiographic density.

Variable Mas Technique Chart

A variable KV technique chart may not be practical for all x-ray machines. Certain older machines do not allow for kilovoltage variation in steps of 1 or 2 KV that are necessary for an accurate use of a variable KV chart. Unfortunately, the timing interval of most x-ray machines does not permit the accurate use of a variable mas technique chart.

A compromise between a variable KV and a variable mas chart works best for equipment that does not have short KV selection intervals. For example, if KV settings may be made only in 10 KV intervals, increased radiographic density may be attained for each centimeter of increased patient thickness by adding small increases of mas to the exposure technique.

In order to modify the variable KV chart in Table 4–3 for use with an x-ray machine with this KV interval limitation, an interval of 10 KV increase is chosen, such as from 1 to 5 cm of patient thickness (Table 4–6). From Table 4–1, the approximate mas change that has the approximate equivalence of the 10 KV change can be determined. In this case, the KV interval of 10 (for kilovoltage in the range of 51 to 60 KV) is approximately equal to doubling the mas. Therefore, if the mas is raised from 5 to 10 for the thickness interval of 1 to 5 cm, the inability to raise the kilovoltage will be compensated for. The value of 10 mas is then used for the 5 cm thickness line. The mas values for the 2, 3 and 4 cm thickness lines are estimated according to the milliamperage and timer setting combinations available on the x-ray machine. The remaining centimeter thickness lines may be calculated in a similar manner.

A major disadvantage of the variable mas method of calculating exposure is the neces-

TABLE 4–6

EXAMPLE OF A VARIABLE MAS METHOD TO COMPENSATE FOR AN X-RAY
MACHINE WITH KV SETTING INTERVALS OF 10 (MODIFIED FROM TABLE 4–3)

Thickness (cm)	KV	ma	Time (Seconds)	mas	FFD (Inches)	Grid
1	50	100	1/20	5	36	No
2	50	100	1/15	6.66	36	No
3	50	75	1/10	7.5	36	No
4	50	100	1/12	8.3	36	No
5	50	100	1/10	10	36	No
6	60	100	1/20	5	36	No

sity of using relatively long exposure times to obtain some needed mas values.

High KV Technique Charts

Certain radiographic examinations require the use of relatively high KV technique to demonstrate subtle differences in soft tissue densities or to radiograph structures having marked variation in radiodensity, such as the dorsoventral view of a thorax. In order to penetrate the thoracic vertebrae through the dense cardiac silhouette without overexposing the radiolucent lungs, a relatively low mas, high KV technique should be used (Douglas and Williamson, 1972).

Practical application of this technique is possible by modification of the exposure values on the variable KV chart (Table 4–3). The KV and mas values are determined from the chart after measurement of the thorax. The kilovoltage is then increased by a factor indicated in Table 4–1, depending on the KV range, and the mas value is halved to maintain radiographic density.

For example, examination of a 14 cm thick abdomen using a high KV technique may be accomplished by determining the exposure factors from the variable KV chart (Table 4–3). The 77 KV, 10 mas technique may be altered by increasing the kilovoltage by 14 KV (from Table 1) and halving the mas. The new, high KV exposure factors would then be 91 KV and 5 mas (100 ma at 1/20 sec).

This method is also useful for decreasing exposure times while maintaining radiographic density when examining patients with rapid respiratory movements.

Nonscreen Film Technique Chart

Medical nonscreen film may be used to examine bony parts (such as peripheral limbs) when increased radiographic detail is needed. Table 4–7 is an example of a technique chart constructed for use with nonscreen film. The factors should be determined for each x-ray machine using the trial exposure method.

Common Exposure Causes of Unsatisfactory Radiographs

Periodic readjustment of technique charts is necessary due to the instability of some variable factors and the decreased efficiency of certain x-ray machine components. Common exposure causes of unsatisfactory radiographs are listed in Table 4–8. Consulting this table may aid in differentiating the cause of poor radiographs and in determining if technique chart readjustment is necessary.

TABLE 4–7

NONSCREEN FILM TECHNIQUE CHART
FOR USE ON PERIPHERAL LIMBS

Thickness (cm)	KV	ma	Time (Seconds)	mas	FFD (Inches)
1	50	100	3/20	15	36
2	52	100	3/20	15	36
3	54	100	3/20	15	36
4	56	100	3/20	15	36
5	58	100	3/20	15	36

TABLE 4–8

COMMON EXPOSURE CAUSES OF UNSATISFACTORY RADIOGRAPHS

Low Density
I. UNDEREXPOSURE
  A. Wrong Exposure Factors
    1. Too low kilovoltage
    2. Too low milliamperage
    3. Too short exposure
    4. Too great focal-film distance
  B. Meters out of calibration
  C. Timer out of calibration
  D. Inaccurate setting of meters or timer
  E. Drop in incoming line voltage
    1. Furnaces and blowers on same circuit
    2. Insufficient size of power line or trans-
      formers
  F. Central ray of x-ray tube not directed on
    film
  G. FFD not correct for grid used
  H. One or more rectifiers not functioning

High Density
I. OVEREXPOSURE
  A. Wrong exposure factors
    1. Too high kilovoltage
    2. Too high milliamperage
    3. Too long exposure
    4. Too short focal-film distance
  B. Meters out of calibration
  C. Timer out of calibration
  D. Inaccurate setting of meters or timer
  E. Surge in incoming line voltage

Low Contrast
I. OVERPENETRATION FROM TOO
  HIGH KILOVOLTAGE
  A. Overmeasurement of part to be examined
  B. Incorrect estimate of material or tissue
    density
  C. Meters out of calibration
  D. Meters inaccurately set
  E. Drop in incoming line voltage
  F. Overmeasurement of focal-film distance
II. TOO LONG EXPOSURE
  A. Timer out of calibration
  B. Timer inaccurately set

Lack of Detail or Fuzziness
I. MOTION (TUBE, FILM, SUBJECT)
  A. Inadequate immobilization
  B. Too long exposure
  C. Vibration of floor
  D. Failure to arrest tube vibration after
    positioning before making exposure
II. POOR CONTACT OF INTENSIFY-
  ING SCREENS
III. IMPROPER DISTANCE RELATION-
  SHIP
  A. Object-film distance too great
  B. Target-film distance too short
IV. IMPROPER FOCAL SPOT
  A. Too large
  B. Damaged (cracked or pitted)

REFERENCES

Carlson, W. D.: Veterinary Radiology. 2nd ed. Phila-
delphia, Lea and Febiger, 1967.
Carlson, W. D., and Corley, E. A.: Radiographic
equipment and supplies. *In* Felson, B., Roentgen
Techniques in Laboratory Animals. Philadelphia, W.
B. Saunders Co., 1968.
Douglas, S. W., and Williamson, H. D.: Principles of
Veterinary Radiography. 2nd ed. Baltimore, Wil-
liams and Wilkins Co., 1972.
Eastman Kodak Company: The Fundamentals of Ra-
diography. 11th ed. Rochester, N. Y., 1968.
Harris, N. C., and Hemmerling, E. M.: Introductory

Applied Physics. New York, McGraw-Hill Book
Co., 1955.
Matthews, H. G., and Barnhard, H. J.: Radiographic
technique. *In* Felson, B., Roentgen Technique in
Laboratory Animals. Philadelphia, W. B. Saunders
Co., 1968.
Selman, J.: The Fundamentals of X-ray and Radium
Physics. 5th ed. Springfield, Ill., Charles C Thomas,
1972.
Ticer, J. W., and Evans, J. W.: Production of diagnostic
radiographs in veterinary practice. IV. Technique
chart for small animal radiography. Calif. Vet. *32:*29,
1969.

5

PLANNING AND EQUIPPING YOUR RADIOLOGY DEPARTMENT

Neil Kooyman

X-RAY EQUIPMENT

Equipment requirements for small animal veterinary practice vary considerably, depending on caseload, prevalent patient type, and degree of sophistication desired. An outpatient-type practice that stresses general patient care does not have the same requirements as a larger practice performing more comprehensive care in a hospital environment. Likewise, a practice serving clientele that have predominantly large breeds of dogs as pets does not have the same equipment requirements as a practice serving a population of cat and small dog owners.

Unfortunately, requirements based on need must also be tempered by economics. Generally, the higher the milliamperage and the shorter the timing capabilities of the equipment, the more expensive will be the costs. A balance of requirements and costs must therefore be attained during the planning stage of any construction or upgrading program.

Basic Equipment

Basic radiographic equipment that is necessary to perform routine radiographic examinations includes the x-ray generating system (consisting of controls, high voltage transformer, and x-ray tubes), the x-ray beam localizing system (collimator), the grid, and the handling devices (which include the table, tubestand, and positioning aids).

Controls. The x-ray control system contains all of the circuitry necessary to vary independently the x-ray tube current (ma), the voltage applied across the tube (KV), and the time of exposure. The degree of independence and reproducibility or accuracy of these three parameters and the magnitude of the power to be controlled determine the size and complexity of the components and circuitry. Standard items in the control system are an x-ray tube starter and power circuits for locks, Bucky motor, lights, and other auxiliary equipment. Optional equipment in the control system includes circuits for tube protection, fluoroscopy, spot film device, and photo-timing. The physical size of the control, then, is determined by the space needed to house all the circuits in such a way that they are serviceable. Solid state circuitry has enabled manufacturers to reduce the physical size and weight of the controls, which, in turn, makes installation,

71

servicing, and space-planning less of a problem than in the past.

A typical 300 ma, 125 KV, $1/60$ sec time control is shown in Figure 5–1.

For the modern, nonspecialty small animal practice, a single phase control rated for 200 to 300 ma at 125 KV, with at least $1/60$ sec timing, will provide the necessary range of exposure capabilities for most routine examinations. Some of the features found in this size control which are not usually found in the smaller 30 to 100 ma controls are preset ma stations activated by dial or pushbutton, space charge compensation, accurate KV selection in small increments (1 to 2 KV) over the whole KV range, electronic timing, line voltage compensation, tube protection circuits, ma stabilization, and, in some controls, electronic contacting. With a control of this type, the unpredictable results caused by smaller, less expensive controls is replaced with greater predictability.

Outpatient practices with a preponderance of the caseload consisting of small dogs and cats may find 100 ma control systems to be adequate. This is particularly true when a well-equipped hospital facility is available for referral of larger patients or those requiring complicated internal medical radiographic procedures. A minimal timing capability of $1/60$ or $1/30$ sec is highly recommended with a 100 ma unit, since quality radiography of rapidly breathing patients requires short exposure times. The recently available rare earth phosphor intensifying screens, with their increased speed, allow utilization of faster exposure times, since the mas requirements are decreased. With their use, $1/120$ sec exposures may become routine.

Central hospital facilities and specialty practices usually find minimal ma requirements to be in the 300 to 500 ma range. In this milliamperage range, $1/120$ sec timing is practical and desirable. Solid state or electronic contacting makes the $1/120$ sec timer reliable.

High Voltage Transformer. The high voltage transformer is electrically matched to the control system and is contained in a separate metal enclosure. This enclosure contains the core and windings of the high voltage transformer, the filament transformers for the x-ray tubes, the cable socket changeover switch if more than one tube is to be used, the cable sockets for the high voltage cables, the rectification circuit, and the insulating coil. The size of the enclosure has been reduced recently to about one half its former size and weight due to the use of solid state rectifiers and smaller transformer cores. Along with this reduction in size, the efficiency and reproducibility of output have been increased.

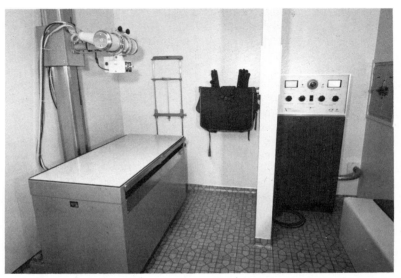

Figure 5–1. A x-ray unit showing the control, table, tubestand, and tube housing with attached collimator. Courtesy of Drs. R. L. Maahs and Robert Conness, San Carlos, California.

X-Ray Tube. The x-ray tube used with high milliamperage controls is commonly a double focus rotating anode tube. Recent improvements in this type of tube have been in the composition and size of the anode and in the radiation shielding of the housing. The renium-tungsten-copper anode is the most common type in use presently and it differs from the solid tungsten-copper anode in its improved ability to dissipate heat. The improved shielding reduces leakage of radiation below the amount allowed by law.

X-Ray Localizing System. The collimation system (Fig. 5–1) aligns and modifies the conical x-ray beam so that it conforms to the size of the film being used or patient part being examined. Manually operated, multi-leaved collimators that provide a light field coincident with the x-ray beam have replaced cones as the means of accomplishing beam shaping. With these collimators, exposures can be reduced to the desired rectangular (or circular in some cases) shape, thereby reducing scatter radiation to the point where split film techniques can be performed without additional lead shielding.

It is a common practice when using a Bucky mechanism or stationary grid cabinet to have the central x-ray beam centered to the cassette by coupling the tubestand to the Bucky or grid cabinet. With the cassette secured in a cassette tray inside the Bucky or grid cabinet under the table, it is difficult to know the exact longitudinal and transverse settings of the collimator that will coincide with film size. To remedy this, the Federal regulations (in effect after 1974) require that sensing devices be used to determine the size of the film in the cabinet tray and to automatically set the collimator opening to this size before an exposure can be made. Although these regulations apply only to medical radiography, the benefits of automatically limiting beam size and thus reducing scatter radiation are desirable in veterinary practice as well.

The use of a Bucky mechanism or stationary grid is necessary in medium-to-thick body part examination. Good clean-up of scatter radiation is obtained with either an 8:1, 80 line per inch stationary grid or a par speed 8:1, 80 line per inch Bucky device. The motion and noise of the older model Bucky mechanism usually do not produce patient excitement while the film is being made since the maximum sound is emitted by this device when the grid travel is terminated, which is after an exposure has been made. Modern reciprocating or recipromatic Bucky mechanisms are relatively quiet and produce no patient excitement problem.

Handling Devices. Handling devices such as the table, tubestand, and positioning aids deserve special consideration when designing an x-ray department. Equipment construction should allow for the following: easy placement of the x-ray tube and film holder in line with the part of the body to be examined; positioning of the patient so that personnel can be in a protected area when the exposure is made (the most improvement is usually needed in this area); and adequate size to accommodate all patients. A table-tubestand combination such as the one shown in Figure 5–1 fulfills essential construction requirements. The tubestand should move the entire length of the table, hold the x-ray tube so that the central x-ray beam is centered to the table and Bucky cabinet, allow the tube to be moved vertically to 40 inches from the table top, and allow the tube to be rotated for horizontal exposures. The tubestand should be attached to the Bucky or grid cabinet so that the central x-ray beam is always centered on the cassette tray for routine exposure technique. This type of table-tubestand combination is made by a number of manufacturers and usually measures about 3 feet in width (including the tubestand) and about 5 feet in length. For veterinary use, this device should be free of dirt-catching edges.

Some available positioning and restraining devices are shown in Figure 5–2. (See Atlas section for further illustration of these devices.) These devices assist in positioning the anesthetized or sedated patient and permit the operator to make exposures from a protected area. The need for a complete restraining-positioning device which will accommodate all patients is obvious.

Special Purpose Equipment

Special purpose radiographic equipment is being used with increased frequency by teaching institutions, specialty practices, and some group practices. Requirements for special equipment used in motion studies

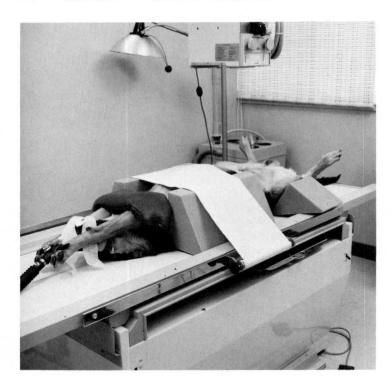

Figure 5–2. Positioning aids. Sponge blocks, sand bags, and compression band shown in use during the examination of an abdomen.

and body section examinations vary considerably with caseload and degree of sophistication desired. Generally, a system for image intensification fluoroscopy is needed in specialty practices and teaching institutions where motion studies are a routine part of internal medical examinations. A method of recording the fluoroscopic image for future detailed study should also be provided. This may be accomplished* with cine photographic filming, videotape or disc recordings, or by the use of a spot filming device. Cine filming and videotaping provide recordings of motion, whereas a spot filming device records a series of single radiographic images.

Rapid sequential filming is usually accomplished with a rapid film changer. This equipment is used to provide a detailed record of dynamic studies.

Body section equipment may be desirable for specialized studies where the details of structure may be obscured by overlying body parts. A general description of these devices is found in Chapter 14.

The generator used for special procedure equipment is generally more complex and contains more protective devices than the ones used for basic radiographic equipment. Milliamperage capabilities as high as 1000 ma, single or three phase, may be required for the extremely short exposure times needed in some rapid film changer studies.

Special tables with four-way moving tops, with space underneath to house either an x-ray tube or imaging system, are normally used for special radiographic procedures (Fig. 5–10). The tubestand or tubestands should be ceiling-mounted to allow freedom of movement on all sides of the table and to save valuable floor space for the ancillary equipment that is often needed.

Image Amplifier Systems. Most dynamic special examinations are not possible without an image amplifier system. Basically, the image amplifier converts the fluoroscopic image at its input surface to an image 3000 to 10,000 times the intensity of a fluoroscopic screen. The image at the output side is then viewed directly by a mirror optical system or by a closed circuit television camera, or is recorded on 16, 35, 70, or 100 mm photographic film. If a video system is used, videotape or core recorders may be used to preserve the dynamic portions of an examination for future review and study.

Slow motion and still frame techniques increase the usefulness of the video recording methods.

Rapid Film Changers. Rapid film changers are used to record dynamic studies radiographically. They find extensive use in cardiovascular studies where radiographic detail is needed. Cassette film changers have exposure rates of up to 2 per second and the cut film changers have exposure rates normally up to 12 exposures per second.

Mobile X-Ray Equipment. Mobile x-ray equipment may be desirable for mixed practices. Two types of mobile equipment are available: the conventional high voltage, single-phase transformer type and the capacitor discharge type. The conventional type is a mobile version of the basic generator and varies in size from a 30 ma, self-contained x-ray tube machine to a 300 ma, 125 KV machine. Increased milliamperage capacity requires that high ampere power sources be available where the machine is operated, thus requiring extensive hospital wiring for great mobility. A capacitor discharge unit alleviates the wiring problem since high voltage applied across the x-ray tube is built up over a Villard-type voltage doubling circuit, thus eliminating the high voltage transformer. When the charge is sufficient, a high kilovoltage exposure can be made. Power input may be provided by conventional 110 volt electrical outlets.

Automatic Film Processors. Automatic film processors are now available in a price range such that a busy practice should seriously consider their use. The large processors, initially used only in major hospitals, have decreased in cost and physical size. (Fig. 5–11). Small processors may fit into existing darkrooms and thus require minimal installation effort and expense (Fig. 5–3). Automatic film processing not only provides consistent results, but also, and more importantly, the availability of a read-

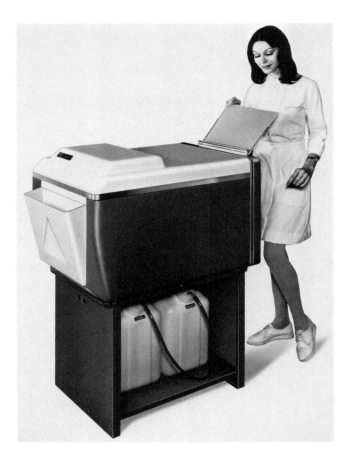

Figure 5–3. Low capacity automatic film processor. Solution replenisher tanks are located under the stand. This type of processor may be installed on a bench top without the stand.

able, diagnostic film with minimal time and effort encourages the use of radiographic examinations.

PLANNING YOUR X-RAY DEPARTMENT

The layout and planning of your x-ray department should start by integrating the location of the department into the overall traffic-flow plan of the clinic or hospital. In general, the department should be adjacent to the patient preparation area and near the surgery area. There should be sufficient isolation so that each area can be used simultaneously. Once the general area is defined, a representative of the company providing the x-ray equipment should be consulted to determine the floor space needed, and a preliminary drawing locating the equipment should be made. Given this preliminary drawing, along with electrical requirements, junction box locations and plumbing requirements, the architect and contractor should be able to integrate the department's location into the total hospital plan.

Floor plans and photographs of existing effectively functional veterinary radiology departments which were economical to build in terms of time and cost of construction are shown in Figures 5–4, 5–7, and 5–9. Department size and equipment capabilities were chosen to illustrate the needs of a small practice, a group practice, and a specialty practice. Dimensions are included only as guidelines for space required.

Generally, two or three junction boxes and a circuit breaker are needed in each x-ray room. Table 5–1 lists the minimum power supply requirements needed for various types of x-ray machines.

Accessory equipment should be located on the drawing during the planning stage. This equipment should include safelights, film bins, cassette transfer box, film dryer, view boxes (both wet and dry), imprinter for labeling film, apron and glove rack, wall cassette holder and cassette storage cabinets.

In order to enhance visualization of the collimator light field, the lighting in the x-ray room should not create a glare on the table top.

The darkroom should be adjacent to the x-ray room so that a cassette transfer box may be used to good advantage. This box may also serve as a cassette storage box.

An exhaust fan and light-tight louvered door vent are desirable darkroom items, especially when the work load is heavy. These items improve working conditions, especially during warm weather or when a film dryer or automatic processor adds heat to the room.

(Text continued on page 86.)

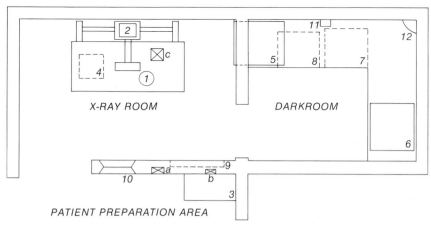

Figure 5–4. Floor plan for a radiology department suitable for a one- or two-man small animal practice. *1*, X-ray table; *2*, tubestand; *3*, x-ray control; *4*, high voltage transformer; *5*, cassette transfer cabinet; *6*, developing tank; *7*, film dryer; *8*, film bin; *9*, illuminator; *10*, leaded window; *11*, imprinter; *12*, safelight; *a*, circuit breaker; *b*, junction box; *c*, floor junction box.

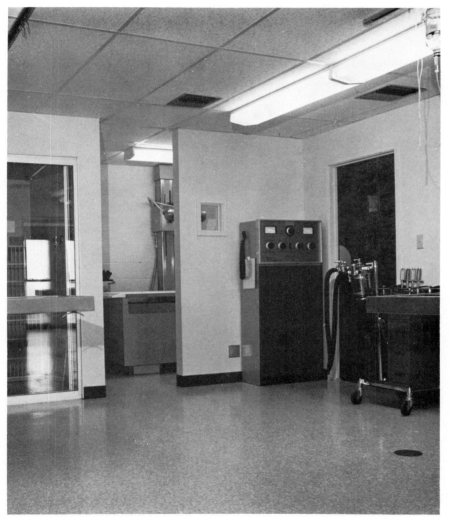

Figure 5–5. View of the x-ray control, leaded window, and door into the x-ray room from the preparation room. Floor plan is as shown in Figure 5–4. Courtesy of Dr. J. E. Rieger, Concord, California.

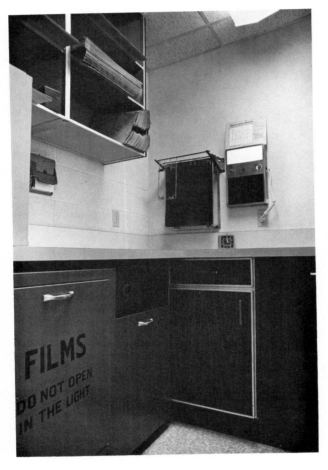

Figure 5–6. View of the darkroom dry bench from the x-ray room. Note the film storage bin and dryer under the bench. Floor plan is as shown in Figure 5–4. Courtesy of Dr. J. E. Rieger, Concord, California.

Figure 5–7. Floor plan for a radiology department suitable for a group practice. *1*, X-ray table; *2*, tubestand; *3*, x-ray control; *4*, high voltage transformer; *5*, cassette transfer cabinet; *6*, automatic processor; *7*, film bin; *8, 9*, illuminator; *10*, leaded window; *11*, imprinter; *a*, circuit breaker; *b*, junction box; *c*, floor junction box.

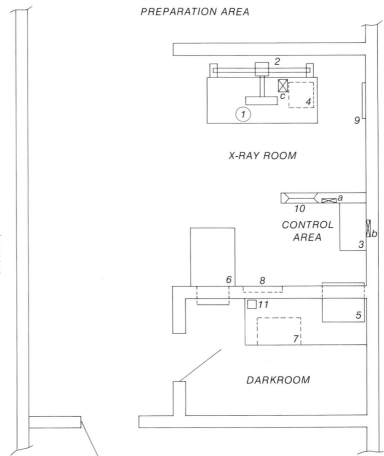

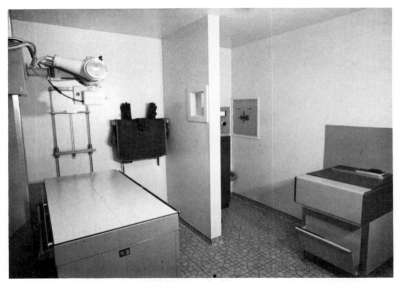

Figure 5–8. View of the x-ray room from hallway. The control is located behind a leaded barrier with a leaded window. The cassette transfer cabinet is located in the wall beside the control. The output of a small automatic processor is installed in the darkroom wall. Floor plan is as shown in Figure 5–7. Courtesy of Drs. R. L. Maahs and Robert Conness, San Carlos, California.

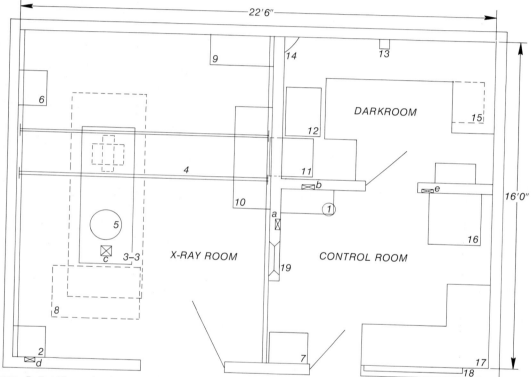

Figure 5–9. Floor plan for a radiology department suitable for a specialty practice. *1,* 300–600 ma x-ray control; *2,* high voltage transformer; *3,* four-way floating table; *4,* overhead tubestand; *5,* image amplifier & television camera under table; *6,* television monitor mounted on wall tracks or cart; *7,* videotape and remote TV monitor; *8,* floor area for film changer; *9,* cardiac monitoring equipment; *10,* sink and storage area; *11,* cassette transfer cabinet; *12,* developing tank covered by hinged counter top; *13,* film imprinter; *14,* safelight; *15,* film bin; *16,* automatic film processor; *17,* film sorting and viewing area; *18,* illuminators; *19,* leaded window; *a,* 70–100 amp circuit breaker, single phase, 220 volt; *b,* wall junction box; *c,* floor junction box; *d,* wall junction box; *e,* 40 amp circuit breaker.

TABLE 5–1
XR4–10 MINIMUM POWER SUPPLY REQUIREMENTS COMING TO X-RAY MACHINES

Classification	Rated Ma. @	Output KvP.	Nominal Line Voltage (see Note IV)	Recommended Distrib. Transformer Capacity (KVA)	Wire Size (AWG) From Distrib. Transformer to Disconnecting Means (See Note III) 50'	100'	200'	Wire Size (AWG) From Disconnecting Means to X-Ray Control For Approx. Length of 15'	Grounding Wire Size (AWG)	X-ray Disconnecting Means — Alternate 1 Switch & Fuse — Switch Rating (AMP)	Fuse Rating (AMP)	Alternate 2 Circuit Breaker Rating (AMP)
SELF-RECTIFIED X-RAY MACHINES For Radiography and Fluoroscopy (including dental, portable, mobile, and stationary types)	10	70	120	*1.5		10		12	14	(15)30	15	15
	15	90–100	120	*1.5		8		10	14	(15)30	20	20
	15	90–100	240	*1.5		12		12	14	(15)30	15	15
	30	85	120	5	8	6	3	10	14	(20)30	30**	30
	30	85	240	5	10	8	6	14	14	30	15**	15
	50–60	85	240	10	8	6	3	8	10	60	50	50
	100	100	240	15	4	2	00	8	10	60	60	60
FULL WAVE RECTIFIED X-RAY MACHINES For Radiography and Fluoroscopy (including mobile and stationary types)	50	100	120	5	6	4	1	10	12	60	40	40
	100	100	240	7.5	8	6	3	10	12	60	40	40
	200	100	240	15	4	2	00	8	10	60	60	60
	200	125	240	25	4	2	00	8	10	60	60	60
	300	150	240	25	2	00	250 MCM	6	8	100	70	70
	300	125	240	37.5	2	00	250 MCM	6	8	100	100	100
	400	125	240	37.5	2	00	250 MCM	4	8	100	100	100
	500	125	240	50	1	000	300 MCM	4	6	200	125	125
	500	150	240	50	0	0000	350 MCM	2	6	200	150	150
	600	125	240	50	0	0000	350 MCM	2	6	200	150	150
	600	150	480	75	6	4	1	6	8	100	100	100
	800	125	480	75	4	2	00	6	6	200	110	110
	1000	100	480	75	4	2	00	6	6	200	110	125

THREE-PHASE X-RAY MACHINES For Radiography and Fluoroscopy (stationary types)											
500	100	240	45	3	0	0000	2	8	100	80	100
700	100	240	75	3	0	0000	0	6	200	110	125
1000	100	240	112.5	1	000	300 MCM	00	6	200	175	175
1000	100	480	112.5	6	4	1	6	8	100	80	100
1250	100	480	150.0	6	3	0	6	6	200	110	125
1500	100	480	150.0	4	2	00	4	6	200	125	125
HALF-WAVE RECTIFIED X-RAY MACHINES											
50	60	240	5	10	8	6	12	14	30	25	30
10	120	120	3	10	8	6	10	14	30	25	30
10	120	240	3	14	12	8	14	14	30	15	15
10	140	120	3	10	8	6	10	14	30	25	30
10	140	240	3	14	12	8	14	14	30	15	15
30	150	240	7.5	6	4	1	8	10	60	40	40

*Any line with 3 per cent regulation will be suitable.

**Use time lag fuses.

( )Suitable attachment plug receptacles of rating indicated may be utilized.

NOTE I   The above specifications are the minimum requirements for a single X-Ray machine of the rating specified.

NOTE II   The maximum recommended daily line voltage variation, due to causes other than the X-Ray equipment load, should not exceed $\pm2\frac{1}{2}$ per cent from the nominal circuit voltage.

NOTE III   The wire sizes "Size Wire (AWG) from Distribution Transformer to X-Ray Disconnecting Means" are based on runs of 50, 100, and 200 feet. If the run is over 200 feet, the manufacturer should be consulted.

NOTE IV   If more than one X-Ray machine is to be used, or additional load is contemplated for the future, larger wire and Transformer size must be specified for satisfactory operation.

NOTE V   The power supply requirements for radiographic and fluoroscopic X-Ray machines are based on an overall line voltage regulation not exceeding 5 per cent as measured at the X-Ray Control at maximum rated output.

NOTE VI   Should the supply line voltage be 208 volts rather than 240 volts, it is recommended that the wire size from the distribution transformer to the disconnect switch be increased to the next larger size.

(From Fischer X-Ray Manual, H. G. Fischer, Inc., Franklin Park, Ill.)

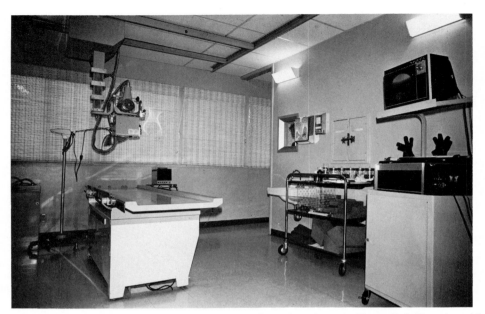

Figure 5–10. View of the x-ray room for the department floor plan shown in Figure 5–9. Note the table with a four-way moving top which contains image intensification and video systems. The TV monitors are seen behind the table and on the right. The large monitor is placed on a cart above a videotape recorder. Note also that the x-ray tube is suspended on a ceiling mounted tubestand. Courtesy of the Berkeley Veterinary Medical Group, Berkeley, California.

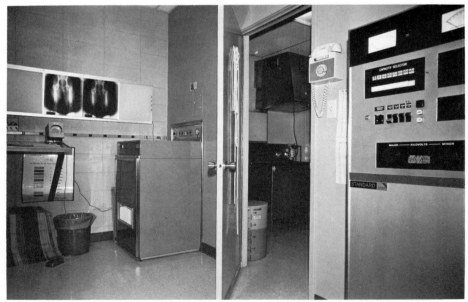

Figure 5–11. View of the control room from the x-ray room for the department shown in Figure 5–9. Note the control on the right and the automatic processor on the left. Processing tanks and dryer mounted overhead are seen through the darkroom door. At times, manual capabilities are desirable for emergency use and for processing some nonscreen film. Courtesy of the Berkeley Veterinary Medical Group, Berkeley, California.

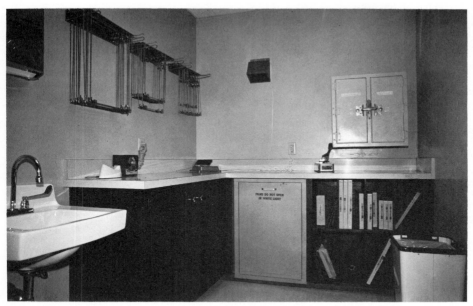

Figure 5–12. View of the dry bench and cassette transfer cabinet for the department shown in Figure 5–9. Courtesy of the Berkeley Veterinary Medical Group, Berkeley, California.

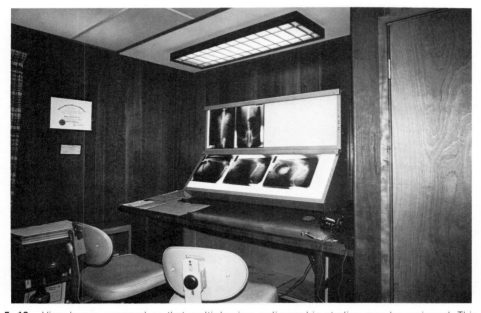

Figure 5–13. View boxes arranged so that multiple-view radiographic studies may be reviewed. This mobile bank of view boxes is surrounded by a slotted table that may be removed to allow transport to a conference room. Courtesy of the Berkeley Veterinary Medical Group, Berkeley, California.

Finally, you should provide a place to sit down and review the finished radiographic study (Fig. 5–13). At least two view boxes are needed so that the multiple view studies may be examined simultaneously. Multiple view box banks are highly desirable, especially for practices in which multiple view special examinations are performed.

REFERENCES

Jaundrell-Thompson, F., and Ashworth, W. J.: X-ray Physics and Equipment. 2nd ed. Philadelphia, F. A. Davis Co., 1965.
Scott, W. G., Ed.: Planning Guide for Radiologic Installations. 2nd ed. Baltimore, Williams and Wilkins, 1966.

6
RADIATION PROTECTION

Louis A. Corwin, Jr.

This chapter will discuss the hazards of radiation from diagnostic X rays, the approximate levels of exposure that are considered safe and the means that the veterinarian and veterinary personnel can employ to minimize exposure. A brief discussion of the regulatory control of veterinary radiology is included.

HAZARDS

In this atomic age, the hazards from ionizing radiation are well defined and the effects of excessive exposure to diagnostic radiation on the older physician and veterinarian have been well publicized. Particularly, indiscriminate use of the fluoroscope with ungloved hands in the fluoroscopic x-ray beam has been shown to produce severe skin damage, including carcinoma, to the exposed areas (Messife et al., 1957). At present, there is also great concern about the more subtle long-term effects from continued exposure to scatter radiation unless a proper radiation safety program is maintained. Possible results of accumulative radiation exposure, besides the long-term skin effects, are inheritable genetic mutation, induction of cataracts and shortening of life from various causes. Protection of the veterinarian, veterinary personnel and the general public can only be accomplished if the practicing veterinarian is aware of the recommended limits of radiation exposure

(maximum permissible doses), the probable dose ranges experienced in radiographic procedures and the ways of minimizing the exposure hazards.

MAXIMUM PERMISSIBLE DOSES (MPD)

Table 6–1 is a summary of the maximum permissible dose levels for radiation workers, which include veterinarians and employees involved in producing radiographic examinations. Exposure dose units are

TABLE 6–1

MAXIMUM PERMISSIBLE DOSE (MPD) FOR VETERINARIAN OR ANY EMPLOYEE INVOLVED IN RADIOGRAPHIC PROCEDURES*

	Week	Year
Whole body: Gonads, bone marrow, lens of eyes	100 mrem†	5,000 mrem
Hands, Forearms, Feet,	1,500 mrem	75,000 mrem

*Recommendations of the International Commission on Radiological Protection. (General Public MPD = 1/10 of stated doses.)
†For X ray, milliroentgens (mr) = millirem (mrem).

87

given in terms of roentgen-equivalents, man (rem), which is the unit used to express human biologic doses resulting from exposure to ionizing radiation. For practical purposes, the measured dose in roentgens of diagnostic X rays is equivalent to rem. In this discussion, the measured dose in milliroentgens (mr or 1/1000 of a roentgen) will be used as equivalent to the millirem unit. The limiting factor in determining the MPD is the radiation exposure to particularly vulnerable or "critical" organs. Since the gonads, the bone marrow and the lenses of the eyes are especially sensitive, particular care should be taken to shield these areas during radiographic procedures. The lenses of the eyes are especially vulnerable since they are not ordinarily shielded by the usual protective gloves and aprons. The MPD for the whole body (including gonads, bone marrow and lenses) is 100 millirems (mrem) per week or 5000 mrem per year for occupationally exposed persons. It should be understood that these are maximum permissible doses. Under proper conditions of practice, these dose levels should never be approached.

EXPOSURE LEVELS

Typical exposure levels in diagnostic radiographic procedures have been calculated (McCullogh and Cameron, 1970; O'Riordan, 1970; Corwin et al., unpublished). Figure 6–1 depicts the situation in which a lateral radiograph of the pelvis of the dog is being produced. The tube head is 40 inches from the table top and the machine factors are 80 KV, 100 ma and 1/10 second or 10 mas. In this situation, a hand exposed to the primary beam on top of the dog would receive about 100 mr per radiograph. At the side of the table, the scatter to the body of the operator, if standing close, could be approximately 5 mr per radiograph. Since radiation intensity decreases to one fourth if the distance between the source (patient's body) and the operator is doubled, further decreased exposure levels may be attained by standing at a maximum distance from the patient if manual restraint is necessary (see Chap. 4). There would also be scatter from the floor if the sides of the table are unshielded. If the 2 mm of aluminum filtration were removed, the exposure levels could be

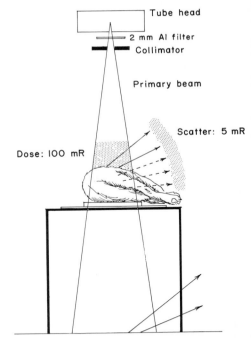

Figure 6–1. Exposure levels in the primary x-ray beam at the top of a dog (32 inches from the x-ray tube) and scattered X rays at the edge of the table. X-ray machine factors were 80 KV and 10 mas. (After O'Riordan, 1970.)

three to four times as high. Without proper collimation and filtration or protective apparel, and with careless technique, the operator could possibly receive the weekly MPD to the whole body from a single radiographic procedure.

Figure 6–2 depicts a typical fluoroscopic situation. The dose level in the primary x-ray beam between the body of the dog and the screen could be of the order of 5000 mr per minute and the scatter from the side of the animal up to 100 mr per minute. Obviously, a few minutes of fluoroscopy exposes the veterinarian to much more radiation than the taking of a single diagnostic radiograph. There is shielding intrinsic to the fluoroscope screen which protects the operator's face, and there should be a lead drape to the side of the screen to protect the operator's body.

It is assumed that protective apparel such as leaded gloves and aprons would be used in the two procedures depicted. However, veterinarians should understand the limitations of this type of shielding. Protective apparel is designed to protect against scatter

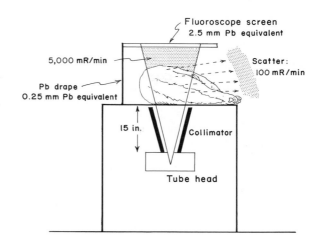

Figure 6-2. Exposure levels in the primary x-ray beam and scattered X rays from a typical fluoroscopic procedure.

radiation which has lower energy than the primary x-ray beam. The lead shielding material in these gloves and aprons usually will reduce the dose of scatter radiation well below one twentieth of the scatter radiation exposure dose. However, the higher energy of the primary x-ray beam may be only attenuated to one fourth by the gloves (Fig. 6-3). Thus, in the typical diagnostic exposure situation, gloved hands in the primary beam could still receive approximately 25 mr from a single radiographic exposure.

Figure 6-3 schematically illustrates the amount of exposure reduction by gloves and aprons from the primary x-ray beam or scatter radiation. It is assumed that the apron and gloves would have a minimum of 0.5 mm of lead equivalency, which would reduce the primary x-ray intensity to approximately one fourth and that of the scatter radiation to a negligible amount.

Published reports on veterinary personnel exposure and surveys of veterinary radiographic installations have shown that nor-

mal exposure to the whole body beneath the protective apron is below measurable levels (Kangstrom and Kilibus, 1972; Unwin, 1970). The exposure to the unprotected areas (head, neck, and elbows) can range between 15 mrem to approximately 100 mrem per week, depending on the work load and the amount of manual restraint performed (Kangstrom and Kilibus, 1972; O'Riordan, 1968; Corwin et al., unpublished). While these exposure levels are still below the MPD levels for the respective body regions, strict radiation safety practices must be maintained to reduce the hazards to an absolute minimum (Jacobsen and van Farowe, 1964).

It should be emphasized that the foregoing MPD levels were established for radiation workers who are working under controlled conditions and wear monitoring devices. The MPD for the general public and for personnel in noncontrolled areas is one tenth of that listed for the radiation worker.

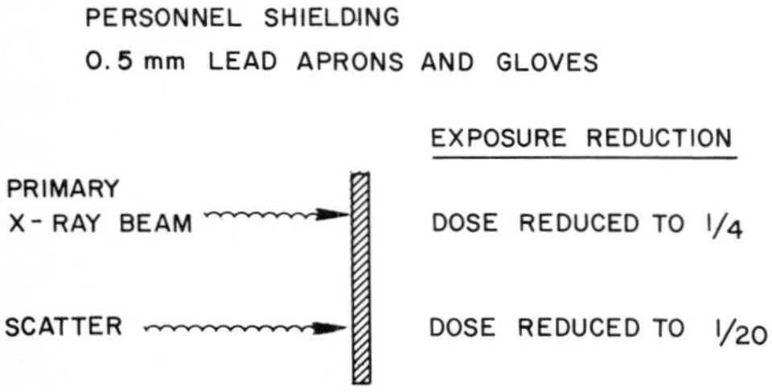

PERSONNEL SHIELDING
0.5 mm LEAD APRONS AND GLOVES

EXPOSURE REDUCTION

PRIMARY
X-RAY BEAM   DOSE REDUCED TO 1/4

SCATTER   DOSE REDUCED TO 1/20

Figure 6-3. Approximate exposure reduction provided by protective apparel.

REGULATORY CONTROL

Legal requirements for the use of diagnostic x-ray machines are under the control of the respective states. These requirements are available from the appropriate state agency, usually the State Health Department. The requirements will vary from state to state but usually have the elements shown in Table 6-2. Most states require registration of a diagnostic x-ray machine

TABLE 6-2

SUMMARY OF RADIATION PROTECTION
RECOMMENDATIONS

Machine:	Properly shielded tube head.
	2 mm aluminum added filtration.
	Rectangular, adjustable collimator and aiming device.
Table:	Permanently mounted fluoroscope screen with shield.
	Shielded table sides.
Personnel:	Lead gloves and apron (0.5 mm lead equivalent).
	Minimum manual restraint.
	Film badge monitoring with monthly report.
	No person under 18 years of age or pregnant female.
Accessories:	Fastest speed screens and film for the procedure.
	Proper radiographic technique and procedures.
Records:	Log to record exposure factors and personnel performing the examination.

and will usually survey the machine and the facility after the initial registration. At that time, specific recommendations may be made regarding the equipment and the operative procedures to aid the veterinarian in following proper radiation safety practices. The National Council on Radiation Protection and most present state health codes would permit occupationally exposed persons (i.e., veterinarians and their employees) to manually restrain and position animal patients for radiography when it is absolutely necessary. However, at this writing, there are state codes in effect or under consideration that prohibit manual restraint of animals during the production of diagnostic radiographs by occupationally exposed personnel. This would imply that the animal owner or other staff personnel not routinely involved in radiographic procedures would have to be used for this purpose. The present federal regulations concerning performance standards for diagnostic x-ray systems (which became effective in August, 1974) are concerned with diagnostic x-ray machines for use on humans and, at the present time, these regulations are usually interpreted as not applying to veterinary medicine (Federal Register, 1972).

RADIATION PROTECTION FACTORS

Equipment

The radiation produced by a diagnostic x-ray machine must be controlled whether the machine is stationary or portable.

Tube Head. Since the x-ray tube emits radiation in all directions, it is important that the tube head be well shielded. Normally, a recently manufactured tube head can be considered safe. If the machine is of an older vintage or if there is a question of radiation leakage, the tube head should be checked by a health physicist or by the radiation safety unit of the State Health Department.

Filtration. At least 2 mm of aluminum filtration equivalent should be added to the primary x-ray beam, usually between the tube window and the collimator, to absorb the softer X rays, which do not contribute to the diagnostic radiograph but do increase exposure to the operator. Without filtrations, the exposure doses may be increased three to four times.

Collimator. The collimator should be an adjustable rectangular type, which can restrict the primary beam to within the size of the cassette. A light source which both acts as an aiming device and indicates the limits of the x-ray beam is particularly desirable. With the addition of this type of collimator, the total equivalent aluminum filtration of the primary beam exceeds the recommended total of 2½ mm of aluminum filtration. To improve the diagnostic quality of the film as well as reduce the scatter radiation exposure to personnel, the collimator should restrict the beam to the area of clinical interest.

Fluoroscope. Hand-held fluoroscopes should never be used. The fluoroscopic unit should be constructed so that the x-ray beam is restricted to the leaded glass screen or the image intensification device. The leaded glass should be at least the equivalent of 1.5 mm of lead with a 0.25 mm lead equivalent drape between the patient and operator. The tube head should be at least 15 inches below the table top, with at least 2.5 mm of aluminum filtration in the primary x-ray beam. If there is a slot for a bucky tray below the table top, it should similarly be shielded by a lead drape.

PERSONNEL

Neither persons under 18 years of age nor pregnant women should be involved in radiographic procedures. No individuals other than the operator and those necessarily involved in the procedure should be in the x-ray room when exposures are being made. All persons in the room should wear protective apparel. Ideally, the gloves and aprons should have a 0.5 mm lead equivalent. Animals should not be manually restrained for radiography. Chemical restraint, such as short-acting anesthetics or tranquilizers, combined with supporting and restraining devices, should be employed as much as possible. If, in the judgment of the clinician, the animal cannot tolerate pharmaceutical restraint, personnel wearing protective gloves and aprons may do so. However, they should position themselves as far away from the primary x-ray beam and the patient as possible. The operator's body should not be exposed to the primary x-ray beam even if shielded, since the type of shielding used will not adequately protect against the more penetrating energy of the primary x-ray beam.

Ideally, the animal would be restrained adequately by supporting devices. The operator should be in a shielded booth or behind a shielding screen or at least 6 feet from the x-ray table when the exposure is made (Fig. 6–4).

Fluoroscopic procedures should be performed in a similar manner, with the operator taking particular care not to expose any part of the body or hands to the primary x-ray beam even though wearing protective gloves and apron. Since fluoroscopy is extremely hazardous, because of the potentially high exposures, it should be performed only by qualified personnel and then only when needed to obtain specific diagnostic information. Fluoroscopy should never be used as a substitute for a non-motion radiographic examination. Fluoroscopic procedures should be carefully planned in advance so that the fluoroscope is turned on only for brief periods and the total time kept to an absolute minimum.

Personnel monitoring devices should be worn at all times by any individuals who may be involved in the radiographic procedures. Ideally, two film badges should be worn, one under the protective apparel at

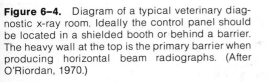

Figure 6–4. Diagram of a typical veterinary diagnostic x-ray room. Ideally the control panel should be located in a shielded booth or behind a barrier. The heavy wall at the top is the primary barrier when producing horizontal beam radiographs. (After O'Riordan, 1970.)

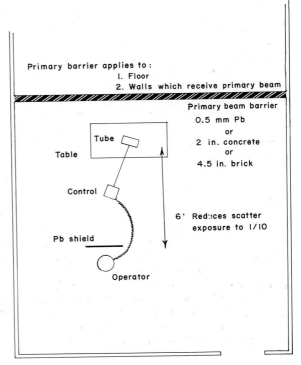

the belt level, to monitor whole body exposure, and the other above the protective apparel at the neckline, to estimate the exposure to the skin of the head and neck and the lenses of the eyes. If there is a fairly heavy workload, the use of protective goggles might be considered. Even ordinary glass eyeglasses will provide protection from the scatter radiation.

Film badges can be obtained from commercial firms who provide this service for a nominal cost. For the average veterinary practice, the film badges should be exchanged once a month. For practices with a low radiology workload, replacement of the badges once every three months is probably adequate.

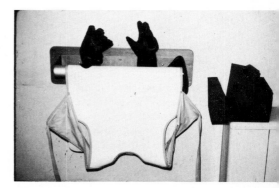

Figure 6–5. Wall rack for proper storage of gloves and aprons in diagnostic x-ray room. Note also foam cushions which aid in positioning to minimize manual restraint.

Accessory Equipment

The use of the highest speed screen and fastest film compatible with the radiographic detail requirements will reduce the amount of radiation needed to produce a diagnostic radiograph and, therefore, reduce the exposure to the personnel involved. Proper radiographic technique and darkroom procedures will ensure a quality radiograph and reduce the number of repeat studies, thereby reducing the amount of exposure per examination.

Protective aprons should never be folded flat, since the lead shielding material tends to separate after repeated bendings. A rack should be provided in the diagnostic x-ray room for proper storage of the aprons (Fig. 6–5). Gloves may be placed on the rack or stored with open-ended cans placed in the gauntlet to permit drying and prevent cracking of the material (Fig. 6–6). All protective apparel should be inspected periodically for defects.

Records

A permanent log should be maintained for each radiographic examination. The date, names of the patient and personnel involved, and the milliamperage, kilovoltage and exposure time should be recorded. Besides providing useful information that may be used as a check against the technique chart, this record provides an indication of the workload and the amount of radiation to

which individuals are exposed. It also provides a guide to permit distributing the workload among all the personnel available so that no one individual is exposed excessively.

Installation

The diagnostic x-ray room should be located away from the traffic flow and in particular away from areas where clients or the general public might be inadvertently exposed. Radiology workload in the average veterinary hospital usually does not require extensive shielding; however, there should be some provision for a primary barrier (Fig. 6–4). This may be any wall or surface through which the primary beam can be

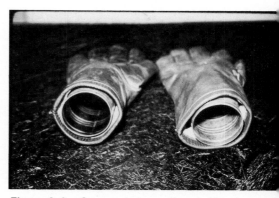

Figure 6–6. Open-ended cans inserted in gloves to allow drying and prevent cracking of shielding material.

directed. A satisfactory amount of shielding is provided by lead and some usual building materials. No barrier wall is necessary if horizontal x-ray beams are directed toward an outside wall. It is recommended that the exposure control be located so that the operator is at least 6 feet from the table at the time the exposure is made, and preferably behind a screen barrier.

REFERENCES

Corwin, L. A., Jr., Lee, P. K., and Larsen, S. J.: Exposure dose to dog gonads in radiography for canine hip dysplasia. Unpublished data, 1975.

Corwin, L. A., Jr., and Lee, P. K.: Exposure levels to personnel in veterinary diagnostic radiography. Unpublished data, 1975.

Council of State Governments: Suggested State Regulations for Control of Radiation. Council of State Governments, 1313 E. 60th St., Chicago, Ill.

Jacobsen, G. A., and van Farowe, D. E.: Survey of x-ray protection practice among Michigan veterinarians. J.A.V.M.A., *145*:783, 1964.

Kangstrom, L. E., and Kilibus, A.: Radiation safety in small animal radiography. Acta Radiol. Suppl., *319*:147, 1972.

McCullough, C. E., and Cameron, J. R.: Exposure rates from diagnostic x-ray units. Brit. J. Radiol., *43*:448, 1970.

Messife, J., Troisi, F. M., and Kleinfield, M.: Radiological hazards due to x-radiation in veterinarians. Amer. Med. Ass. Archiv. Industr. Hlth., *16*:48, 1957.

National Council on Radiation Protection and Measurements: Radiation Protection in Veterinary Medicine. Report No. 36, NCRP Publications, Washington, D.C., 1970.

O'Riordan, M. C.: Occupational exposure to x-rays in veterinary practices. Vet. Rec., *82*:22, 1968.

O'Riordan, M. C.: Examination of a veterinary practice for radiation hazards. J. Small Anim. Pract., *11*:515, 1970.

Regulations for the Administration and Enforcement of the Radiation Control for Health and Safety Act of 1968. Title 42, Part 78. Federal Register, Vol. 37, No. 158, August 15, 1972.

Unwin, D. D.: Radiation protection in a veterinary practice. J. Small Anim. Pract., *11*:523, 1970.

AN ATLAS OF RADIOGRAPHIC POSITIONING AND TECHNIQUE

GENERAL PRINCIPLES

Positioning small animal patients for radiography is a complex and often exacting task that requires the proper means of restraint (chemical and physical), knowledge of anatomy and clinical disease, and a great deal of ingenuity. Proper positioning alone, however, will not guarantee the production of diagnostic radiographs. Careful attention to proper exposure factors as they apply to the specific patient is also necessary.

TECHNIQUE CHART

A usable technique chart should be established for every x-ray machine (Chap. 4). This chart should be easy to use and require minimal alteration in exposure factors for the production of specific radiographs. Alteration of exposure factors to compensate for the changes in contrast and density caused by specific pathologic, physiologic or extraneous factors should be made prior to positioning the patient for radiographic examination.

The proper use of a technique chart demands measurement of each part being radiographed with a caliper that is graduated in centimeters. The thickest region on the part being examined should always be measured (e.g., caudal rib cage for thoracic or cranial abdomen examinations).

Generally, increased exposure is required for examining patients that have an increased amount of x-ray absorbing tissue for a given thickness. For example, patients with pulmonary edema, hemorrhage or contusion, pneumonia, pleural effusion, severe cardiomegaly or diaphragmatic hernia require greater exposure than a patient with a normally aerated thoracic cavity of a given thickness. The increased exposure can be obtained by increasing either the mas or KV. Since short exposure times are desirable (especially when radiographing dyspneic patients), increasing the KV is the preferred method. The magnitude by which KV is increased depends upon the severity of the pathologic process, which may be determined by physical examination of the patient in most cases. An increase of from 5 to 10 KV is usually sufficient. If the pathologic state is severe and the thorax is over 10 cm thick, a grid should be used (see Chap. 4, Table 4–2).

Pathologic states such as pneumothorax or emphysema require decreased exposure. Either decreasing the mas by decreasing the time of exposure or decreasing the KV will lower the exposure. A decrease of from 5 to 10 KV is usually sufficient.

In abdominal examinations, the presence of peritoneal fluid necessitates increased exposure. Increased exposure is also necessary for examining patients with severe obesity or marked enlargement of an abdominal organ, such as the uterus (with pyometra or normal pregnancy). An increase of from 5 to 10 KV is usually sufficient.

When examining patients that have a positive contrast agent in an organ system (as in such studies as esophagram, the G.I. series, the urogram and the angiogram), the exposure should be increased slightly. The addition of 5 to 7 KV or mas increases of one half (for example, from 5 to 7.5) will usually increase contrast and allow better visualization of structures.

Negative contrast studies, such as pneumoperitoneography and pneumocystography, require decreased exposure to maintain adequate radiographic density. This is usually accomplished by subtracting 5 to 7 KV from the value indicated on the technique chart.

When radiographing structures with an increased amount of x-ray absorbing bone per centimeter of thickness, such as the skull of brachycephalic dogs, increased exposure is needed for the production of adequate radiographic density. This is usually accomplished by adding 5 to 10 KV to the value indicated on the technique chart for a given centimeter of thickness or by increasing the mas value by one half.

Radiographs of patients with a decreased amount of bone per centimeter of thickness, such as immature cats or patients with osteoporotic states, require a decreased exposure. This is usually accomplished by decreasing the KV by 5 to 7 from the value indicated on the technique chart for a given centimeter of thickness.

The superimposition of radiodense materials (such as a plaster cast) on the part being examined requires increased exposure. The average dry plaster cast requires doubling the mas or adding 10 to 15 KV to the value indicated on the technique chart. Wood, plastic, or aluminum splints and dry bandage material usually do not require increased exposure values when the thickness of the part being examined is measured to include these materials.

Table 7–1 lists some common alterations in exposure technique used to compensate for various pathologic, physiologic or extraneous factors.

NORMAL ANATOMY AND TERMINOLOGY

Knowledge of the normal anatomy and descriptive terminology is necessary for proper patient positioning. Descriptions of various positional relationships of structures being radiographed are illustrated in this

TABLE 7–1

COMMON ALTERATIONS IN TECHNIQUE CHART VALUES USED TO COMPENSATE FOR VARIOUS PATHOLOGICAL, PHYSIOLOGICAL, OR EXTRANEOUS FACTORS

Conditions Requiring Exposure Alterations	Method of Altering Exposure
A. Increased Exposure	
1. Increased amount of bone per centimeter of thickness, such as brachycephalic dog skulls.	Add 5 to 10 KV or increase mas by one half.
2. Pleural fluid, pulmonary hemorrhage, contusion, edema, pneumonia, severe cardiomegaly, or diaphragmatic hernia.	Add 5 to 10 KV. If thorax is over 10 cm thick, a grid should be used (see Chap. 4, Table 4–2).
3. Peritoneal fluid, severe obesity, or marked organ enlargement, such as of the uterus.	Add 5 to 10 KV.
4. Positive contrast medium in organ system.	Add 5 to 7 KV.
5. Plaster cast.	Double mas or add 10 to 15 KV.
B. Decreased Exposure	
1. Decreased amount of bone per centimeter of thickness, such as in immature cats or in osteoporotic states.	Subtract 5 to 7 KV.
2. Pneumothorax or emphysema.	Subtract 5 to 10 KV.
3. Pneumoperitonography, pneumocystography, and other negative contrast examinations.	Subtract 5 to 7 KV.

atlas section. The positional terminology used in this section is that adopted by a joint committee from the American Association of Veterinary Anatomists and the Educators in Veterinary Radiologic Science (Habel et al., 1963).

The terms "dorsal" and "ventral" are used to describe the top and bottom, respectively, of the head, neck, thorax, abdomen, pelvis and tail while the animal is in the normal quadrupedal position. "Anterior" and "posterior" are used to describe the front and the back, respectively, of the limbs. "Lateral" refers to the outside and "medial" to the inside of the limbs.

Description of a specific radiographic position is given by the direction of the x-ray beam through the part being examined. For example, an anteroposterior (AP) view of a carpus indicates that the x-ray beam passed from the anterior to the posterior surface to reach the x-ray film. Conversely, a posteroanterior (PA) view of a carpus indicates that the x-ray beam passed from the posterior to the anterior surface to reach the x-ray film.

Lateral views of the limbs are given specific designations to indicate either the right or left limb and the direction of the x-ray beam. For example, a left lateromedial view would be produced by passing the x-ray beam from the lateral to the medial surface of the left limb (either front or rear).

Oblique views of the limbs should similarly identify the direction of the x-ray beam and designate the left or right limb. "Lateral" or "medial" is used to describe the location of the x-ray film. For example, an anteroposterior medial oblique (APMO) view would be produced by passing the x-ray beam obliquely from the anterolateral surface medially to the posteromedial surface. The x-ray film is located on the posteromedial surface. An anteroposterior lateral oblique (APLO) view would be produced with the x-ray film on the posterolateral aspect of the limb, with the x-ray beam entering the limb from the anteromedial aspect.

A dorsoventral (DV) view of the head, neck, thorax or abdomen would indicate that the x-ray beam passed from the dorsal surface to the ventral surface, and a ventrodorsal (VD) view would indicate that the beam passed from the ventral surface to the dorsal surface to reach the x-ray film.

Lateral views of the head, neck, thorax or abdomen are termed right or left, depending upon where the film is placed. A right lateral view of the abdomen would be a radiograph produced with the film on the right side and the x-ray beam passing from the left to the right side of the patient. This is accomplished by laying the patient on its right side, or the patient may be in the standing, erect (standing on rear limbs) or inverted position (suspended by rear limbs).

Oblique views of the head, neck, thorax or abdomen are designated to indicate the side of the midline that was placed next to the film and the direction of the x-ray beam. For example, a left dorsoventral (LDVO) view would indicate that the film was placed on the left ventral aspect and that the beam was passed from the right dorsal aspect to the left ventral aspect.

If the patient is not in the recumbent position, its posture should be described as standing, erect or inverted.

An erect ventrodorsal (EVD) view of the abdomen would be produced by standing the patient on its rear limbs and passing the x-ray beam from the ventral to the dorsal aspect in a horizontal plane.

Figure 7–1 illustrates the descriptive terminology used for the head, neck, thorax, abdomen and tail. Figure 7–2 illustrates the descriptive terminology used for the limbs.

Ossification Centers and Bony Fusion. Knowledge of the age at which ossification centers appear and the age at which these structures fuse to adjacent structures is desirable when interpreting radiographs of the immature patient. Table 7–2 lists a summary of available data for the canine. The age at fusion varies with breed, and therefore considerable ranges are listed for some sites.

POSITIONING

Positioning small animal patients for radiographic examination demands the judicious use of an anesthetic or sedative and the aid of various positional and restraint devices. Chemical sedation or anesthesia is desirable when positioning patients in pain or those that are apprehensive. Properly relaxed small animal patients may be positioned with the aid of sponge blocks, ropes, tape, compression bands or head positioning devices.

Only a small percentage of small animal patients should be restrained manually. This method of restraint should be used only when the use of chemical restraint is contraindicated. Strict adherence to radiation safety principles must be observed, especially when manual restraint is necessary (see Chap. 6).

Care must be taken to include all essential anatomical regions in the primary beam when positioning patients. For example, if the radius and ulnar segment are being examined, the elbow and carpal joints should be included.

Angular relationships between the primary x-ray beam and the part being examined must be correct for proper projection onto the film. This is particularly true of skull and vertebral examination. Proper positioning may prevent certain artifacts. For example, when examining the lateral projection of an elbow joint in the immature patient, moderate flexion will avoid the superimposition of the medial epicondylar epiphyseal plate of the humerus on the anconeal process, thereby decreasing the possibility of misdiagnosing an ununited anconeal process.

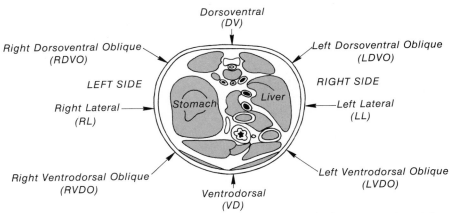

Figure 7–1. Transverse section of the canine abdomen. The arrows indicate the direction of the x-ray beam. Descriptive terminology and abbreviations are indicated for each projection.

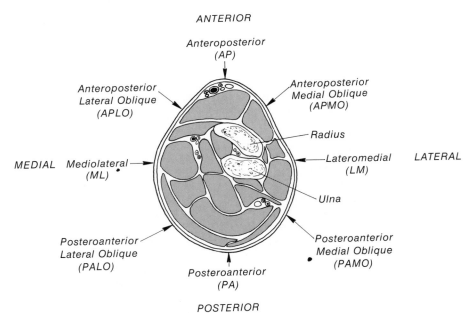

Figure 7–2. Transverse section of the canine forelimb at the level of the radius and ulna. The arrows indicate the direction of the x-ray beam. Descriptive terminology and abbreviations are indicated for each projection.

TABLE 7–2

AGE AT APPEARANCE OF OSSIFICATION CENTERS AND OF BONY FUSION IN THE IMMATURE CANINE

Anatomical Site	Age at Appearance of Ossification Center	Age When Fusion Occurs	Anatomical Site	Age at Appearance of Ossification Center	Age When Fusion Occurs
Scapula			Ilium	Birth	4–6 mo
Body	Birth		Ischium	Birth	4–6 mo
Tuber scapulae	7 wk	4–7 mo	Os acetabulum	7 wk	5 mo
			Iliac crest	4 mo	1–2 yr
Humerus			Tuber ischii	3 mo	8–10 mo
Diaphysis	Birth	—	Ischial arch	6 mo	12 mo
Proximal epiphysis	1–2 wk	10–13 mo	Caudal symphysis pubis	7 mo	5 yr
Distal epiphysis		6–8 mo to shaft	Symphysis pubis		5 yr
Medial condyle	2–3 wk	6 wk to lateral condyle	*Femur*		
Lateral condyle	2–3 wk		Diaphysis	Birth	
Medial epicondyle	6–8 wk	6 mo to condyles	Proximal epiphysis (head)	2 wk	7–11 mo
			Trochanter major	8 wk	6–10 mo
Radius			Trochanter minor	8 wk	8–13 mo
Diaphysis	Birth	—	Distal epiphysis		8–11 mo to shaft
Proximal epiphysis	3–5 wk	6–11 mo	Trochlea	2 wk	3 mo condyles to trochlea
Distal epiphysis	2–4 wk	8–12 mo	Medial condyle	3 wk	
Ulna			Lateral condyle	3 wk	
Diaphysis	Birth		*Patella*	9 wk	
Olecranon	8 wk	6–10 mo	*Tibia*		
Distal epiphysis	8 wk	8–12 mo	Diaphysis	Birth	
Carpus			Condyles		
Ulnar	4 wk		Medial	3 wk	6 wk to lateral
Radial	3–4 wk		Lateral	3 wk	6–12 mo to shaft
Central	4–5 wk		Tuberosity	8 wk	6–8 mo to condyles
Intermediate	3–4 wk				6–12 mo to shaft
Accessory			Distal epiphysis	3 wk	8–11 mo
Body	2 wk		Medial malleolus	3 mo	5 mo
Epiphysis	7 wk	4 mo	*Fibula*		
First	3 wk		Diaphysis	Birth	
Second	4 wk		Proximal epiphysis	9 wk	8–12 mo
Third	4 wk		Distal epiphysis	2–7 wk	7–11 mo
Fourth	3 wk		*Tarsus*		
Sesamoid bone	4 mo		Tibial	Birth–1 wk	
Metacarpus			Fibular	Birth–1 wk	
Diaphysis	Birth		Tuber calcis	6 wk	3–8 mo
Distal epiphysis (2–5)*	4 wk	6 mo	Central	3 wk	
Proximal epiphysis (1)*	5 wk	6 mo	First	4 wk	
			Second	4 wk	
Phalanges			Third	3 wk	
First phalanx			Fourth	2 wk	
Diaphysis (1–5)*	Birth		Metatarsus and pelvic limb phalanges are approximately the same as the metacarpus and pectoral limb phalanges.		
Distal epiphysis (2–5)*	4 wk	6 mo			
Distal epiphysis (1)*	6 wk	6 mo			
Second phalanx					
Diaphysis (2–5)*	Birth				
Proximal epiphysis (2–5)*	5 wk	6 mo			
Second phalanx absent or fused with first in first digit.			*Sesamoids*		
Third phalanx			Fabellar	3 mo	
Diaphysis	Birth		Popliteal	3 mo	
Volar sesamoids	2 mo		Plantar phalangeal	2 mo	
Dorsal sesamoids	4 mo		Dorsal phalangeal	5 mo	
Pelvis					
Pubis	Birth	4–6 mo			

*Digit numbers.

REFERENCES

Carlson, W. D.: Veterinary Radiology. 2nd ed. Philadelphia, Lea and Febiger, 1967.

Chapman, W. L.: Appearance of ossification centers and epiphyseal closures—determined by radiographic techniques. Thesis. Fort Collins, Colorado, Colorado State University, 1963.

Crouch, J. E.: Text-Atlas of Cat Anatomy. Philadelphia, Lea & Febiger, 1969.

Douglas, S. W., and Williamson, H. D.: Principles of Veterinary Radiography. 2nd ed. Baltimore, Williams & Wilkins Co., 1972.

Habel, R. E., Barrett, R. B., Diesem, C. D., and Roenigk, W. J.: Nomenclature for radiologic anatomy. J.A.V.M.A., *142*:38, 1963.

Miller, M. E., Christensen, G. C., and Evans, H. E.: Anatomy of the Dog. Philadelphia, W. B. Saunders Co., 1953.

Schebitz, H., and Wilkens, H.: Atlas of Radiographic Anatomy of Dog and Horse. Berlin, Paul Parey, 1964.

Sisson, S., and Grossman, J. D.: The Anatomy of the Domestic Animals. 4th ed. Philadelphia, W. B. Saunders Co., 1953.

SCAPULA AND SHOULDER JOINT

Posteroanterior (PA) View. The patient is placed in dorsal recumbency (supine), and the sternum is rotated (approximately 30°) away from the side being examined in such a manner that the vertical x-ray beam is passed between the scapula and rib cage (Figs. 8–1 and 8–2). The limb is fully extended. For scapular examinations, x-ray beam collimation and film size should be large enough to allow visualization of the entire blade of the scapula and shoulder joint. The central x-ray beam should transect the midscapula. For shoulder joint examination, the x-ray beam should be centered at the joint.

Figure 8–3 illustrates the radiographic anatomy of the mature canine scapula and shoulder joint in the PA projection. Excessive abduction of the humerus may result in an artifactual subluxation of the shoulder joint since a moderate degree of joint laxity is normal. When positioning the scapula, shoulder joint and humerus in the PA projection, this artifact may be avoided by aligning the scapula and humerus.

Mediolateral (ML) View. The patient is placed in lateral recumbency, and the limb to be examined is placed adjacent to the film. The scapula may be placed over the caudal cervical region (Fig. 8–4) or superimposed over the cranial thorax (Fig. 8–6).

Visualization of the distal aspect of the scapula and shoulder joint is best accomplished by placing the scapula over the caudal cervical region. This is the best position for survey radiographs of the scapular and shoulder region. The limb should be extended and placed at an angle of approximately 45° from the spinal column. This places the shoulder joint over soft tissue, thereby avoiding superimposition over the bony structures of the sternum and ribs. The contralateral limb should be flexed and placed over the cranial aspect of the thorax. The normal radiographic anatomy of the mature canine scapula in this projection is shown in Figure 8–5. The normal radiographic anatomy of the mature canine shoulder joint is shown in Figure 8–8.

If the scapular blade is to be visualized in its entirety, the scapula should be superimposed over the cranial thorax. This places the thin structure of the bone over the radiolucent lung fields and allows better visualization of the borders. The contralat-

(*Text continued on page 108.*)

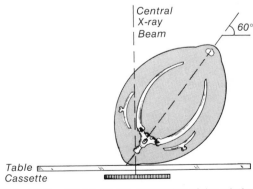

Figure 8–1. Diagrammatic illustration of the relationship of the scapular blade and thoracic wall to the central x-ray beam when producing a PA view of the scapula and shoulder joint. Note that the sagittal plane of the thoracic cavity is placed at an angle of 60 degrees to the x-ray film surface.

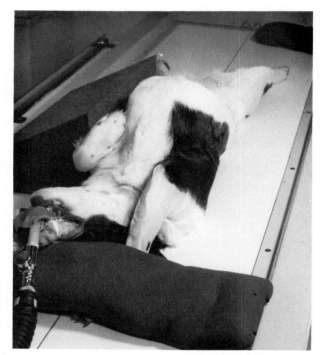

Figure 8–2. Position for the PA view of the scapula and shoulder joint.

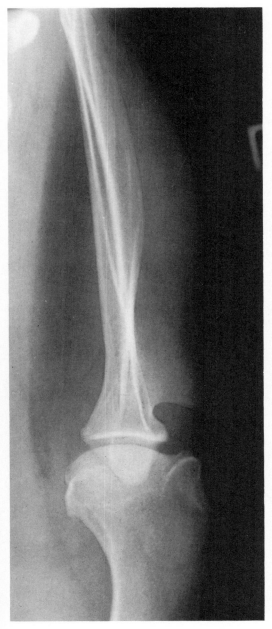
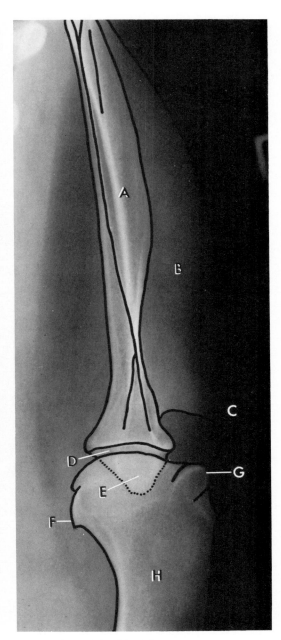

Figure 8–3. PA view of the canine scapula and shoulder joint.
A. Scapula
B. Spine of scapula
C. Acromion
D. Glenoid cavity
E. Scapular and coracoid tuberosities
F. Lesser tubercle
G. Greater tubercle
H. Humerus

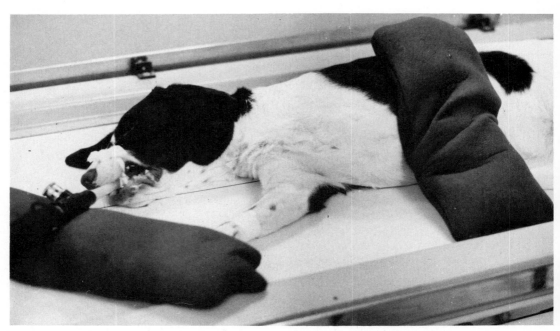

Figure 8–4. Position for the ML view of the scapula and shoulder joint.

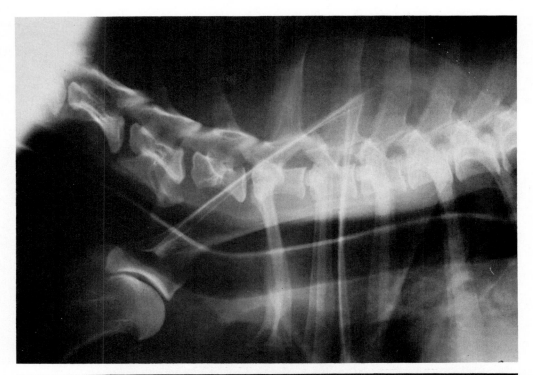

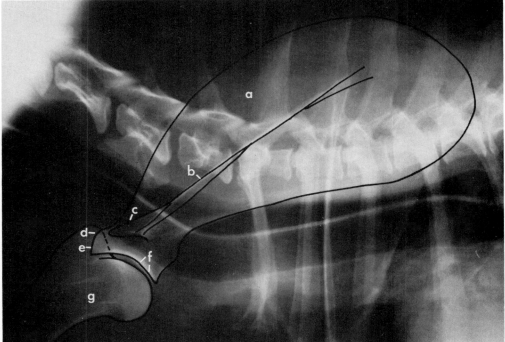

Figure 8–5. ML view of the canine scapula.

    a. Scapula
    b. Spine of scapula
    c. Acromion
    d. Coracoid process
    e. Scapular tuberosity
    f. Glenoid cavity
    g. Humerus

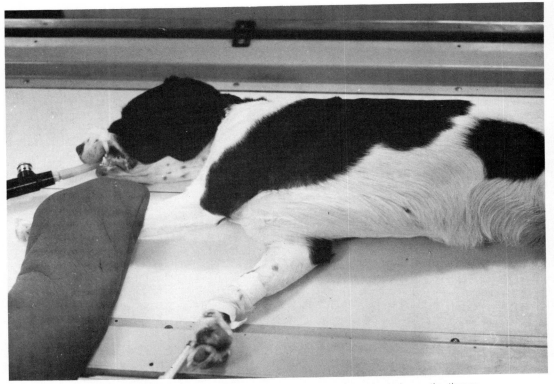

Figure 8–6. Position for the ML view of the scapula projected over the thorax.

eral limb should be extended and placed over the cervical region (Fig. 8–6). The normal radiographic anatomy of the mature canine scapula in this projection is shown in Figure 8–7.

The mediolateral projection of the immature canine shoulder includes two epiphyseal plates that are often misdiagnosed as pathological processes. The ossification center of the scapular tuberosity appears between the fifth and the eighth week of age and is seen on the mediolateral view lying just anterior to the glenoid fossa (Hare, 1959b). The ossification center soon becomes wedge-shaped (Fig. 8–9) and unites with the body of the scapula between four and six months after birth (Hare, 1959b; Chapman, 1963). This normal structure should not be misdiagnosed as a fracture.

The proximal epiphysis of the humerus appears during the first two weeks of life and unites with the diaphysis at 10 to 15 months of age (Hare, 1959b; Chapman, 1963). Figure 8–10 illustrates the normal appearance of the epiphyseal plate (physis) of the proximal humerus in a six month old dog. At this age, the anterior aspect of the plate appears widened on the mediolateral view. This normal structure must not be considered an avulsion fracture.

Mature feline shoulder radiographs show well mineralized clavicles (Fig. 8–11). Occasionally, vestiges of these structures are seen in the canine and should be considered normal.

SHOULDER ARTHROGRAPHY

Arthrography is the radiographic demonstration of articular surfaces and joint capsule outlines after introduction of either positive or negative contrast medium into the joint space. Positive contrast medium is superior to negative or double (both positive and negative) medium in canine shoulder joints for the demonstration of articular or capsular defects (Suter and Carb, 1969).

(*Text continued on page 116.*)

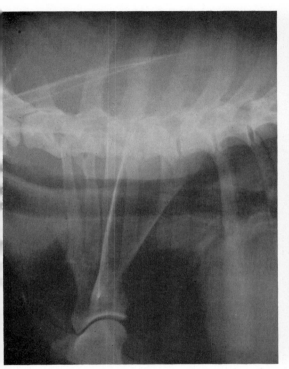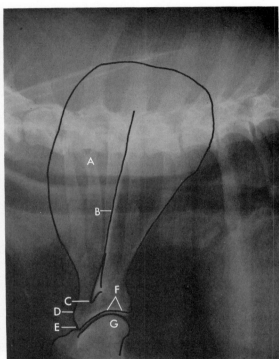

Figure 8–7. ML view of the canine scapula projected over the thorax.

    A. Scapula
    B. Spine of scapula
    C. Acromion
    D. Coracoid process
    E. Scapular tuberosity
    F. Glenoid cavity
    G. Humerus

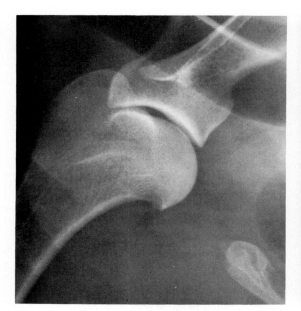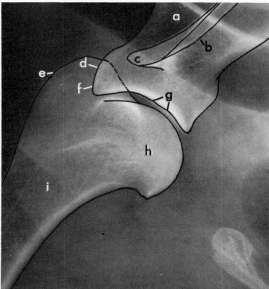

Figure 8–8. ML view of the canine shoulder joint.
a. Scapula
b. Spine of scapula
c. Acromion
d. Coracoid process
e. Greater tubercle
f. Scapular tuberosity
g. Glenoid cavity
h. Humeral head
i. Humerus

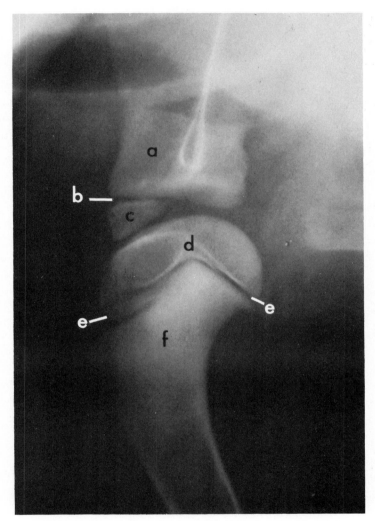

Figure 8–9. ML view of a 3 month old canine shoulder joint.
  a. Scapula
  b. Scapular tuberosity epiphyseal plate
  c. Scapular tuberosity
  d. Epiphysis of proximal humerus (head)
  e. Epiphyseal plate of proximal humerus (physis)
  f. Metaphysis of proximal humerus

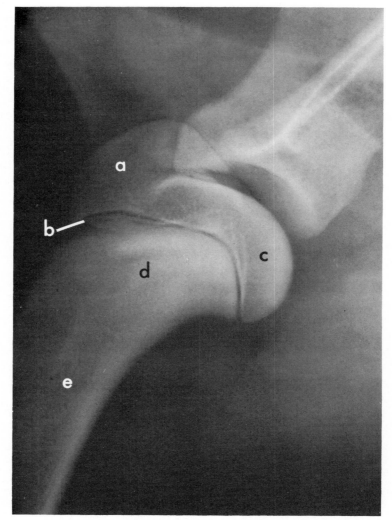

Figure 8–10.   ML view of an immature canine shoulder.
a. Greater tubercle
b. Proximal humeral physis
c. Proximal humeral epiphysis
d. Humeral metaphysis
e. Humeral diaphysis

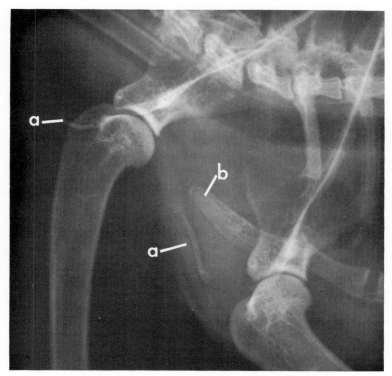

Figure 8–11. ML view of a mature feline shoulder.
a. Clavicles
b. Manubrium of sternum

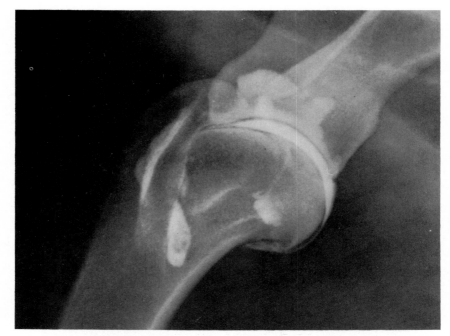

Figure 8–12. ML view of a canine shoulder arthrogram.

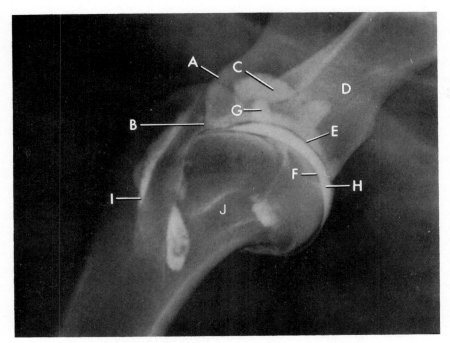

Figure 8–12. ML view of a canine shoulder arthrogram.
A. Coracoid process
B. Scapular tuberosity
C. Acromion
D. Scapula
E. Articular cartilage of glenoid cavity
F. Articular cartilage of humeral head
G. Contrast medium in subscapular pouch of joint capsule
H. Contrast medium in shoulder joint cavity
I. Contrast medium in tendon sheath of biceps muscle
J. Humeral head

Indications. Shoulder arthrography aids in demonstrating radiolucent articular cartilage defects and joint capsule abnormalities that are not visualized on noncontrast radiographs. The extent of cartilaginous and subchondral bone defects may also be demonstrated with a greater degree of accuracy using arthrography. This information may aid in establishing a diagnosis and in planning a therapeutic regimen.

Method. Anesthesia is induced and an area of approximately 8 cm square is clipped, prepared surgically, and draped. As with all arthrocentesis procedures, asepsis must be maintained. The acromion is palpated with a gloved finger, and a one inch, 20 gauge needle (with syringe attached) is introduced approximately 1 cm distally. The needle is directed distally and posteriorly into the shoulder joint. Aspiration of a small amount of synovia confirms the proper location. The syringe is then removed from the needle, and a second syringe containing 4 to 5 ml of sodium diatrizoate solution (Hypaque sodium, 50%, Winthrop Laboratories) is attached. Inject the medium with moderate pressure to avoid reflux of medium around the needle. Withdraw the needle and flex and extend the joint a few times to allow thorough mixing of the medium and synovia. Place the affected shoulder adjacent to the x-ray film and produce mediolateral (Fig. 8–12) and posteroanterior (Fig. 8–13) views. The radiographs should be produced within one minute after injection since prolongation of the interval between injection and radiography allows partial absorption of the contrast medium, which reduces the detail at the cartilage-synovia interface.

Considerable variation is found in the normal appearance of the canine shoulder arthrogram. Various degrees of subscapular pouch enlargement and biceps muscle tendon sheath distention may occur without corresponding clinical signs. Large outpouching defects of the area of the infraspinatus and supraspinatus muscles are associated with clinical signs of shoulder lameness and may indicate tear of the joint capsule (Suter and Carb, 1969). Articular surfaces should be well delineated and free from defects. Such defects are commonly seen in cases of osteochondrosis dissecans where marginal detachment of the articular cartilage has occurred.

HUMERUS

Posteroanterior (PA) View. The patient is placed in dorsal recumbency (supine), and the sternum is rotated slightly away from the limb being examined until a true PA projection is obtained (Fig. 8–14). The central x-ray beam is placed at midhumerus. The x-ray beam should be collimated to include both the shoulder and elbow joints. In large dogs, proper exposure of the proximal humerus usually results in overexposure of the distal end. In these cases, two exposures may be necessary. Cats and most dogs may be radiographed adequately with one exposure.

Figure 8–15 illustrates the normal radiographic anatomy of a mature canine humerus in PA projection.

Mediolateral (ML) View. The patient is placed in lateral recumbency, with the limb to be examined placed adjacent to the film. (Fig. 8–16). The shoulder is extended and the axis of the limb is placed at an angle of approximately 45 degrees from the axis of the spinal column. The sternum is elevated a few centimeters above the table with radiolucent sponges. This prevents overlying radiodensities in the region of the proximal humerus. The x-ray beam collimation and film size should be large enough to include the shoulder and elbow joints.

Figure 8–17 illustrates the normal radiographic anatomy of the mature canine humerus in ML projection.

ELBOW JOINT

Anteroposterior (AP) View. The patient is placed in ventral recumbency (prone) with the limb extended and pulled forward (Fig. 8–18). The head should be rotated away from the elbow joint. The elbow joint must be in a true AP plane, with the olecranon placed at equal distances from the medial and lateral humeral epicondyles. This is most easily accomplished by elevating the contralateral elbow slightly. Both elbow joints should not be radiographed simultaneously because malpositioning due to elbow rotation will make radiographic interpretation difficult.

Figure 8–19 illustrates the normal radiographic anatomy of the AP view of a mature canine elbow.

(*Text continued on page 124.*)

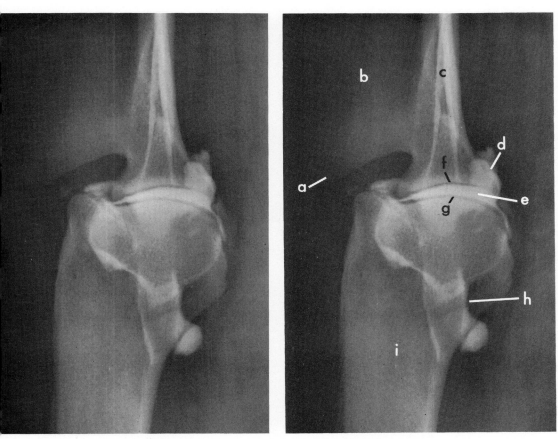

Figure 8–13. PA view of a canine shoulder arthrogram.
a. Acromion
b. Spine of scapula
c. Scapula
d. Subscapular pouch
e. Contrast medium in shoulder joint
f. Articular cartilage of the glenoid cavity
g. Articular cartilage of humeral head
h. Contrast medium in tendon sheath of biceps muscle
i. Humerus

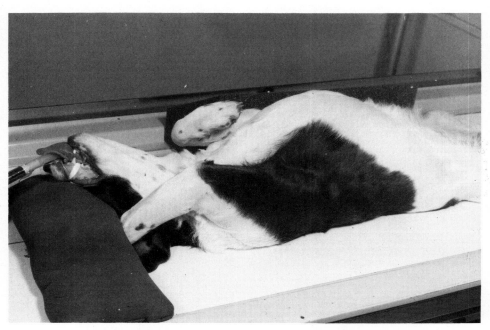

Figure 8–14. Position for the PA view of the humerus.

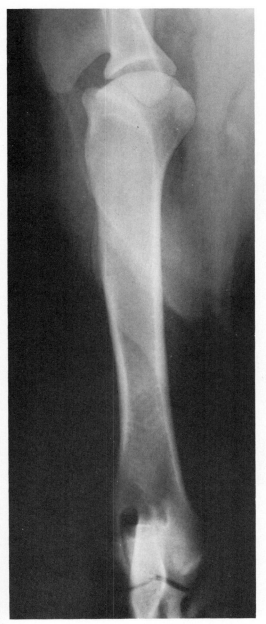
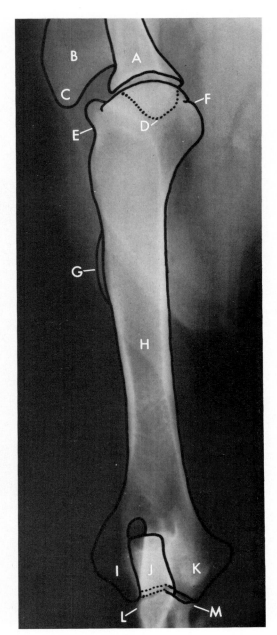

Figure 8–15. PA view of a mature canine humerus.
A. Scapula
B. Spine of scapula
C. Acromion
D. Scapula and coracoid tuberosities
E. Greater tubercle
F. Lesser tubercle
G. Deltoid tuberosity
H. Humeral diaphysis
I. Lateral condyle
J. Olecranon of ulna
K. Medial condyle
L. Head of radius
M. Medial aspect of ulnar coronoid process

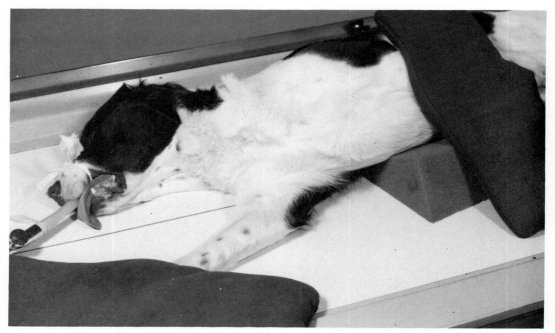

Figure 8–16. Position for the ML view of the humerus.

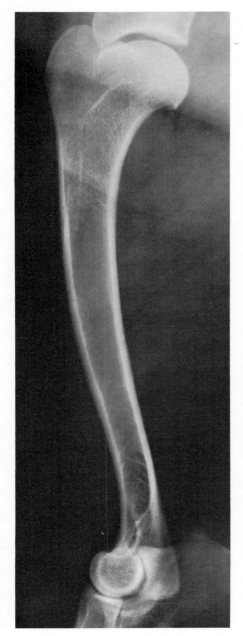
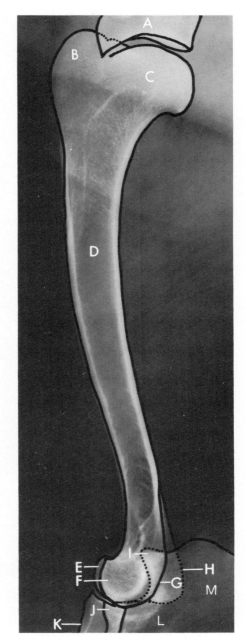

Figure 8–17. ML view of the canine humerus.

    A. Scapula
    B. Greater tubercle
    C. Humeral head
    D. Humeral diaphysis
    E. Medial condyle
    F. Lateral condyle
    G. Lateral epicondyle
    H. Medial epicondyle
    I. Anconeal process
    J. Coronoid process
    K. Radius
    L. Ulna
    M. Olecranon

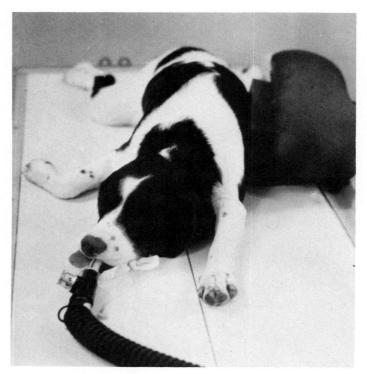

Figure 8–18. Position for the AP view of the elbow.

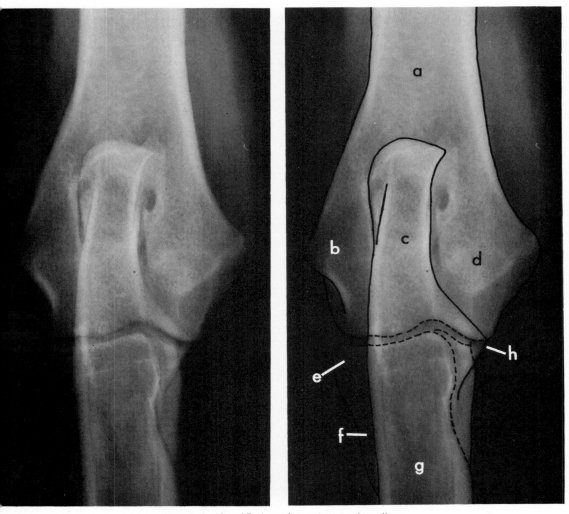

Figure 8–19. AP view of a mature canine elbow.
  a. Humerus
  b. Lateral condyle
  c. Olecranon
  d. Medial condyle
  e. Head of radius
  f. Radius
  g. Ulna
  h. Medial aspect of ulnar coronoid process

The medial aspect of the distal feline humerus contains the supracondyloid foramen, which may be visible on AP or AP lateral oblique (film placed on the posterolateral aspect to profile the anteromedial aspect tangentially to the x-ray beam) views of the elbow region (Fig. 8–20).

Mediolateral (ML) View. The patient is placed in lateral recumbency with the elbow joint to be examined placed adjacent to the film. The elbow joint may be either extended (Fig. 8–21) or flexed (Fig. 8–23). The flexed position is used specifically to examine the anconeal process. The contralateral limb is flexed and placed over the thorax. The sternum may need to be elevated slightly to avoid superimposition of the thoracic bony structures, especially for examination of the flexed position.

Figure 8–22 illustrates the normal radiographic anatomy of a mature canine elbow in the extended position. Figure 8–24 illustrates the normal appearance of the anconeal process when the elbow is radiographed in the flexed position.

The center of ossification for the medial humeral epicondyle appears between the sixth and eighth week of life and unites with the medial condyle during the sixth to eighth month of life (Hare, 1959b; Chapman, 1963). During this period, a distinct epiphyseal plate (physis) is visible radiographically on lateral projection (Fig. 8–25). Note the superimposition of the medial epicondylar epiphyseal plate on the anconeal process. This should not be mistaken for an ununited anconeal process. To avoid this superimposition, the ML projection of the elbow joint in patients less than six months of age should be produced in a flexed position.

RADIUS AND ULNA

Anteroposterior (AP) View. The patient is placed in sternal recumbency with the limb to be examined pulled forward and the head rotated toward the contralateral side (Fig. 8–26). If a true AP projection of the elbow is obtained, the carpus will be projected in a moderately oblique manner, because there is usually a moderate degree of supination (rotated laterally) of the distal limb. On the other hand, if a true AP projection of the carpus is obtained, the elbow joint may be shown in a slightly oblique projection. Generally, it is preferable to position the elbow

joint in a true AP projection when examining the radius and ulna. Specific evaluation of the elbow or carpal joints should not be attempted on survey radiographs of the radius and ulna.

The x-ray beam should be collimated to include both the elbow and carpal joints. The central x-ray beam is placed at the mid-diaphyseal region.

Figure 8–27 illustrates the normal radiographic anatomy of the mature canine radius and ulna in AP projection. Figure 8–28 illustrates the normal radiographic anatomy of the mature feline radius and ulna in AP projection. Notice the normal appearance of the distal radioulnar articulation (a) in the feline.

Mediolateral (ML) View. The patient is placed in lateral recumbency with the limb being radiographed placed adjacent to the film (Fig. 8–29). The contralateral limb is flexed and pulled back over the cranial thorax. The x-ray beam is collimated to include both the elbow and carpal joints. The central x-ray beam is placed at the mid-diaphyseal region. Slight flexion of the elbow and carpus usually does not interfere with interpretation of the radiograph. Specific evaluation of the elbow or carpal joint should not be attempted on survey radiographs of the radius and ulna.

Figure 8–30 illustrates the normal radiographic anatomy of the mature canine radius and ulna in lateral projection.

CARPUS

Anteroposterior (AP) View. The patient is placed in sternal recumbency with the limb to be examined pulled forward (Fig. 8–31). Allow the elbow to abduct slightly so that the natural supination of the distal limb will not cause the carpus to be projected in an oblique manner. The x-ray beam is centered at the carpus.

Figure 8–32 illustrates the normal radiographic anatomy of the mature canine carpus in AP projection. Figure 8–33 illustrates the normal radiographic anatomy of a four month old canine carpus in AP projection. The normal distal radial epiphysis (c) should not be confused with the radial carpal bone (d) in immature patients. Notice that the distal ulnar epiphyseal plate (physis) is cone-shaped and that the proximal edge of the epiphysis produces a radio-

(*Text continued on page 138.*)

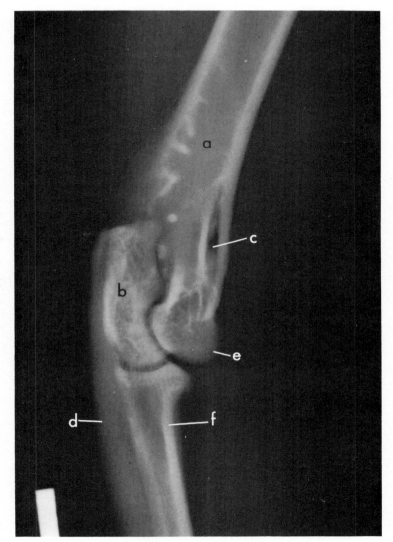

Figure 8–20. APLO view of a feline elbow.
a. Humerus
b. Olecranon
c. Supracondyloid foramen
d. Ulna
e. Medial humeral condyle
f. Radius

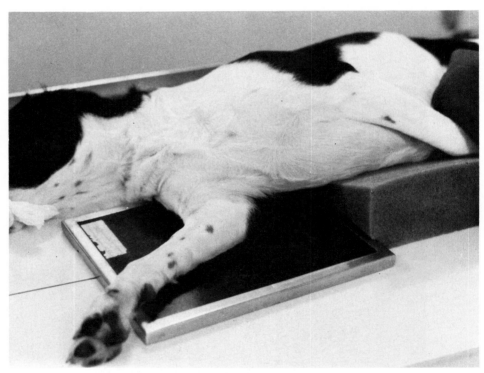

Figure 8–21. Position for the ML view of the elbow.

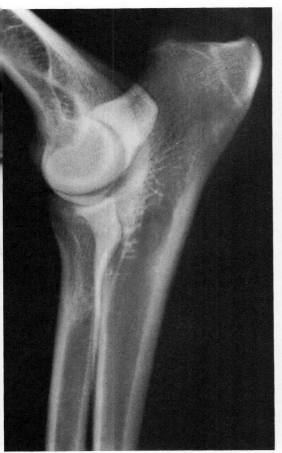
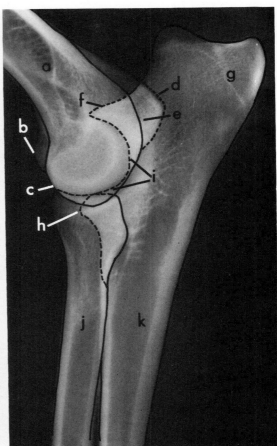

Figure 8–22. ML view of a mature canine elbow.
    a. Humerus
    b. Medial condyle
    c. Lateral condyle
    d. Medial epicondyle
    e. Lateral epicondyle
    f. Anconeal process
    g. Olecranon
    h. Coronoid process
    i. Trochlear notch
    j. Radius
    k. Ulna

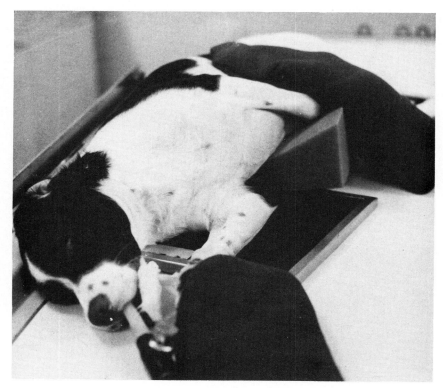

Figure 8–23. Position for flexed ML view of the elbow.

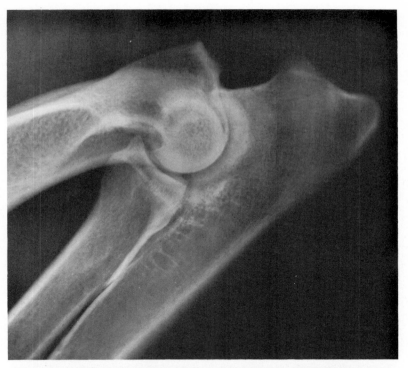

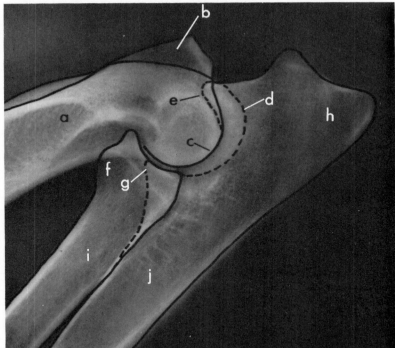

Figure 8–24. Flexed ML view of a mature canine elbow.

    a. Humerus
    b. Medial epicondyle
    c. Medial condyle
    d. Lateral condyle
    e. Anconeal process
    f. Radial tuberosity
    g. Coronoid process
    h. Olecranon
    i. Radius
    j. Ulna

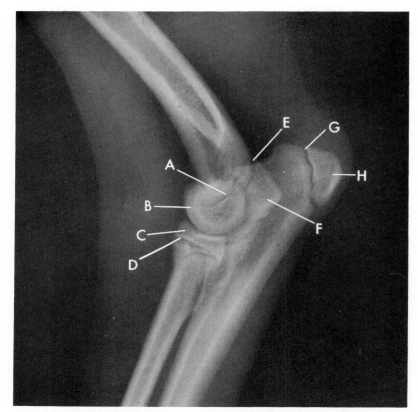

Figure 8–25. ML view of an immature canine elbow (5 mo. old miniature poodle).
A. Physis of humeral condyles
B. Humeral condyles (superimposed)
C. Proximal radial epiphysis
D. Proximal radial physis
E. Medial humeral epicondylar physis
F. Medial humeral epicondylar
G. Olecranon physis
H. Olecranon epiphysis

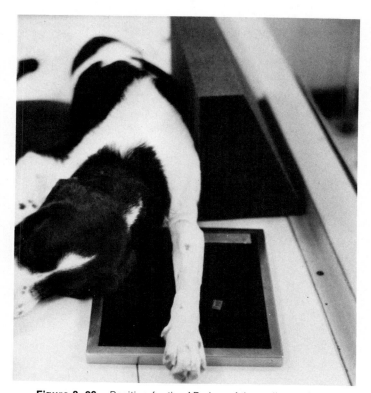

Figure 8-26. Position for the AP view of the radius and ulna.

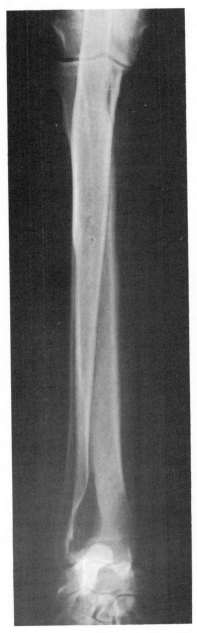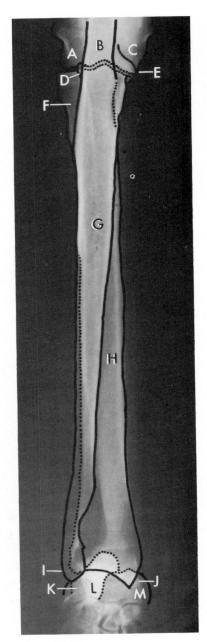

Figure 8–27. AP view of the mature canine radius and ulna.
A. Lateral condyle of humerus
B. Olecranon
C. Medial condyle of humerus
D. Lateral aspect of coronoid process
E. Medial aspect of coronoid process
F. Head of radius
G. Ulna
H. Radius
I. Styloid process of ulna
J. Styloid process of radius
K. Ulnar carpal bone
L. Accessory carpal bone
M. Radial carpal bone

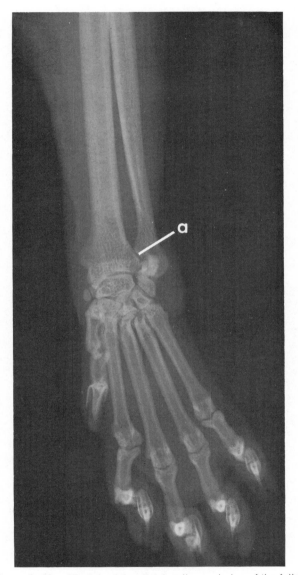

Figure 8–28. AP view of the distal radius and ulna of the feline.
a. Distal radioulnar articulation

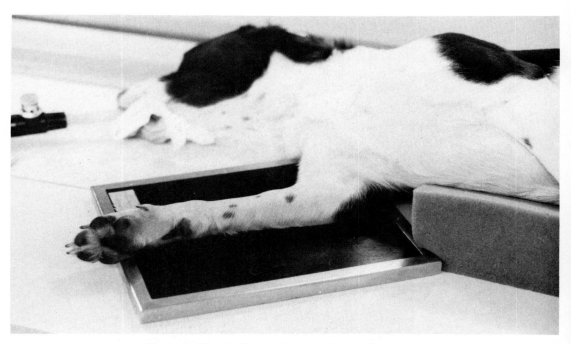

Figure 8–29. Position for ML view of the radius and ulna.

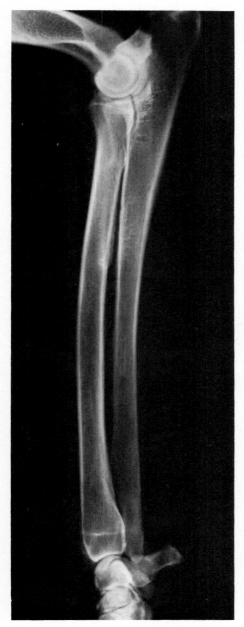
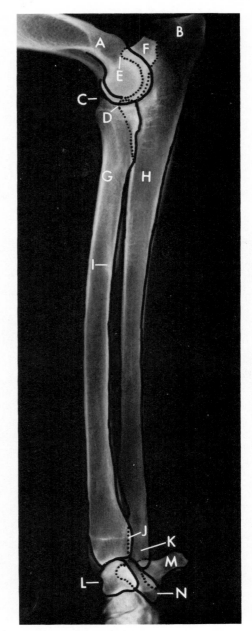

Figure 8–30. ML view of the mature canine radius and ulna.

A. Humerus
B. Olecranon
C. Radial tuberosity
D. Coronoid process
E. Anconeal process
F. Medial epicondyle
G. Radius
H. Ulna
I. Nutrient foramen of radius
J. Distal radioulnar articulation
K. Styloid process of ulna
L. Radial carpal bone
M. Accessory carpal bone
N. Ulnar carpal bone

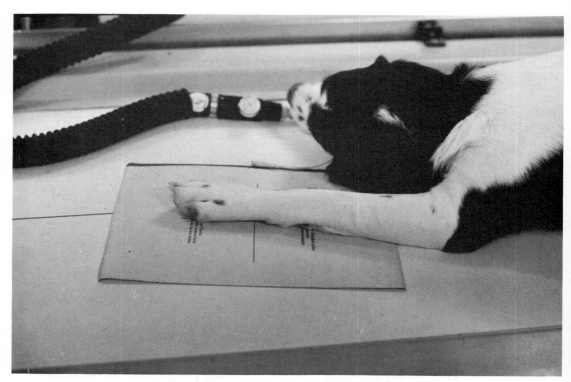

Figure 8–31. Position for AP view of the carpus.

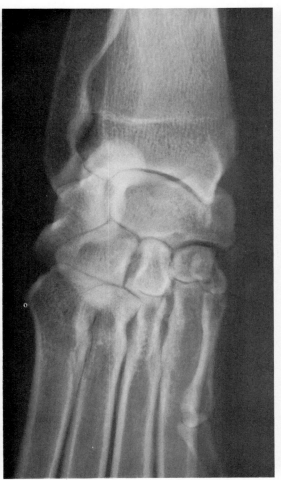
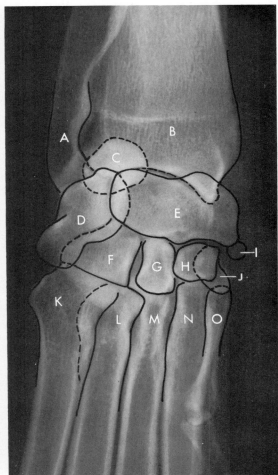

Figure 8–32. AP view of the mature canine carpus.

A. Ulna
B. Radius
C. Accessory carpal bone
D. Ulnar carpal bone
E. Radial carpal bone
F. 4th carpal bone
G. 3rd carpal bone
H. 2nd carpal bone
I. Sesamoid bone in the tendon of abductor pollicis longus muscle
J. 1st carpal bone
K. 5th metacarpal bone
L. 4th metacarpal bone
M. 3rd metacarpal bone
N. 2nd metacarpal bone
O. 1st metacarpal bone

lucent line across the distal metaphysis (Fig. 8–33).

Mediolateral (ML) View. The patient is placed in lateral recumbency and the limb to be examined is placed adjacent to the film (Fig. 8–34). The contralateral limb is flexed and pulled back over the thorax. The x-ray beam is centered over the carpal joint.

Figure 8–35 illustrates the normal radiographic anatomy of the mature canine carpus in ML projection.

Flexed Mediolateral (ML) View. The patient is placed in lateral recumbency and the limb to be examined is placed adjacent to the film (Fig. 8–36). The joint is flexed and the contralateral limb is pulled back over the thorax. The x-ray beam is centered over the carpal joint.

This position is useful at times to delineate the source of chip fractures or to examine the anterior aspects of the carpal joint surfaces.

Figure 8–37 illustrates the normal radiographic anatomy of the mature canine carpus in the flexed ML projection.

Anteroposterior Lateral Oblique (APLO) View. The patient is placed in sternal recumbency and the limb to be examined is pulled forward. The carpus is then supinated (anterior surface rotated laterally) approximately 45 degrees (Fig. 8–38). The x-ray beam is then centered on the carpal joint. The projection is a lateral oblique one because the film is placed on the lateral aspect of the limb.

The APLO view is used to examine the anterolateral and posteromedial aspects of the carpus, and the lateral projection of the first, the second and possibly the third metacarpal bones.

Figure 8–39 illustrates the normal radiographic anatomy of the APLO view of a mature canine carpus.

Posteroanterior Lateral Oblique (PALO) View. The patient is placed in lateral recumbency with the limb being examined placed adjacent to the film, which is placed on the lateral aspect of the limb. The limb is supinated (dorsal surface rotated laterally) approximately 45 degrees (Fig. 8–40). The x-ray beam is centered at the carpus.

The PALO view is used to examine the anteromedial and posterolateral aspects of the carpal joint and the lateral projection of the distal ulna and the fourth and fifth metacarpal bones.

Figure 8–41 illustrates the normal radio-

graphic anatomy of the PALO view of the mature canine carpus.

METACARPUS

Anteroposterior (AP) View. The patient is placed in sternal recumbency and the limb to be examined is pulled forward (Fig. 8–42). The x-ray beam is centered at the junction of the proximal two thirds to the distal one third of the metacarpal bones. Specific examination of the carpus should not be made using this position, because obliquity of the x-ray beam may cause a false narrowing of the carpal articular spaces. This view may be used for the AP projection of the digits because the natural flexion or extension of the metacarpal-phalangeal and intraphalangeal joints usually prevents adequate evaluation of joint space even with specific centering of the x-ray beam at the joint space of interest. These spaces are best examined in the lateral projection.

Figure 8–43 illustrates the normal radiographic anatomy of the AP view of the mature canine metacarpal region.

Mediolateral (ML) View. The patient is placed in lateral recumbency and the limb being examined is placed adjacent to the film (Fig. 8–44). The contralateral limb is pulled back and placed over the thorax. The x-ray beam is centered at the junction of the proximal two thirds to the distal one third of the metacarpal bones. Figure 8–45 illustrates the normal radiographic anatomy of the ML view of the mature canine metacarpal region.

DIGITS

Anteroposterior (AP) View. The AP projection of the digits is similar to the AP view of the metacarpal region. Special positioning usually is not necessary.

Mediolateral (ML) View. The patient is placed in lateral recumbency and the limb to be examined is pulled forward and placed on the film. The specific digit to be examined is pulled anteriorly and fixed in this position with tape (Fig. 8–46). The x-ray beam is centered at the distal end of the first phalanx. If the joint spaces are to be evaluated, the digit must be kept parallel to the film.

Figure 8–47 illustrates the normal radio-

(*Text continued on page 154.*)

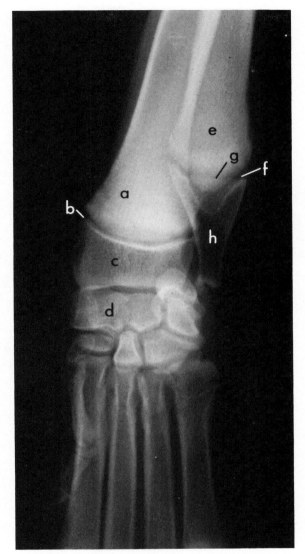

Figure 8–33. AP view of a 4 month old canine carpal region.
- a. Distal radial metaphysis
- b. Distal radial epiphyseal plate (physis)
- c. Distal radial epiphysis
- d. Radial carpal bone
- e. Distal ulnar metaphysis
- f. Distal ulnar epiphyseal plate (physis)
- g. Lucent line produced by proximal edge of the ulnar epiphysis
- h. Distal ulnar epiphysis

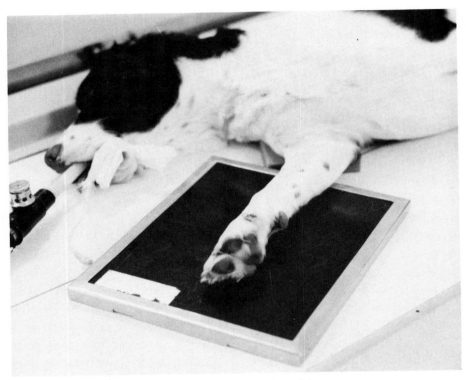

Figure 8–34. Position for ML view of the carpus.

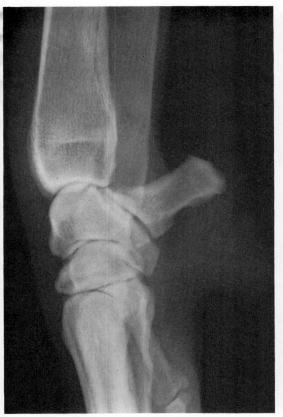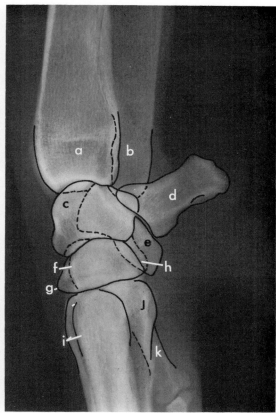

Figure 8–35. ML view of the mature canine carpus.
a. Radius
b. Ulna
c. Radial carpal bone
d. Accessory carpal bone
e. Ulnar carpal bone
f. 2nd carpal bone
g. 3rd carpal bone
h. 4th carpal bone
i. 2nd, 3rd, and 4th metacarpal bones superimposed
j. 5th metacarpal bone
k. 1st metacarpal bone

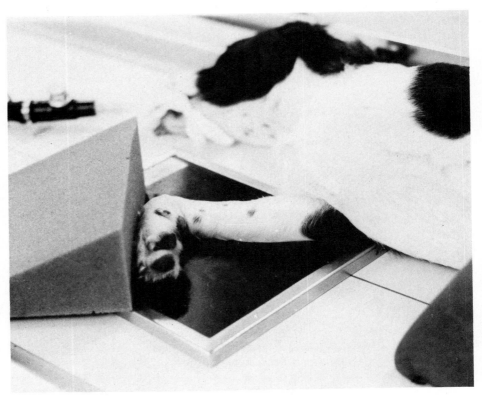

Figure 8–36. Position for the flexed ML view of the carpus.

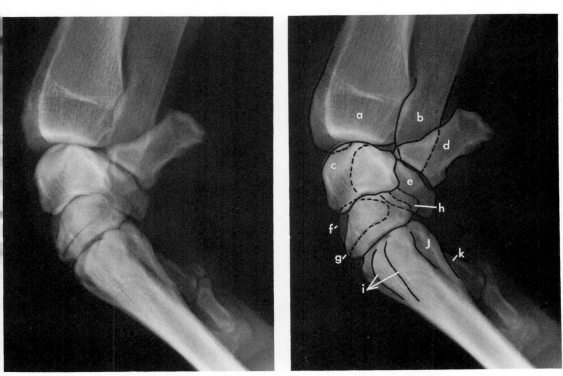

Figure 8–37. Flexed ML view of the mature canine carpus.

   a. Radius
   b. Ulna
   c. Radial carpal bone
   d. Accessory carpal bone
   e. Ulnar carpal bone
   f. 2nd carpal bone
   g. 3rd carpal bone
   h. 4th carpal bone
   i. 2nd, 3rd, and 4th metacarpal bones superimposed
   j. 5th metacarpal bone
   k. 1st metacarpal bone

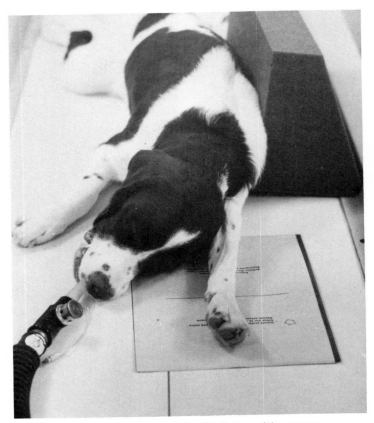

Figure 8–38. Position for APLO view of the carpus.

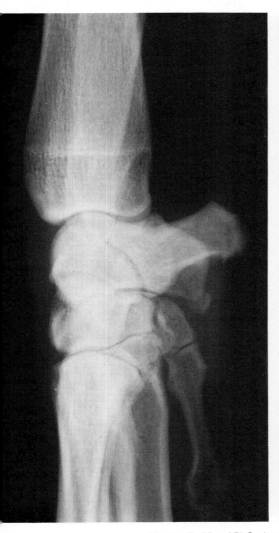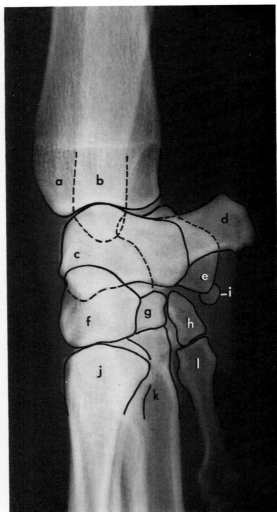

Figure 8–39. APLO view of the mature canine carpus.
a. Radius
b. Ulna
c. Radial carpal bone
d. Accessory carpal bone
e. Ulnar carpal bone
f. 4th carpal bone
g. 3rd carpal bone
h. 1st carpal bone
i. Sesamoid bone in the tendon of abductor pollicis longus muscle
j. 4th and 5th metacarpal bones superimposed
k. 2nd metacarpal bone
l. 1st metacarpal bone

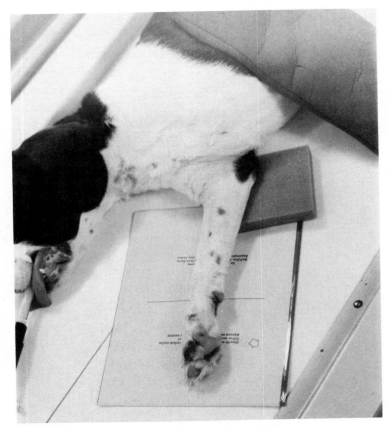

Figure 8–40. Position for PALO view of the carpus.

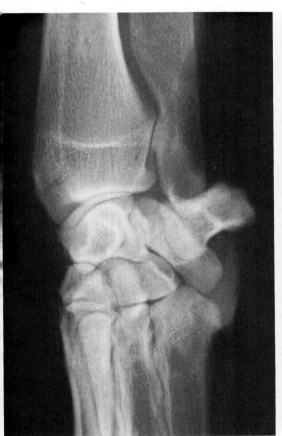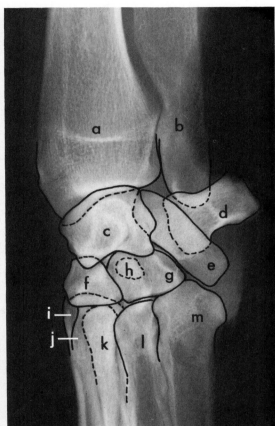

Figure 8–41. PALO view of the mature canine carpus.

a. Radius
b. Ulna
c. Radial carpal bone
d. Accessory carpal bone
e. Ulnar carpal bone
f. 2nd carpal bone
g. 4th carpal bone
h. Sesamoid bone in the tendon of abductor pollicis longus muscle
i. 2nd metacarpal bone
j. 3rd metacarpal bone
k. 1st metacarpal bone
l. 4th metacarpal bone
m. 5th metacarpal bone

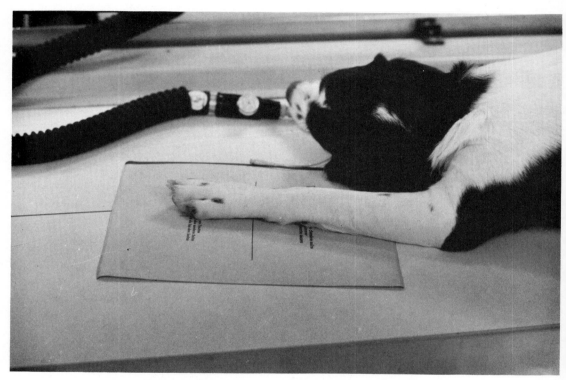

Figure 8–42. Position for AP view of the metacarpal region.

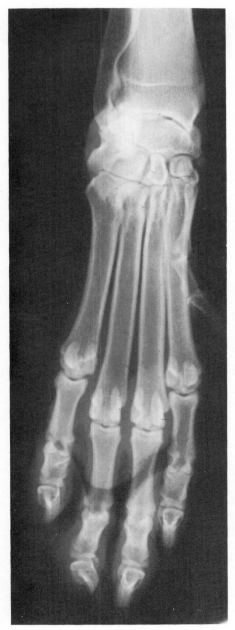

Figure 8–43. AP view of the mature canine metacarpal region.

A. Ulna
B. Radius
C. Accessory carpal bone
D. Ulnar carpal bone
E. Radial carpal bone
F. 4th carpal bone
G. 3rd carpal bone
H. 2nd carpal bone
 I. Sesamoid bone in the tendon of abductor pollicis longus muscle
J. 1st carpal bone
K. 5th metacarpal bone

L. 4th metacarpal bone
M. 3rd metacarpal bone
N. 2nd metacarpal bone
O. 1st metacarpal bone
P. 1st and 2nd phalanx (fused), 1st digit
Q. 3rd phalanx, 1st digit
R. Palmar sesamoid bones at metacarpo-phalangeal articulation of 4th digit
S. 1st phalanx, 4th digit
T. 2nd phalanx, 4th digit
U. 3rd phalanx, 4th digit
V. Ungual crest of 3rd phalanx

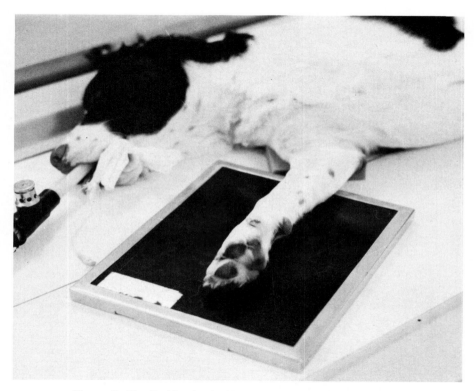

Figure 8–44. Position for the ML view of the metacarpal region.

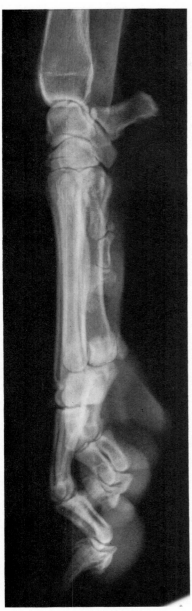

Figure 8–45. ML view of the mature canine metacarpal region.

A. Radius
B. Ulna
C. Radial carpal bone
D. Accessory carpal bone
E. Ulnar carpal bone
F. 2nd carpal bone
G. 3rd carpal bone
H. 4th carpal bone
I. 1st metacarpal bone
J. Palmar sesamoid bones at meta-
   carpophalangeal articulation of
   1st digit

K. 1st and 2nd phalanx, 1st digit
L. 3rd phalanx, 1st digit
M. 5th metacarpal bone
N. Dorsal sesamoid bone at meta-
   carpophalangeal articulation of
   5th digit
O. Palmar sesamoid bone at meta-
   carpophalangeal articulation of
   5th digit
P. 1st phalanx, 5th digit
Q. 2nd phalanx, 5th digit
R. 3rd phalanx, 5th digit
S. Ungual crest of 3rd phalanx

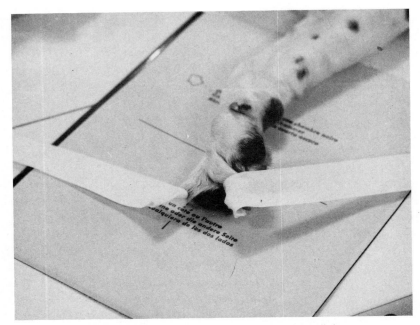

Figure 8–46. Position for the ML view of the digits.

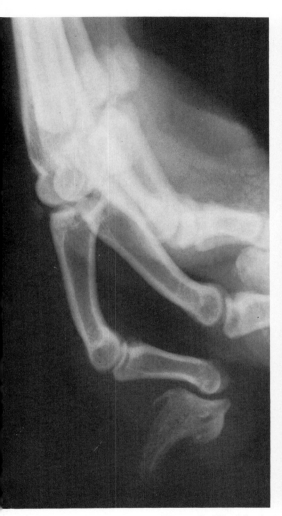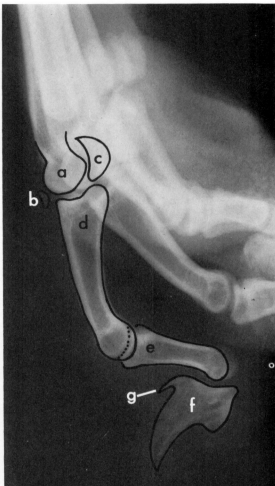

Figure 8–47. ML view of the mature canine digits.

a. 3rd metacarpal bone
b. Dorsal sesamoid bone
c. Palmar sesamoid bones at metacarpophalangeal
   articulation of the 3rd digit
d. 1st phalanx of the 3rd digit
e. 2nd phalanx of the 3rd digit
f. 3rd phalanx of the 3rd digit
g. Ungual crest of the 3rd phalanx

graphic anatomy of the ML view of the mature canine digit.

REFERENCES

Carlson, W. D.: Veterinary Radiology. 2nd ed. Philadelphia, Lea and Febiger, 1967.

Chapman, W. L.: Appearance of ossification centers and epiphyseal closures—determined by radiographic techniques. Thesis. Fort Collins, Colorado, Colorado State University, 1963.

Crouch, J. E.: Text-Atlas of Cat Anatomy. Philadelphia, Lea & Febiger, 1969.

Douglas, S. W., and Williamson, H. D.: Principles of Veterinary Radiography. 2nd ed. Baltimore, Williams & Wilkins Co., 1972.

Habel, R. E., Barrett, R. B., Diesem, C. D., and Roenigk, W. J.: Nomenclature for radiologic anatomy. J.A.V.M.A., *142*:38, 1963.

Hare, W. C. D.: Radiographic anatomy of the canine pectoral limb. Part I. Fully developed limb. J.A.V.M.A., *135*:265, 1959*a*.

Hare, W. C. D.: Radiographic anatomy of the canine pectoral limb. Part II. Developing limb. J.A.V.M.A., *135*:305, 1959*b*.

Miller, M. E., Christensen, G. C., and Evans, H. E.: Anatomy of the Dog. Philadelphia, W. B. Saunders Co., 1964.

Schebitz, H., and Wilkens, H.: Atlas of Radiographic Anatomy of Dog and Horse. Berlin, Paul Parey, 1964.

Sisson, S., and Grossman, J. D.: The Anatomy of the Domestic Animals. 4th ed. Philadelphia, W. B. Saunders Co., 1953.

Suter, P. F., and Carb, A. V.: Shoulder arthrography in dogs—radiographic anatomy and clinical application. J. Sm. An. Pract., *10*:407, 1969.

9
PELVIC
LIMB
POSITIONING

PELVIS AND HIP JOINT

Ventrodorsal (VD) View—Hips Extended.
The patient is placed in dorsal recumbency
(supine), and the femurs are extended, abducted and placed parallel to a line extended
along the vertebral column. The hip joints
are fully extended, and anterior aspects of
the femurs are rotated medially (Fig. 9–1)
so that the patellas are projected over the
midportion of the distal femur (Fig. 9–2).
The hip joints should be equidistant from
the table top. Slight rotation of the pelvis
causing elevation or depression of either hip
joint will result in an asymmetrical projection of the acetabulums and femoral heads.
When properly positioned, the obturator
foramens, the hip joints, the hemipelves
and the sacroiliac joints appear as mirror
images of each other. With imperfect positioning, the side with the smallest obturator
foramen will show the shallowest appearing
acetabulum (Morgan, 1972a). This side will
be the closest to the film (Smith, 1963).
Positional correction may be accomplished
by elevating the affected side.

When pelvic rotation occurs, the side with
the largest obturator foramen will show an
artifactually deeper acetabulum. For radiographic evaluation of hip joint conformation,
pelvic rotation must be prevented.

If inadequate medial rotation of anterior
aspects of the femurs occurs, the patellas will
be projected laterally, and the fovea capitus
and lesser trochanter will be more prominent (Smith, 1963). If excessive medial rotation occurs, the patellas will be projected
medially, the curvature of the femoral head

will appear unbroken, and neither fovea
capitus nor lesser trochanter will be well
visualized (Morgan, 1972b). These signs
vary considerably in different breeds of
dogs.

Excessive femoral abduction will force
the femoral heads into the acetabulums and
change the profile of the femoral necks. This
may result in a mistaken diagnosis of a
femoral neck valgus deformity (Morgan,
1972a).

Positioning of the dog for a VD extended
hip view of the pelvis is facilitated by the
use of general anesthesia or a tranquilizer
(Morgan, 1972b). Support devices are also
helpful (Olsson, 1962). Positioning devices
may be as simple as a pair of sand bags laid
alongside the patient to maintain the supine
position while the femurs are extended with
ropes. Medial rotation of the patellas and
the parallel relationship of the femurs may
be maintained with tape placed around the
stifle joints. Anesthetized patients in such
devices may be maintained in a single position until the first radiograph is developed.
Positional adjustments may then be made,
using the first film as a reference. Anes-
thesia-produced relaxation does not allow
subluxation of normal hip joints (Dixon,
1972).

The VD extended hip position is most
commonly used to evaluate the canine hip
joints for dysplasia (Whittington et al.,
1961; Riser, 1962). For the radiographic
demonstration of hip joint laxity, an object
(wedge) is placed between the femurs while
the animal is in the VD extended hip position (Bardens, 1972). This wedge acts as a

155

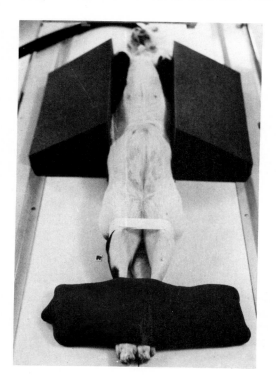

Figure 9-1. Position for VD view of the pelvis with femurs extended.

fulcrum when medial pressure is applied to the distal aspects of the limbs. Since this technique involves many variables, it should not be used for routine radiographic examination of the hip joints.

Figure 9–2 illustrates the normal radiographic anatomy of a mature canine pelvis in VD extended hip view.

Ventrodorsal (VD) View — Hips Flexed (Frog-Legged Position). The patient is placed in dorsal recumbency (supine), and the femurs are flexed and abducted so that the stifle joints are lateral to the abdomen (Fig. 9–3). The femurs are placed at an angle of approximately 45 degrees to a line extended from the vertebral column. It is important that the limbs be positioned identically. Excessive, forceful hip flexion may result in caudal pelvic elevation which will cause the pelvis to appear shortened (Olsson, 1962; Lawson, 1963; Smith, 1963). This artifact will cause the acetabulums to appear deeper than they are when properly positioned (Morgan, 1972b).

Figure 9–4 illustrates the normal radiographic anatomy of a mature canine pelvis in VD flexed hip view.

Lateral View. The patient is placed in lateral recumbency with the limb underneath pulled forward and labeled with a lead marker (Fig. 9–5). The upper limb is elevated with a sponge block or sand bag to a position parallel to the table top. This view is most useful for examining suspected pubic or sacral pathology.

Figure 9–6 illustrates the normal radiographic anatomy of a mature canine pelvis in lateral view.

Lateral Oblique View. The patient is placed in lateral recumbency with the limb underneath pulled forward and labeled (Fig. 9–7). A sponge wedge is used to elevate the dorsocaudal aspect of the pelvis approximately 20 degrees from the table in such a manner that there will be no superimposition of the hemipelves and hip joints. This view is used to examine the hemipelves and hip joints in lateral projection.

(*Text continued on page 164.*)

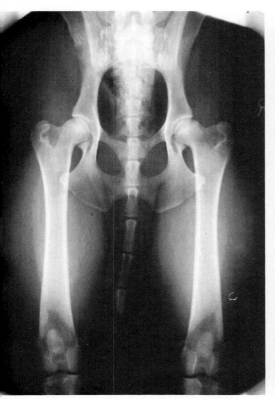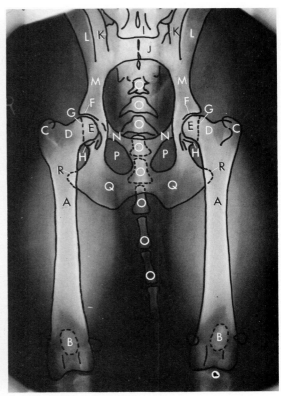

Figure 9–2. VD view of a mature canine pelvis with femurs extended.

    A. Femur
    B. Patella
    C. Greater trochanter
    D. Femoral neck
    E. Femoral head
    F. Cranial acetabular edge
    G. Dorsal acetabular edge
    H. Caudal acetabular edge
    I. 7th lumbar vertebra
    J. Sacrum
    K. Sacroiliac joint
    L. Wing of the ilium
    M. Ilium
    N. Pubis
    O. Coccygeal vertebrae
    P. Obturator foramen
    Q. Ischium
    R. Ischiatic tuberosity

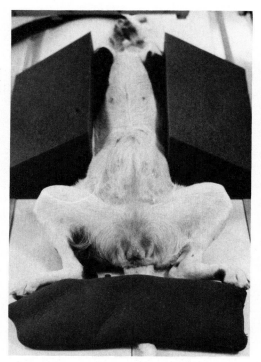

Figure 9–3. Position for VD view of the pelvis with femurs flexed.

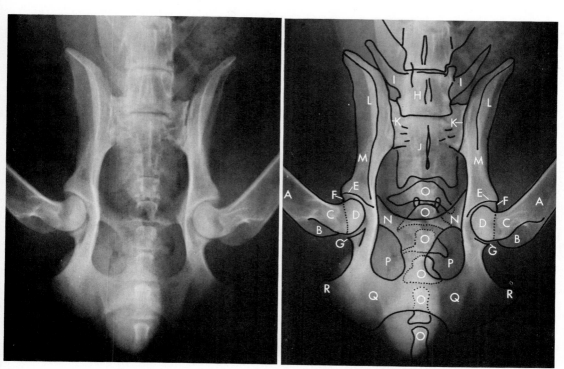

Figure 9–4. VD view of a mature canine pelvis with femurs flexed.
A. Femur
B. Greater trochanter
C. Femoral neck
D. Femoral head
E. Cranial acetabular edge
F. Dorsal acetabular edge
G. Caudal acetabular edge
H. 7th lumbar vertebra
I. Lateral processes of 7th lumbar vertebra
J. Sacrum
K. Sacroiliac joint
L. Wing of the ilium
M. Ilium
N. Pubis
O. Coccygeal vertebrae
P. Obturator foramen
Q. Ischium
R. Ischiatic tuberosity

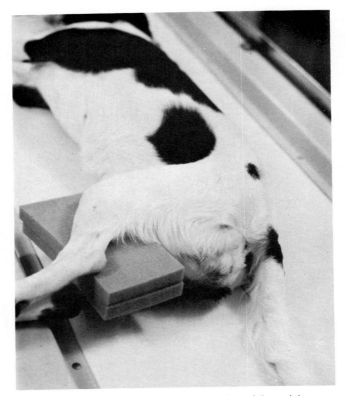

Figure 9–5. Position for the lateral view of the pelvis.

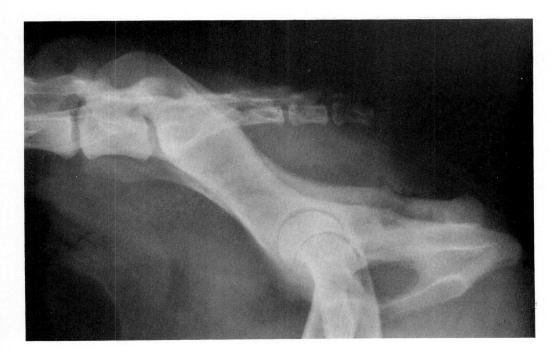

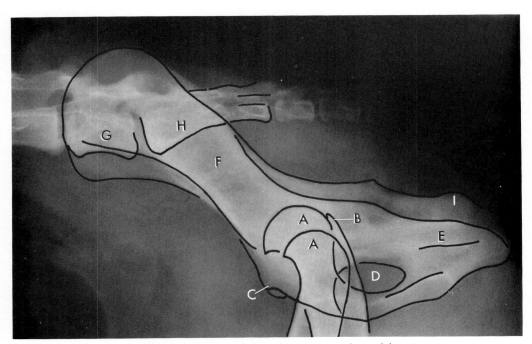

Figure 9–6. Lateral view of a mature canine pelvis.

    A. Femoral heads
    B. Greater trochanter
    C. Pubis
    D. Obturator foramen
    E. Ischium
    F. Ilium
    G. 7th lumbar vertebra
    H. Sacrum
    I. Ischiatic tuberosity

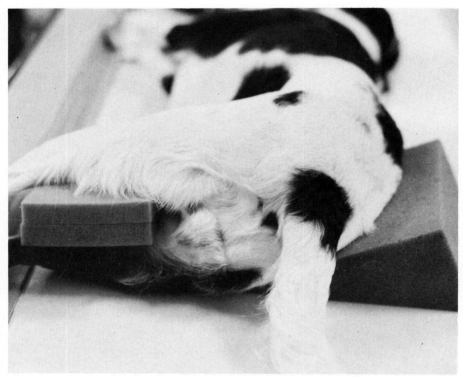

Figure 9–7. Position for the lateral oblique view of the canine pelvis.

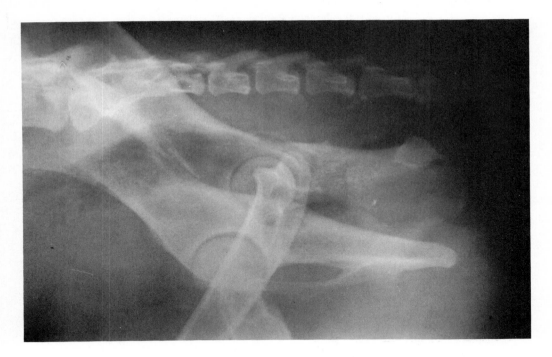

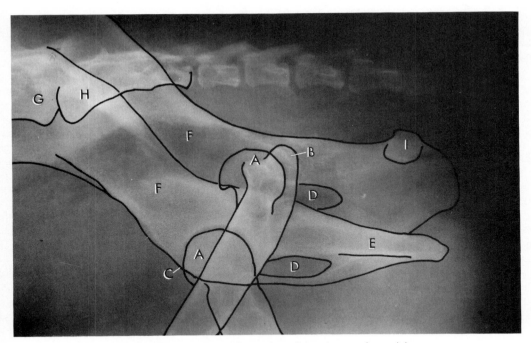

Figure 9–8. Lateral oblique view of a mature canine pelvis.

A. Femoral heads
B. Greater trochanter
C. Pubis
D. Obturator foramen
E. Ischium
F. Ilium
G. 7th lumbar vertebra
H. Sacrum
I. Ischiatic tuberosity

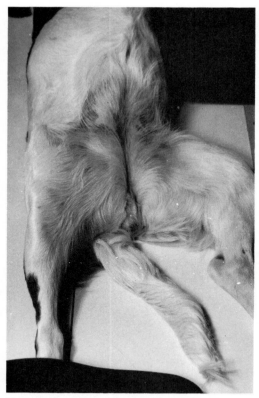

Figure 9-9. Position for the AP view of the femur.

Figure 9-8 illustrates the normal radiographic anatomy of a mature canine pelvis in lateral oblique view.

FEMUR

Anteroposterior (AP) View. The patient is placed in dorsal recumbency (supine) and the limb to be examined is extended (Fig. 9-9). The x-ray beam is centered at midfemur. The beam collimation and film size should be large enough to include the hip and stifle joints. Slight abduction of the limb will aid in obtaining a proper AP alignment.

To prevent underexposure, measurement for exposure calculation should be made at the proximal femur. In some breeds of dogs, this exposure may cause excessive density of the distal femur and stifle joint, thus requiring two radiographs for adequate examination.

Figure 9-10 illustrates the normal radiographic anatomy of a mature canine femur in the AP view.

Mediolateral (ML) View. The patient is placed in lateral recumbency with the limb to be examined placed on the table. The upper leg is abducted and rotated out of the line of the x-ray beam (Fig. 9-11). The x-ray beam is centered midfemur. The beam collimation and film size should be large enough to include the hip and stifle joints.

Measurement for exposure calculation should be made at the proximal femur. In some breeds of dogs, this exposure may cause excessive density of the distal femur, and two radiographs may be required for adequate examination.

Figure 9-12 illustrates the normal radiographic anatomy of a mature canine femur in the ML view.

STIFLE JOINT

Posteroanterior (PA) View. The patient is placed in ventral recumbency (prone) and the limb to be examined is pulled caudally into a position of maximum extension. The contralateral limb is flexed and elevated with a sand bag or sponge wedge (Fig. 9-13). The degree of elevation will control the rotation of the stifle joint being examined. Palpation of the tibial tuberosity of the limb assists in determining the proper degree of limb rotation necessary for exact PA projection. The x-ray beam is centered at the joint space.

Weight-bearing studies using a horizontal x-ray beam centered at the joint space may be useful in evaluating chronic joint disease in small animals (Morgan, 1972a). Because of the difficulty in obtaining an accurate positional relationship between the joint space and the x-ray beam, such studies should be limited to cases that fail to show diagnostic radiographic signs on routine radiographs.

Figure 9-14 illustrates the normal radiographic anatomy of a mature canine stifle joint in the PA view.

Mediolateral (ML) View. The patient is placed in lateral recumbency and the joint to be examined is placed adjacent to the film. The contralateral limb is flexed and abducted (Fig. 9-15). The tarsal joint is elevated with a sponge pad so that the tibia is parallel to the film surface. The x-ray beam is centered at the joint space.

Figure 9-16 illustrates the normal radiographic anatomy of a mature canine stifle joint in the ML view.

(*Text continued on page 173.*)

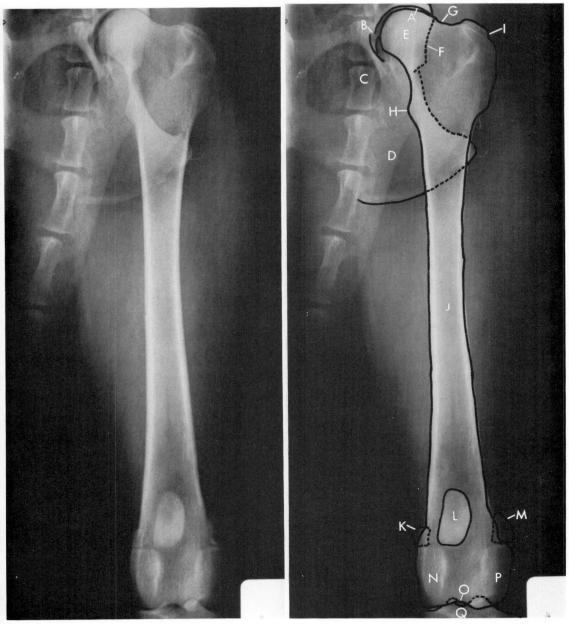

Figure 9–10. AP view of a mature canine femur.

A. Cranial acetabular edge
B. Acetabular notch
C. Obturator foramen
D. Ischium
E. Femoral head
F. Dorsal acetabular edge
G. Femoral neck
H. Lesser trochanter
I. Greater trochanter

J. Femoral diaphysis
K. Medial fabella in tendon of gastrocnemius muscle
L. Patella
M. Lateral fabella in tendon of gastrocnemius muscle
N. Medial condyle
O. Intercondyloid fossa
P. Lateral condyle
Q. Tibia

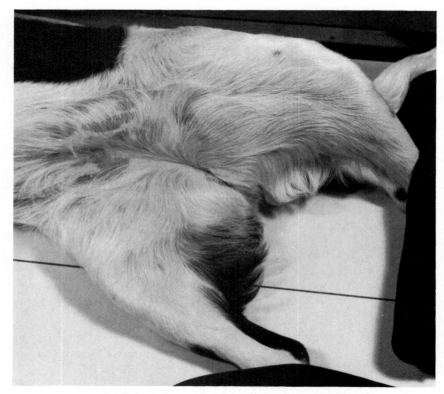

Figure 9–11. Position for the ML view of the femur.

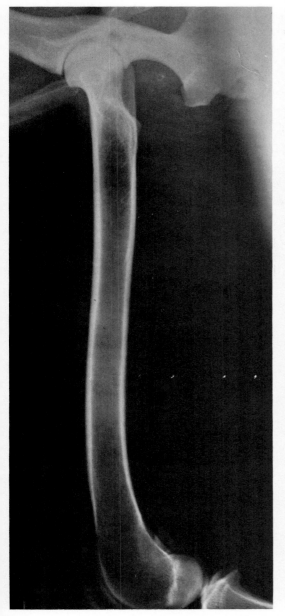

Figure 9–12. ML view of a mature canine femur.

A. Acetabulum
B. Ilium
C. Pubis
D. Ischium
E. Femoral head
F. Greater trochanter
G. Lesser trochanter
H. Femoral diaphysis

I. Patella
J. Femoral condyles superimposed
K. Lateral fabella in tendon of gastrocnemius muscle
L. Medial fabella in tendon of gastrocnemius muscle
M. Fabella in tendon of popliteus muscle
N. Fibula
O. Tibia

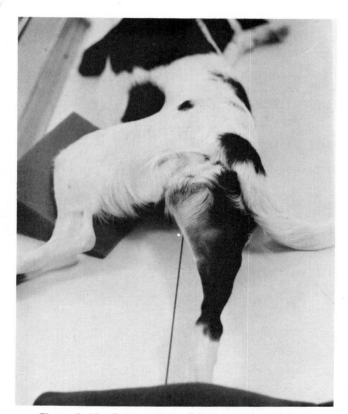

Figure 9–13. Position for the PA view of the stifle joint.

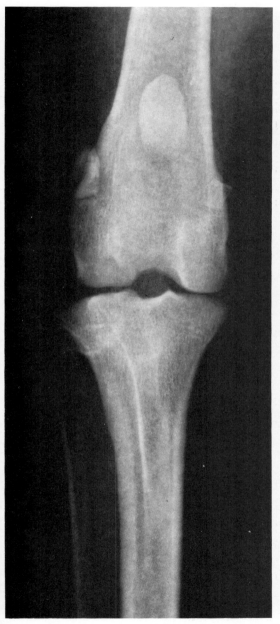
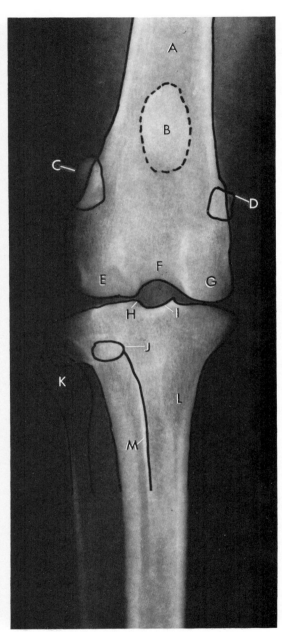

Figure 9–14. PA view of a mature canine stifle joint.

A. Femur
B. Patella
C. Lateral fabella in tendon of gastrocnemius muscle
D. Medial fabella in tendon of gastrocnemius muscle
E. Lateral condyle
F. Intercondyloid fossa
G. Medial condyle

H. Lateral intercondyloid tubercle
I. Medial intercondyloid tubercle
J. Fabella in tendon of popliteus muscle
K. Fibula
L. Tibia
M. Tibial crest

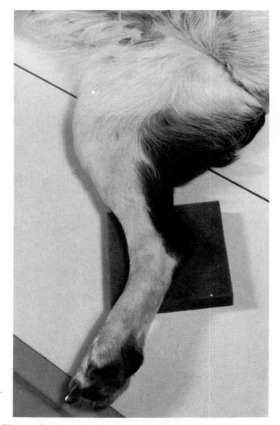

Figure 9–15. Position for the ML view of the stifle joint.

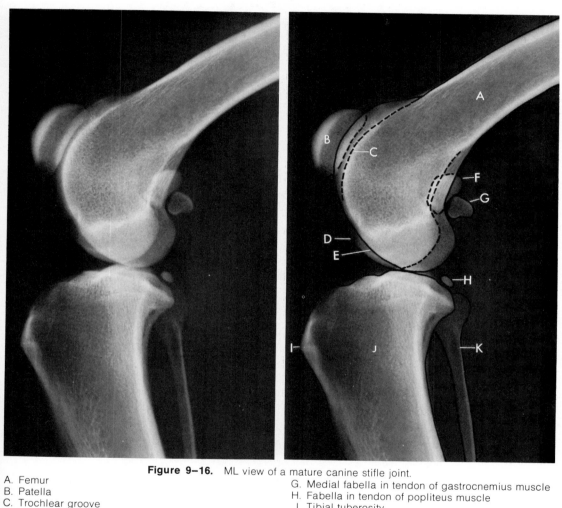

Figure 9–16. ML view of a mature canine stifle joint.

A. Femur
B. Patella
C. Trochlear groove
D. Lateral condyle
E. Medial condyle
F. Lateral fabella in tendon of gastrocnemius muscle
G. Medial fabella in tendon of gastrocnemius muscle
H. Fabella in tendon of popliteus muscle
I. Tibial tuberosity
J. Tibia
K. Fibula

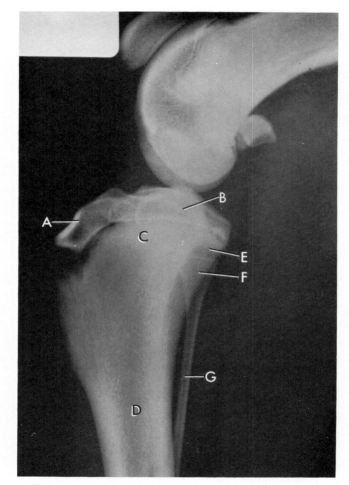

Figure 9–17. ML view of an immature canine stifle region.

A. Epiphysis of tibial tuberosity
B. Epiphysis of proximal tibia
C. Metaphysis of proximal tibia
D. Diaphysis of tibia
E. Epiphysis of proximal fibula
F. Metaphysis of proximal fibula
G. Diaphysis of fibula

Figure 9–17 illustrates the normal radiographic anatomy of a six month old canine stifle joint region. Note that the distal aspect of the tibial tuberosity physis (the epiphyseal plate) appears as a widened radiolucent space between the tuberosity epiphysis (*A*) and the proximal tibial metaphysis (*C*). This normal structure must not be mistaken for an avulsion fracture. The tibial tuberosity epiphysis appears during the third month of life and unites with the proximal tibial epiphysis (*B*) during the eighth or ninth month; together, they unite with the tibial diaphysis during the tenth to twelfth month (Hare, 1960*b*).

Tangential View. The patient is placed in dorsal recumbency and the joint to be examined is flexed maximally and abducted. The hip is then flexed until the femur is perpendicular to the table surface (Fig. 9–18). The film cassette or envelope is placed adjacent to the anterior surface of the femoral segment, and the x-ray beam is directed in a plane parallel to the table top and centered at the distal end of the femur. This examination is useful in examining the depth of the intercondylar groove.

Figure 9–19 illustrates the normal radiographic anatomy of a mature canine stifle joint in the tangential view.

TIBIA AND FIBULA

Posteroanterior (PA) View. The patient is placed in ventral recumbency (prone) and the limb to be examined is pulled caudally into a position of maximum extension. The contralateral limb is flexed and elevated with a sand bag or sponge wedge (Fig. 9–20). The degree of elevation will control the rotation of the tibia being examined. Palpation of the tibial crest of the limb assists in determining the proper degree of limb rotation necessary for exact PA projection.

The x-ray beam should be collimated to include both the stifle and tarsal joints. The central x-ray beam is placed at the mid-diaphyseal region.

Figure 9–21 illustrates the normal radiographic anatomy of the mature canine tibia and fibula in the PA view.

Mediolateral (ML) View. The patient is placed in lateral recumbency and the tibia to be examined is placed adjacent to the film.

The contralateral limb is flexed and abducted (Fig. 9–22).

The x-ray beam is collimated to include both the stifle and tarsal joints. The central x-ray beam is placed at the mid-diaphyseal region.

Figure 9–23 illustrates the normal radiographic anatomy of the mature canine tibia and fibula in the ML view.

TARSUS

Anteroposterior (AP) View. The patient is placed in ventral recumbency, and the limb to be examined is flexed at the hip and extended at the stifle and tarsal joints in such a manner that the limb lies alongside the patient (Fig. 9–24). The limb is slightly abducted and the tarsal joint is aligned in a true AP projection. The x-ray beam is centered at the proximal intratarsal joint.

Figure 9–25 illustrates the normal radiographic anatomy of the mature canine tarsus in an AP projection.

Mediolateral (ML) View. The patient is placed in lateral recumbency and the limb to be examined is placed adjacent to the film. The tibial-tarsal articulation is moderately flexed (Fig. 9–26). The contralateral limb is retracted caudally. The x-ray beam is centered at the proximal intratarsal joint.

Figure 9–27 illustrates the normal radiographic anatomy of the mature canine tarsus in ML projection.

Anteroposterior Medial Oblique (APMO) View. The patient is placed in dorsal recumbency and the limb to be examined is fully extended behind the patient (Fig. 9–28). The anterior surface of the tarsus is rotated medially (supinated) approximately 45 degrees and the film is placed under the tarsus in contact with posteromedial surface of the joint. The x-ray beam is centered at the proximal intratarsal joint.

The oblique view of the tarsus is most easily produced in the AP projection where controlled limb rotation can be readily accomplished.

Figure 9–29 illustrates the normal radiographic anatomy of the mature canine tarsus in the APMO projection.

Anteroposterior Lateral Oblique (APLO) View. The patient is placed in dorsal recumbency and the limb to be examined is

(*Text continued on page 186.*)

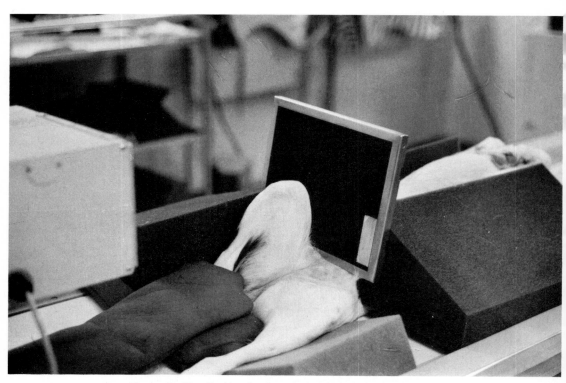

Figure 9–18. Position for the tangential view of the stifle joint.

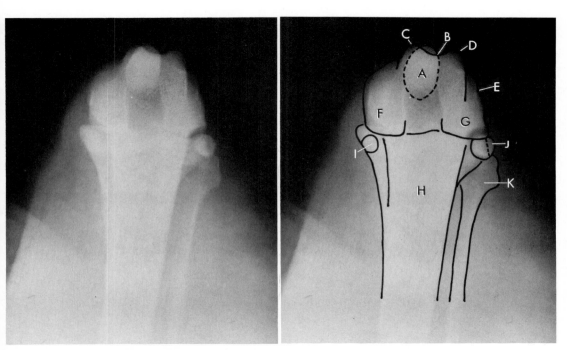

Figure 9–19. Tangential view of the mature canine stifle joint.

A. Patella
B. Trochlear groove
C. Medial ridge of trochlear groove
D. Lateral ridge of trochlear groove
E. Femur
F. Medial condyle of femur
G. Lateral condyle of femur
H. Tibia
I. Medial fabella in tendon of gastrocnemius muscle
J. Lateral fabella in tendon of gastrocnemius muscle
K. Fibula

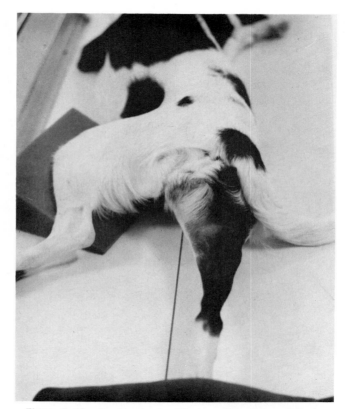

Figure 9–20. Position for the PA view of the tibia and fibula.

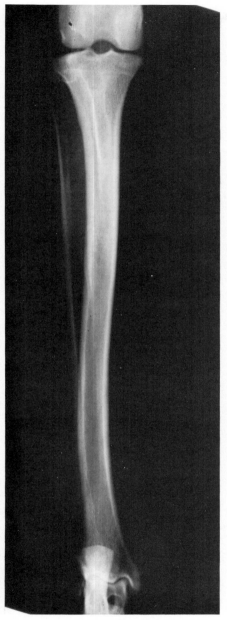

Figure 9–21. PA view of the mature canine tibia and fibula.

A. Lateral condyle of femur
B. Intercondyloid fossa
C. Medial condyle of femur
D. Lateral intercondyloid tubercle
E. Medial intercondyloid tubercle
F. Fibula
G. Tibial crest

H. Nutrient foramen
I. Tibia
J. Lateral malleolus
K. Calcaneal process of fibular tarsal bone
L. Medial malleolus
M. Medial trochlear ridge of tibial tarsal bone

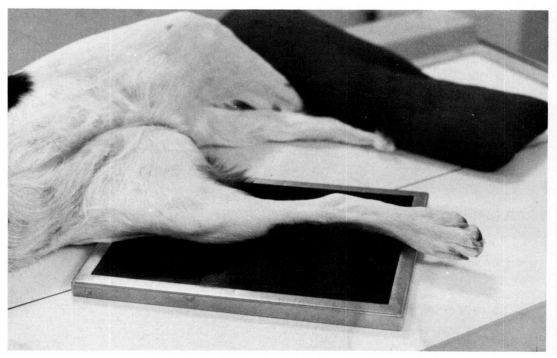

Figure 9–22. Position for the ML view of the tibia and fibula.

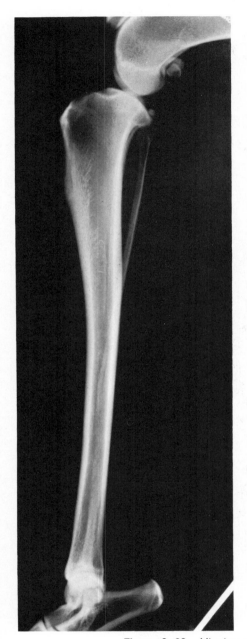

Figure 9–23. ML view of a mature canine tibia and fibula.

A. Femur
B. Patella
C. Lateral condyle
D. Medial condyle
E. Lateral fabella in tendon of gastrocnemius muscle
F. Medial fabella in tendon of gastrocnemius muscle
G. Fabella in tendon of popliteus muscle
H. Tibial tuberosity
I. Tibial crest
J. Tibia
K. Fibula
L. Tibial tarsal bone
M. Distal fibula and trochlea of tibial tarsal bone
N. Fibular tarsal bone

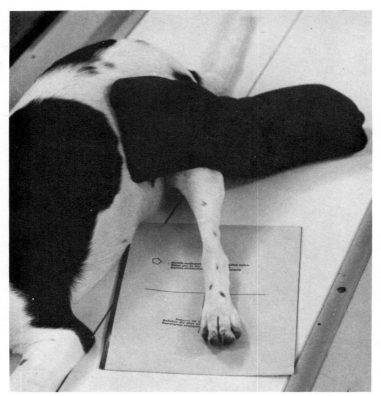

Figure 9–24. Position for the AP view of the canine tarsus.

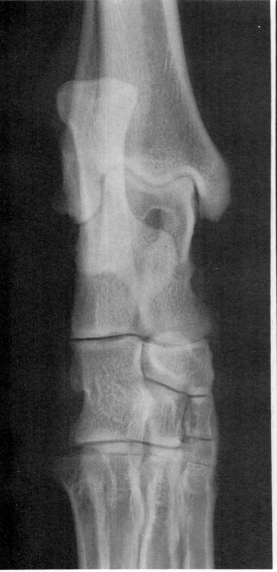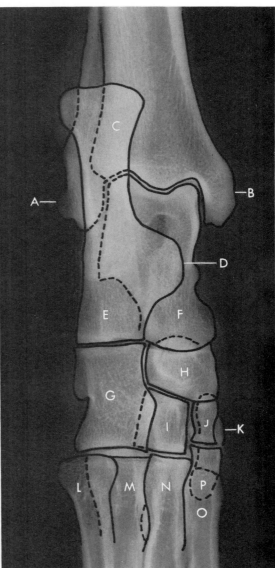

Figure 9–25. AP view of a mature canine tarsus.

A. Lateral malleolus (fibula)
B. Medial malleolus (tibia)
C. Calcaneal process of fibular tarsal bone
D. Sustentaculum tali of fibular tarsal bone
E. Fibular tarsal bone
F. Tibial tarsal bone
G. 4th tarsal bone
H. Central tarsal bone

I. 3rd tarsal bone
J. 2nd tarsal bone
K. 1st tarsal bone
L. 5th metatarsal bone
M. 4th metatarsal bone
N. 3rd metatarsal bone
O. 2nd metatarsal bone
P. 1st metatarsal bone

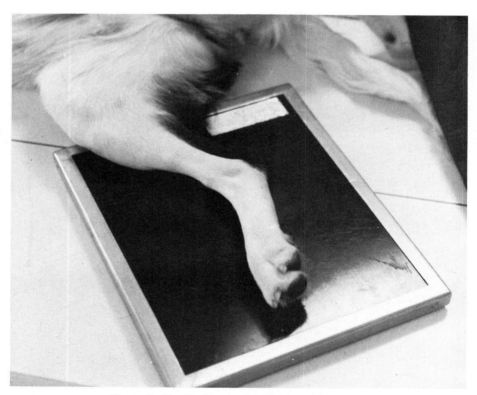

Figure 9–26. Position for the ML view of the tarsus.

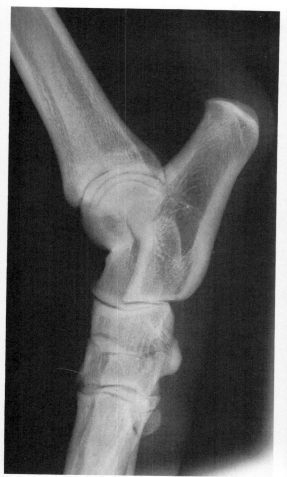 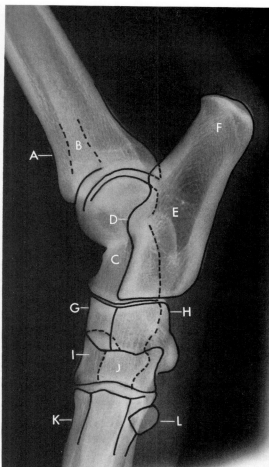

Figure 9–27. ML view of a mature canine tarsus.

A. Tibia
B. Fibula
C. Tibial tarsal bone
D. Cochlear process of fibular tarsal bone
E. Tibial tarsal bone
F. Calcaneal process of fibular tarsal bone
G. Central tarsal bone
H. 4th tarsal bone
I. 3rd tarsal bone
J. 2nd tarsal bone
K. 3rd metatarsal bone
L. 1st metatarsal bone

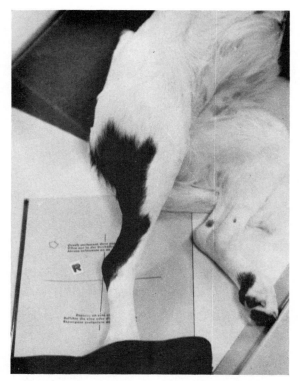

Figure 9–28. Position for APMO view of the tarsus.

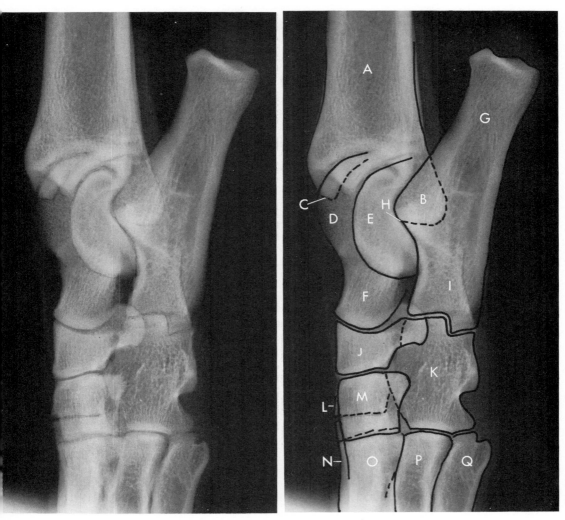

Figure 9–29. APMO view of a mature canine tarsus.

A. Tibia
B. Lateral malleolus (fibula)
C. Medial malleolus
D. Medial trochlear ridge
E. Lateral trochlear ridge
F. Tibial tarsal bone
G. Calcaneal process of fibular tarsal bone
H. Cochlear process of fibular tarsal bone
I. Fibular tarsal bone
J. Central tarsal bone
K. 4th tarsal bone
L. 2nd tarsal bone
M. 3rd tarsal bone
N. 2nd metatarsal bone
O. 3rd metatarsal bone
P. 4th metatarsal bone
Q. 5th metatarsal bone

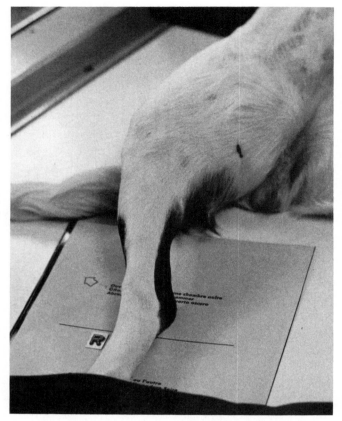

Figure 9–30. Position for APLO view of the tarsus.

fully extended behind the patient (Fig. 9–30). The anterior surface of the tarsus is rotated laterally (pronated) approximately 45 degrees, and the film is placed under the posterolateral surface of the joint. The x-ray beam is centered at the proximal intratarsal joint.

Figure 9–31 illustrates the normal radiographic anatomy of the mature canine tarsus in the APLO projection.

METATARSUS

Anteroposterior (AP) View. The patient is placed in ventral recumbency, and the limb to be examined is flexed at the hip and extended at the stifle and tarsal joints in such a manner that the limb lies alongside the patient (Fig. 9–32). The limb is slightly abducted and the metatarsal region is aligned in a true AP projection. The x-ray beam is centered at the mid-metatarsal region.

Figure 9–33 illustrates the normal radiographic anatomy of the mature canine metatarsal region in an AP projection.

Mediolateral (ML) View. The patient is placed in lateral recumbency and the limb to be examined is placed adjacent to the film. The metatarsal region is moderately flexed (Fig. 9–34). The contralateral limb is retracted caudally. The x-ray beam is centered at the mid-metatarsal region.

Figure 9–35 illustrates the normal radiographic anatomy of the mature canine metatarsal region in ML projection.

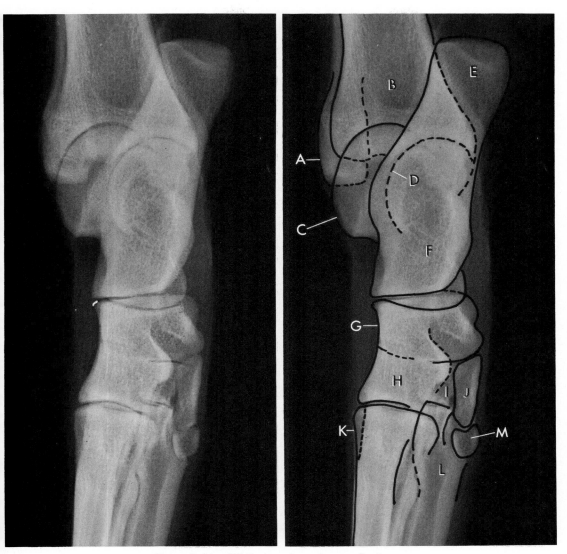

Figure 9-31. APLO view of a mature canine tarsus.

A. Lateral malleolus (fibula)
B. Tibia
C. Lateral trochlear ridge
D. Medial trochlear ridge
E. Calcaneal process of fibular tarsal bone
F. Fibular tarsal bone
G. 4th tarsal bone

H. 3rd tarsal bone superimposed on 4th
I. 2nd tarsal bone
J. 1st tarsal bone
K. 5th metatarsal bone
L. 2nd metatarsal bone
M. 1st metatarsal bone

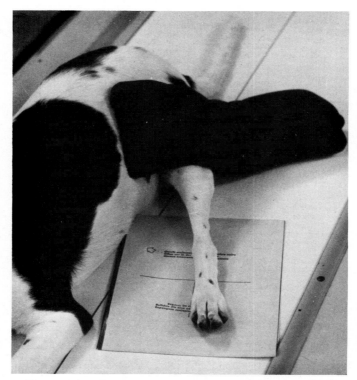

Figure 9–32. Position for the AP view of the metatarsal region.

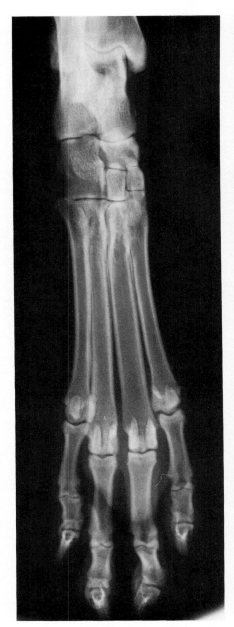
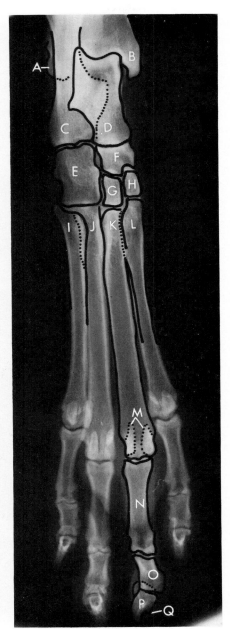

Figure 9–33. AP view of a mature canine metatarsal region.

A. Lateral malleolus (distal fibula)
B. Medial malleolus (distal tibia)
C. Fibular tarsal bone
D. Tibial tarsal bone
E. 4th tarsal bone
F. Central tarsal bone
G. 3rd tarsal bone
H. 2nd tarsal bone
I. 5th metatarsal bone

J. 4th metatarsal bone
K. 3rd metatarsal bone
L. 2nd metatarsal bone
M. Plantar sesamoid bones at metatarsophalangeal articulation of 3rd digit
N. 1st phalanx, 3rd digit
O. 2nd phalanx, 3rd digit
P. 3rd phalanx, 3rd digit
Q. Ungual crest, 3rd phalanx

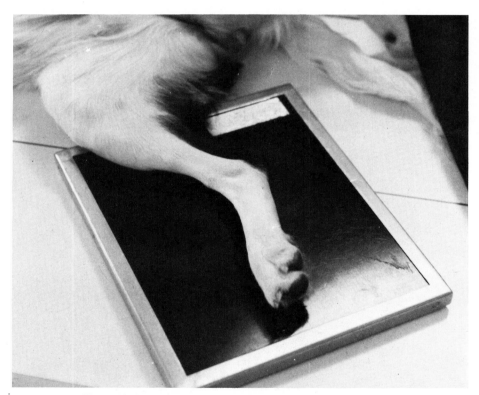

Figure 9–34. Position for the ML view of the metatarsal region.

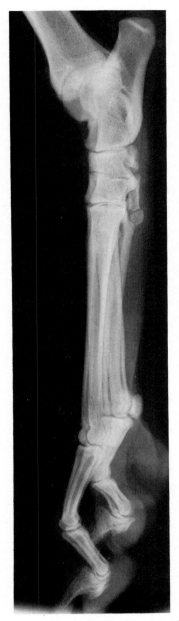
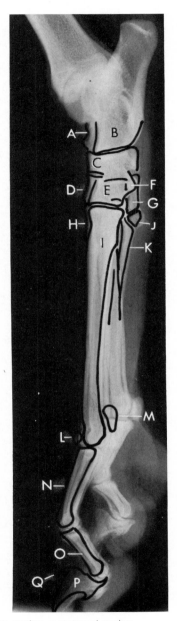

Figure 9–35. ML view of a mature canine metatarsal region.

A. Tibial tarsal bone
B. Fibular tarsal bone
C. Central tarsal bone
D. 3rd tarsal bone
E. 2nd tarsal bone
F. 4th tarsal bone
G. 1st tarsal bone
H. 4th metatarsal bone
I. 3rd metatarsal bone

J. 1st metatarsal bone
K. 2nd metatarsal bone
L. Dorsal sesamoid bone
M. Plantar sesamoid bones at the metatarsophalangeal articulation of the 3rd digit
N. 1st phalanx, 3rd digit
O. 2nd phalanx, 3rd digit
P. 1st phalanx, 3rd digit
Q. Ungual crest, 3rd phalanx

REFERENCES

Bardens, J. W.: Palpation for the detection of dysplasia and wedge technique for pelvic radiography. Proceedings of the 39th Annual Meeting, American Animal Hospital Association, Las Vegas, Nevada, 1972, p. 468.

Carlson, W. D.: Veterinary Radiology. 2nd ed. Philadelphia, Lea & Febiger, 1967.

Dixon, R. T.: The effect of limb positioning on the radiographic diagnosis of canine hip dysplasia. Vet. Rec., 91:644, 1972.

Douglas, S. W., and Williamson, H. D.: Principles of Veterinary Radiography. 2nd ed. Baltimore, Williams & Wilkins Co., 1972.

Hare, W. C. D.: Radiographic anatomy of the canine pelvic limb. Part I. Fully developed limb. J.A.V.M.A., 136:542, 1960a.

Hare, W. C. D.: Radiographic anatomy of the canine pelvic limb. Part II. Developing limb. J.A.V.M.A., 136:603, 1960b.

Lawson, D. D.: The radiographic diagnosis of hip dysplasia in the dog. Vet. Rec., 75:445, 1963.

Miller, M. E., Christensen, G. C., and Evans, H. E.: Anatomy of the Dog. Philadelphia, W. B. Saunders Co., 1964.

Morgan, J. P.: Radiography in Veterinary Orthopedics. Philadelphia, Lea & Febiger, 1972a.

Morgan, J. P.: Radiographic diagnosis of hip dysplasia in skeletally mature dogs. In Canine Hip Dysplasia Symposium and Workshop, St. Louis, Missouri, October, 1972b.

Olsson, S. E.: Roentgen examination of the hip joints of German shepherd dogs. Advanc. Sm. An. Pract., 3:117, 1962.

Riser, W. H.: Producing diagnostic pelvic radiographs for canine hip dysplasia. J.A.V.M.A., 141:600, 1962.

Schebitz, H., and Wilkens, H.: Atlas of Radiographic Anatomy of Dog and Horse. Berlin, Paul Parey, 1964.

Sisson, S., and Grossman, J. D.: The Anatomy of the Domestic Animals. 4th ed. Philadelphia, W. B. Saunders Co., 1953.

Smith, R. N.: The normal radiological anatomy of the hip joint of the dog. J. Sm. An. Pract., 4:1, 1963.

Whittington, K., Banks, W. C., Carlson, W. D., Hoerlein, B. F., Husted, P. W., Leonard, E. F., McClave, P. L., Rhodes, W. H., Riser, W. H., and Schnelle, G. B.: Report of the panel on canine hip dysplasia. J.A.V.M.A., 139:791, 1961.

CERVICAL VERTEBRAE

Extended Lateral View. Proper radiographic examination of the vertebral column can only be performed on patients that are relaxed, having been given either general anesthesia or sedation. This is particularly true for the lateral view of the cervical region.

The patient is placed in lateral recumbency and the forelimbs are retracted over the cranial thorax (Fig. 10–1). The vertebrae are elevated from the x-ray table with dry sponge pads so that the cervical and the thoracic vertebrae are on the same level.

The occipital-atlantal joint is moderately flexed (at approximately 45 degrees to the vertebral column) and the cranial aspect of the head is elevated to eliminate skull obliquity.

The x-ray beam is centered mid-cervically in small dogs. The x-ray beam should be collimated to include the caudal skull and the first few thoracic vertebrae and to exclude most cervical soft tissue. In large dogs (over 40 lb), it is generally preferable to produce two radiographs, one with the central x-ray beam at the C2–3 interspace and another at the C5–6 interspace. This technique will prevent obliquity of the intervertebral spaces at the edges of the x-ray beam and will also allow an increased exposure necessary to properly examine the relatively thick caudal cervical region without overexposing the cranial cervical region.

Figure 10–2 illustrates the normal radiographic anatomy of mature canine cervical vertebrae in lateral view.

Flexed Occipital-Atlantal Articulation— Lateral View. The occipital-atlantal articulation may be flexed approximately 90 degrees to the vertebral column for studies of suspected odontoid process (dens) luxation. Positioning is the same as for the extended lateral cervical view except for the flexion (Fig. 10–3). The x-ray beam is centered at the joint.

Figure 10–4 illustrates the normal radiographic anatomy of a mature canine in flexed occipital-atlantal lateral view.

Atlantal-Axial Articulation—Lateral Oblique View. The patient is placed in lateral recumbency and the lower mandible and sternum are elevated 20 degrees (Fig. 10–5). The x-ray beam is centered at the atlantal-axial articulation. This examination is useful for evaluating suspected odontoid process (dens) pathology other than luxation. The oblique projection artifactually elevates the process from the floor of the atlas and rotates the usually superimposed wings of the atlas from the plane of the process.

Figure 10–6 illustrates the normal radiographic anatomy of a mature canine atlantal-axial region in oblique lateral view.

Flexed Cervical Region—Lateral View. The patient is placed in lateral recumbency, and the forelegs are retracted caudally. A rope or cord loop is placed around the mandible just caudal to the canine teeth, and the free end of the line is placed between the forelegs. Gentle traction on the free end of this line will produce a continuous cervical arch (Fig. 10–7).

The cervical vertebral bodies are elevated above the table with sponges to the level of

(Text continued on page 200.)

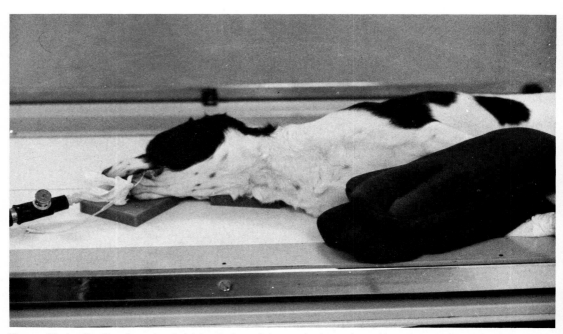

Figure 10–1. Position for extended lateral view of the cervical vertebrae. Note the sponge pads elevating the midcervical region and cranial skull.

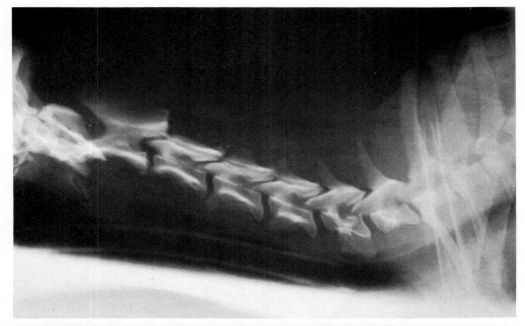

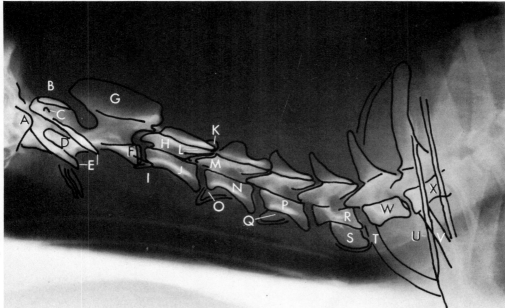

Figure 10–2. Extended lateral view of the canine cervical vertebrae.

A. Occipital condyle
B. Dorsal arch of the atlas (C_1)
C. Transverse foramen
D. Dens
E. Wings of the atlas
F. Body of the axis (C_2)
G. Spinous process of the axis
H. Neural canal
I. Transverse process of the axis
J. Body of C_3
K. Tubercle of the caudal articular process of C_3
L. Caudal articular process of C_3

M. Cranial articular process of C_4
N. Body of C_4
O. Transverse processes of C_4
P. Body of C_5
Q. Transverse processes of C_5
R. Body of C_6
S. Transverse processes of C_6
T. Blade of the scapula
U. Spine of the scapula
V. 1st rib
W. Body of C_7
X. Body of T_1

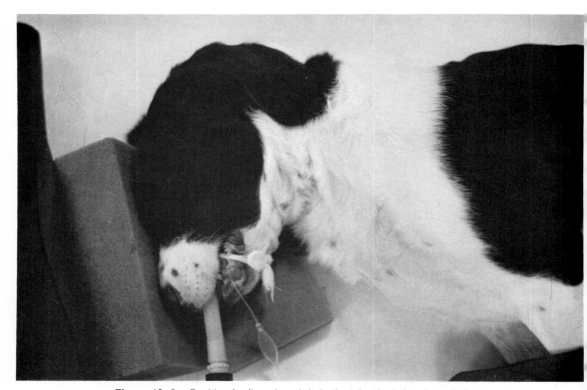

Figure 10–3. Position for flexed occipital-atlantal articulation, lateral view.

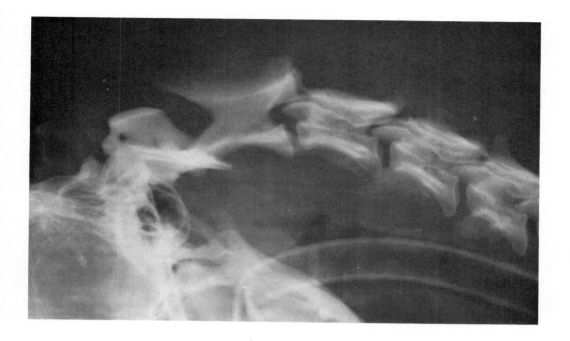

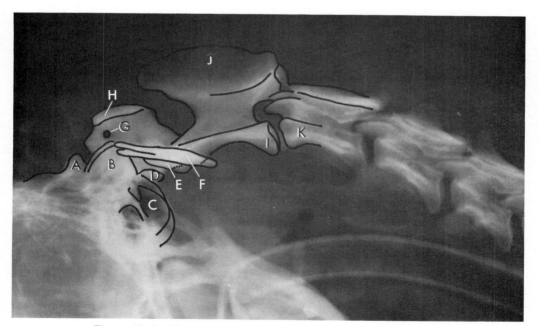

Figure 10–4. Flexed canine occipital-atlantal articulation, lateral view.

A. Nuchal tubercle
B. Occipital condyles
C. Tympanic bullae
D. Ventral arch (floor) of the atlas (C_1)
E. Dens
F. Lateral processes of the atlas (C_1)

G. Transverse foramen
H. Dorsal arch of atlas (C_1)
I. Body of axis (C_2)
J. Spinous process of axis (C_2)
K. Body of C_3

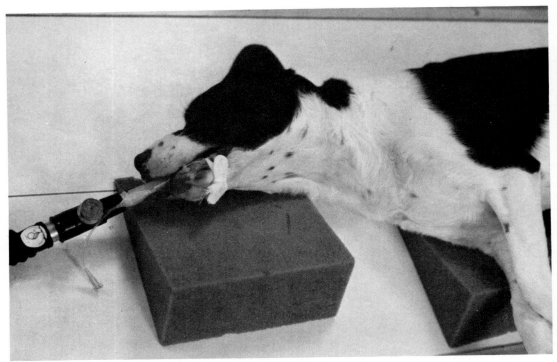

Figure 10–5. Position for atlantal-axial articulation, lateral oblique view.

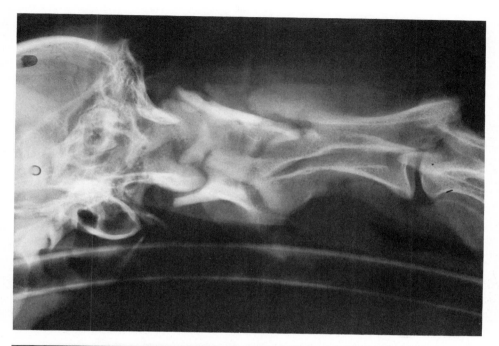

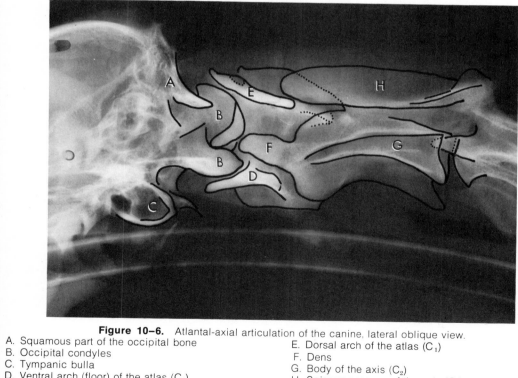

Figure 10–6. Atlantal-axial articulation of the canine, lateral oblique view.

A. Squamous part of the occipital bone
B. Occipital condyles
C. Tympanic bulla
D. Ventral arch (floor) of the atlas (C_1)
E. Dorsal arch of the atlas (C_1)
F. Dens
G. Body of the axis (C_2)
H. Spinous process of the axis (C_2)

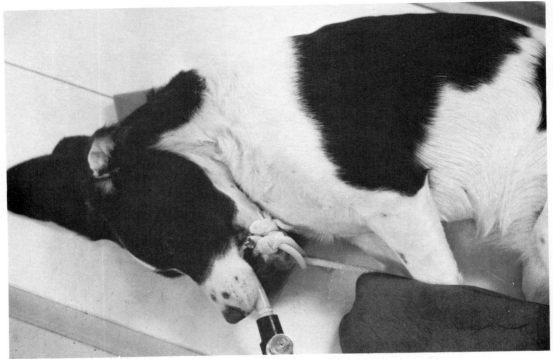

Figure 10–7. Position for flexed lateral view of the cervical vertebrae.

the thoracic vertebral bodies. The x-ray beam is centered at the C4–5 interspace. This examination is useful in cases of suspected cervical vertebral instability (CVI).

Figure 10–8 illustrates the normal radiographic anatomy of a mature canine cervical region in the flexed lateral view.

Ventrodorsal (VD) View. The patient is placed in dorsal recumbency with the forelimbs secured lateral to the thoracic walls (Fig. 10–9). The central x-ray beam is placed at the mid-cervical region and angled cranially approximately 15 degrees. If the caudal cervical vertebrae are of particular interest, this angle should be increased to 20 degrees. These angles most nearly approximate the angles of the intervertebral disc spaces in the cervical region. Measurement to determine the proper exposure should be made in the mid-cervical region in small dogs in order to adequately expose both the cranial and caudal aspects of the cervical vertebrae. A lead marker should be used to identify the left and right sides. The tracheal tube should be removed prior to exposure in

order to avoid confusing overlying images. The x-ray beam is collimated to exclude excessive soft tissue.

Figure 10–10 illustrates the normal radiographic anatomy of mature canine cervical vertebrae in VD view.

THORACIC VERTEBRAE

Lateral View. The patient is placed in lateral recumbency and the forelimbs are extended to lie cranial to the thorax (Fig. 10–11). The sternum is elevated above the table to the level of the thoracic vertebrae in order to avoid obliquity. At times, moderate obliquity may be necessary for proper visualization of the intervertebral foramen if rib overlay becomes a problem. However, the initial examination should be performed without obliquity.

The x-ray beam is centered at the region of suspected pathology. If a survey examination is preferred, the x-ray beam is centered at the T6–7 interspace. The x-ray
(*Text continued on page 204.*)

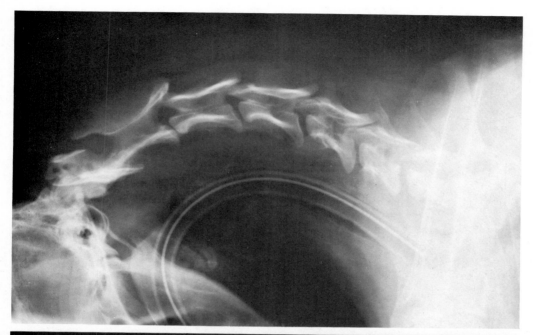

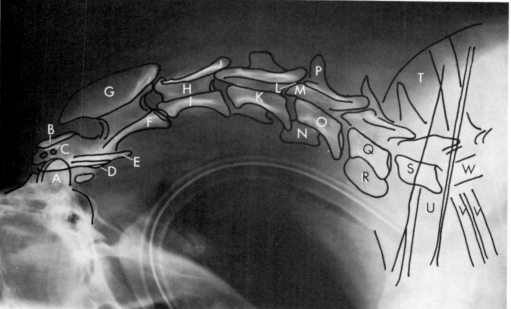

Figure 10–8. Flexed lateral view of the canine cervical vertebrae.

A. Occipital condyle
B. Dorsal arch of the atlas (C_1)
C. Transverse foramen
D. Dens
E. Wings of the atlas
F. Body of the axis (C_2)
G. Spinous process of the axis
H. Neural canal
I. Body of C_3
J. Tubercle of the caudal articular process of C_3
K. Body of C_4
L. Caudal articular process of C_4

M. Cranial articular process of C_5
N. Transverse process of C_5
O. Body of C_5
P. Spinous processes of C_5
Q. Body of C_6
R. Transverse process of C_6
S. Body of C_7
T. Scapulas
U. Spine of the scapulas
V. 1st ribs
W. Body of T_1

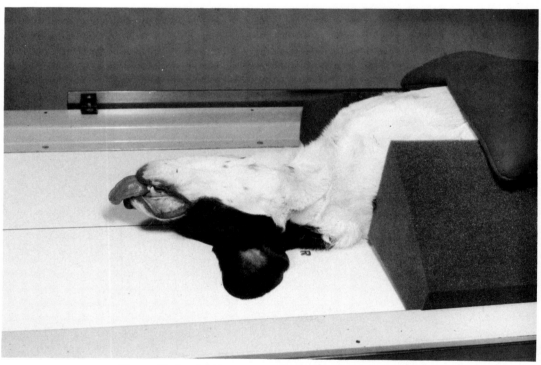

Figure 10–9. Position for VD view of the cervical vertebrae.

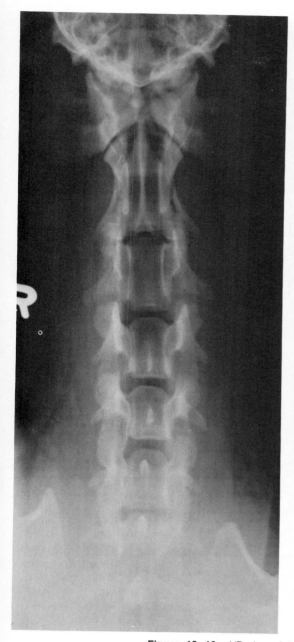

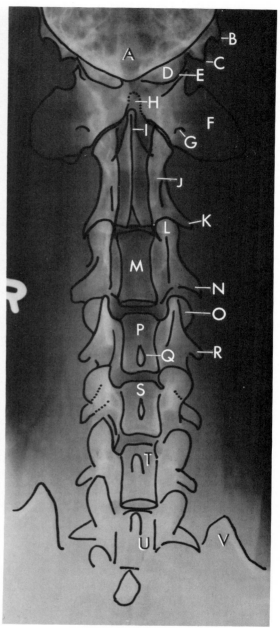

Figure 10–10. VD view of the canine cervical vertebrae.

A. Skull
B. Mastoid process
C. Jugular process
D. Occipital condyle
E. Occipital-atlantal articulation
F. Wings of the atlas (C_1)
G. Transverse foramen
H. Dens
I. Spinous process of the axis (C_2)
J. Axis (C_2)
K. Transverse process of the axis

L. Cranial articular process of C_3
M. C_3
N. Transverse process of C_3
O. Caudal articular process of the C_{3-4} articulation
P. C_4
Q. Spinous process of C_4
R. Transverse process of C_4
S. C_5
T. C_6
U. C_7
V. Scapula

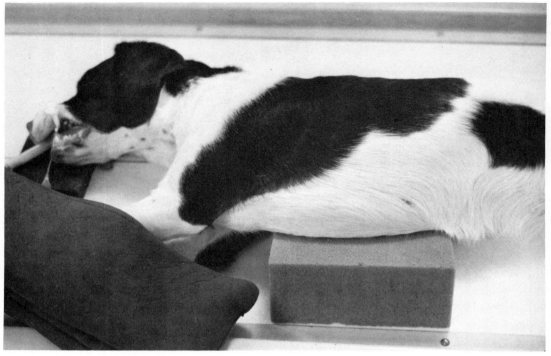

Figure 10–11. Position for lateral view of the thoracic vertebrae.

beam is collimated to exclude excessive soft tissue.

Figure 10–12 illustrates the normal radiographic anatomy of mature canine thoracic vertebrae in lateral view.

Ventrodorsal (VD) View. The patient is placed in dorsal recumbency and the forelimbs are extended and placed beside the cervical region (Fig. 10–13). Moderate thoracic obliquity (approximately 5 degrees) is usually necessary to avoid sternebral overlay, especially in large dogs.

The x-ray beam is centered at the T6–7 interspace and collimated to exclude soft tissue.

Vertebral radiographs in the VD projection are produced without a parallel relationship between the x-ray film and the axis of the vertebral bodies because of the varying heights of the dorsal spinous processes in the thorax. This produces artifactual narrowing of some intervertebral spaces.

Figure 10–14 illustrates the normal radiographic anatomy of mature canine thoracic vertebrae in VD view.

LUMBAR VERTEBRAE

Lateral View. The patient is placed in lateral recumbency with the sternum elevated above the table to a height equal to that of the thoracic vertebrae (Fig. 10–15). In patients with a wide rib spring and a relatively narrow abdominal region, the lumbar vertebrae are elevated with a dry sponge to the level of the thoracic vertebrae. The upper rear limb should be elevated to avoid obliquity of the caudal lumbar vertebrae. Measurement for determining exposure should be made at the thickest part (usually the cranial aspect) to avoid underexposure.

The x-ray beam is centered at the level of suspected pathology. For survey radiographs, the x-ray beam is centered at the thoracolumbar junction, and a second radiograph is produced with the beam at the L3–4 interspace.

Figure 10–16 illustrates the normal radiographic anatomy of mature canine lumbar vertebrae in lateral view.

Ventrodorsal (VD) View. The patient is
(*Text continued on page 210.*)

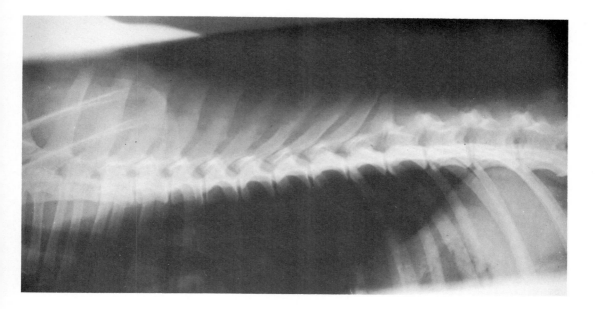

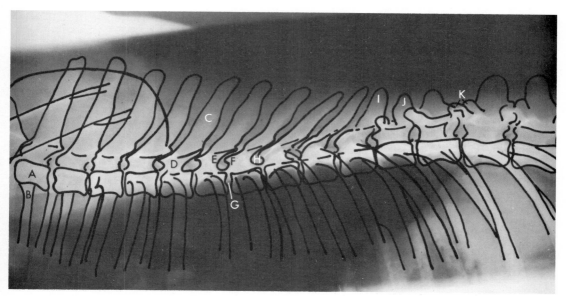

Figure 10–12. Lateral view of the canine thoracic vertebrae.

A. Body of T_1
B. 1st ribs
C. Spinous process of T_5
D. Neural canal
E. Caudal articular process of T_6
F. Cranial articular process of T_7
G. Intervertebral disc space between T_{6-7}
H. Intervertebral foramen between T_{7-8}
I. Spinous process of T_{10}
J. Spinous process of T_{11}
K. Articular processes

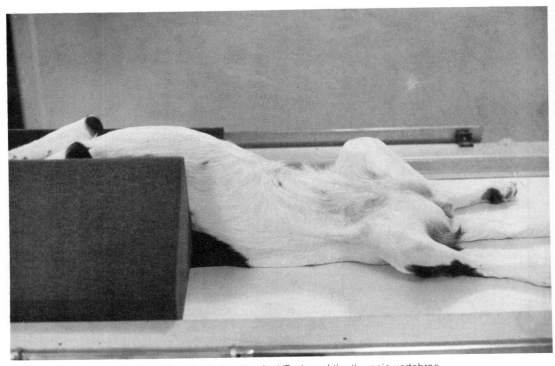

Figure 10–13. Positioning for VD view of the thoracic vertebrae.

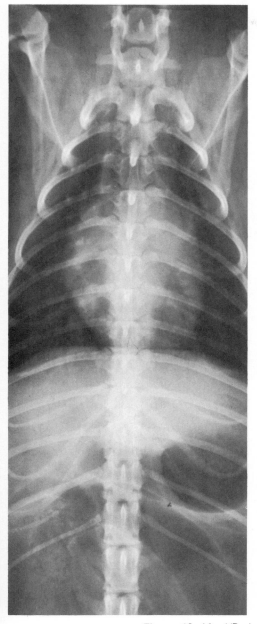
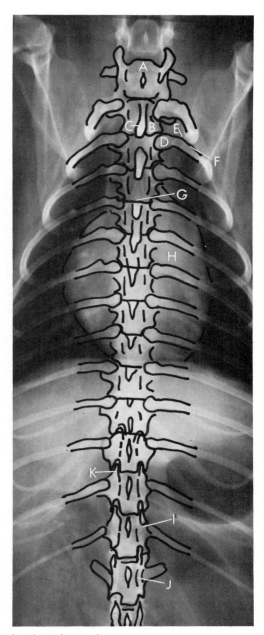

Figure 10–14. VD view of the canine thoracic vertebrae.

A. C_7
B. T_1
C. Spinous process of T_1
D. Head of 2nd rib
E. Tubercle of 2nd rib
F. 2nd rib

G. Intervertebral disc space between T_{3-4}
H. Heart
I. T_{13}
J. L_1
K. Cranial articular process of T_{12}

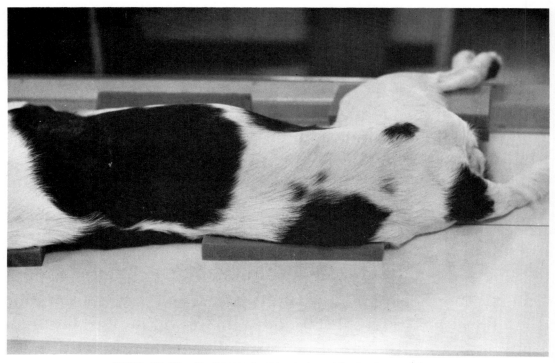

Figure 10–15. Positioning for lateral view of the lumbar vertebrae.

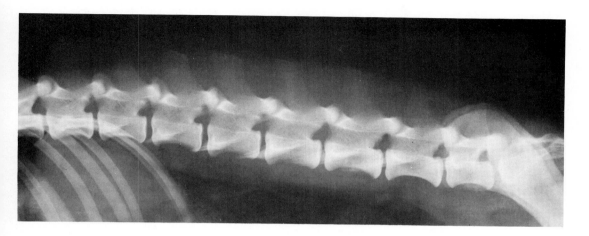

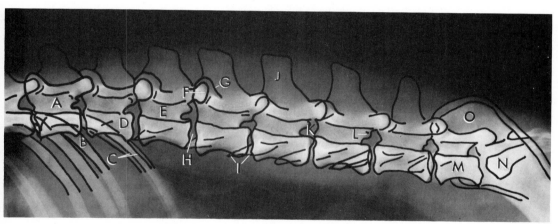

Figure 10–16. Lateral view of the canine lumbar vertebrae.

A. T_{13}
B. 12th rib
C. 13th rib
D. L_1
E. Neural canal
F. Caudal articular process of L_2
G. Cranial articular process of L_3
H. Intervertebral disc space between L_{2-3}

I. Transverse processes of L_4
J. Spinous process of L_4
K. Intervertebral foramen between L_{4-5}
L. Accessory process
M. L_7
N. Sacrum
O. Wings of the ilia

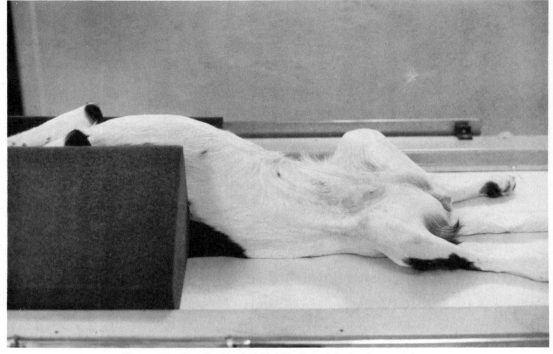

Figure 10–17. Positioning for VD view of the lumbar vertebrae.

placed in dorsal recumbency and the x-ray beam is centered at the level of suspected pathology or at the L3–4 interspace for survey radiographs (Fig. 10–17). Measurement for determining exposure should be made at the thickest part (usually the cranial aspect) to avoid underexposure. The x-ray beam is collimated to exclude excessive soft tissue.

Figure 10–18 illustrates the normal radiographic anatomy of mature canine lumbar vertebrae in VD view.

SACRUM

Lateral View. The patient is placed in lateral recumbency with the upper rear limb elevated to avoid obliquity (Fig. 10–19). The x-ray beam is centered at mid-sacrum. Exposure factors must be approximately doubled in dogs weighing over 40 lb in order to compensate for the increased tissue density provided by the superimposed iliac wings.

Figure 10–20 illustrates the normal radiographic anatomy of mature canine sacrum in lateral view.

Ventrodorsal View (VD). The patient is placed in dorsal recumbency and the rear limbs are placed in semiflexion (Fig. 10–21). The x-ray beam is centered at mid-sacrum and directed cranially approximately 30 degrees to coincide with the angle of the lumbosacral intervertebral space.

Figure 10–22 illustrates the normal radiographic anatomy of mature canine sacrum in VD view.

COCCYGEAL VERTEBRAE

Lateral View. The patient is placed in lateral recumbency and the tail is extended (Fig. 10–23). A cassette is placed beneath the tail and elevated above the table with a block to the level of the lumbar and sacral vertebrae. The x-ray beam is centered at the region of pathology.

Figure 10–24 illustrates the normal radiographic anatomy of mature canine coccygeal vertebrae in lateral view.

Ventrodorsal View (VD). The patient is placed in dorsal recumbency and the tail is

(*Text continued on page 218.*)

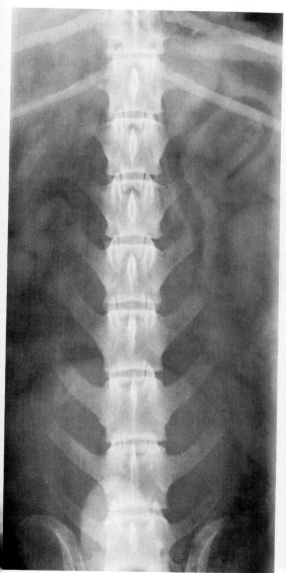
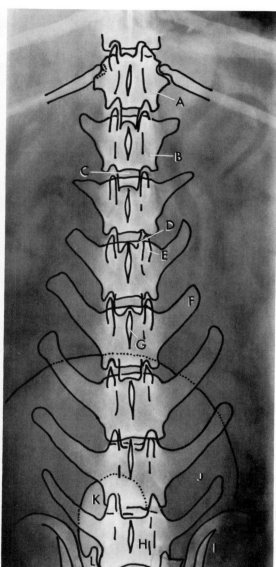

Figure 10–18. VD view of the canine lumbar vertebrae.

A. T_{13}
B. L_1
C. Intervertebral disc space between L_{1-2}
D. Caudal articular process of L_2
E. Cranial articular process of L_3
F. Transverse process of L_4

G. Spinous process of L_4
H. L_7
I. Wing of the ilium
J. Urinary bladder
K. Prepuce
L. Sacrum

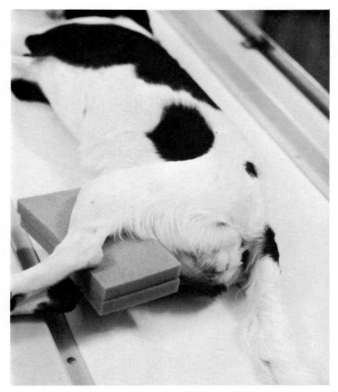

Figure 10–19. Positioning for lateral view of the sacrum.

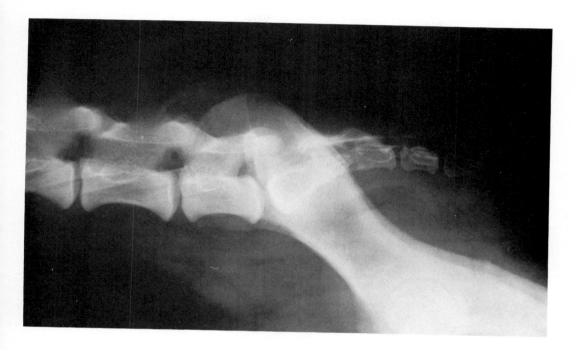

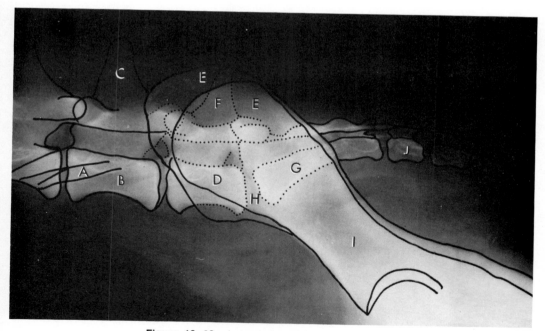

Figure 10–20. Lateral view of the canine sacrum.

A. Transverse processes of L_6
B. L_6
C. Spinous process of L_6
D. L_7
E. Wings of the ilia

F. Spinous process of L_7
G. Sacrum
H. Lumbosacral joint
I. Ilia superimposed
J. 1st coccygeal vertebra

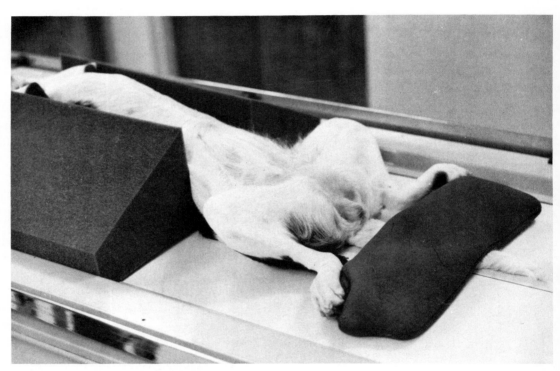

Figure 10–21. Positioning for VD view of the sacrum.

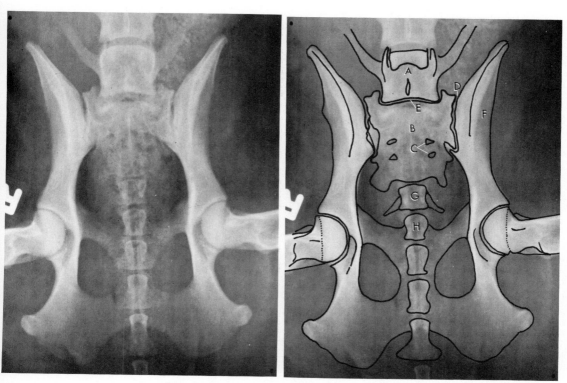

Figure 10–22. VD view of the canine sacrum.

A. L₇
B. Sacrum
C. Sacral foramina
D. Sacroiliac joint
E. Lumbosacral joint
F. Wing of the ilium
G. 1st coccygeal vertebra
H. 2nd coccygeal vertebra

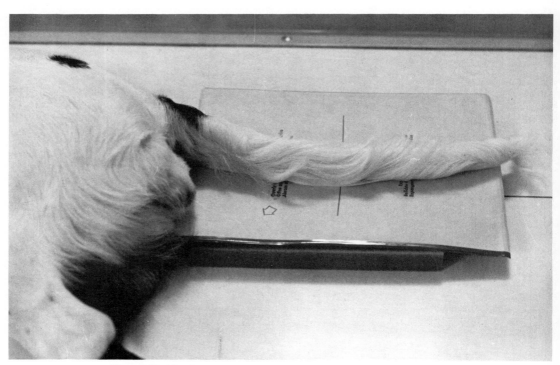

Figure 10–23. Positioning for lateral view of the coccygeal vertebrae.

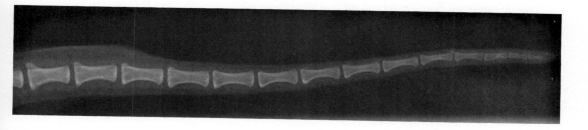

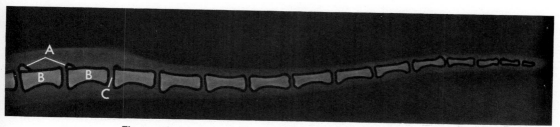

Figure 10–24. Lateral view of the canine coccygeal vertebrae.
    A. Cranial articular processes
    B. Coccygeal vertebral bodies
    C. Intervertebral space

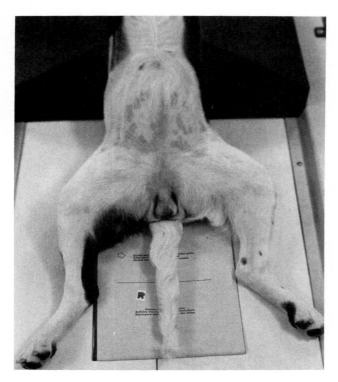

Figure 10–25. Positioning for VD view of the coccygeal vertebrae.

extended (Fig. 10–25). The x-ray beam is centered at the region of pathology.

Figure 10–26 illustrates the normal radiographic anatomy of mature canine coccygeal vertebrae in VD view.

MYELOGRAPHY

Myelography is a radiographic examination performed after the introduction of a contrast medium into the spinal subarachnoid space for the purpose of evaluating intramedullary, extramedullary-intradural, or extradural disease (Suter et al., 1971).

Indications

Myelography is of value in evaluating clinical transverse myelopathies but not disseminated myelopathies or meningopathies (Bailey and Holliday [in press]). These patients usually have herniated intervertebral discs (Morgan et al., 1972; Ticer and Brown, 1974; Morgan, 1972) and may have neoplasms, abscesses, hematomas, congenital malformations or some effect of trauma (Bailey and Holliday [in press]; Morgan, 1972).

Myelography should be performed only on patients that have inconclusive findings on the noncontrast radiographic examination (Hoerlein, 1965; Olsson, 1966; Bailey and Holliday [in press]). When the neurologic examination suggests a diagnosis of a disease that may be amenable to surgical treatment, myelography may be used to confirm the diagnosis and delineate the location of a spinal cord lesion. In these cases, the relative risk involved in the myelographic procedure is acceptable when the information obtained is taken into account (Bullock and Zook, 1967; Morgan et al., 1972; Bailey and Holliday [in press]; Wortman, 1974). A study comparing noncontrast radiographs with myelograms performed for the diagnosis and localization of disc disease concluded that myelograms yielded information unobtainable from the noncontrast studies in almost 70 per cent of cases (Wortman, 1974). This information included diagnoses when the noncontrast radiographs were either nondiagnostic or only sugges-

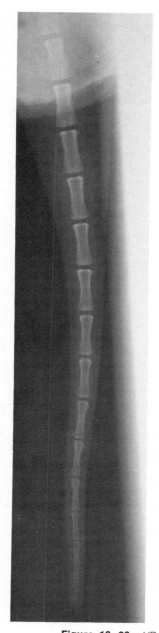
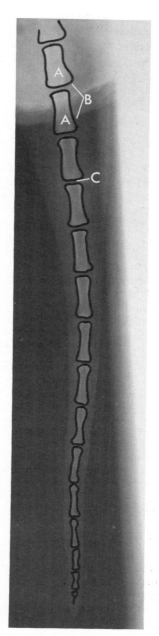

Figure 10–26. VD view of the canine coccygeal vertebrae.
A. Coccygeal vertebral bodies
B. Transverse processes
C. Intervertebral space

tive. Spinal cord edema, hematomyelia (before clinically evident), and laterality of the lesion were also demonstrated myelographically. There was a 30 per cent incidence of complications, of which 75 per cent were transitory convulsions. It is therefore evident that the benefits of myelography outweigh the risks in the canine patient with transverse myelopathy requiring decompressive surgery.

Contraindications

Myelography is not indicated in cases in which a definitive diagnosis can be made on the noncontrast radiographic examination. If disseminated myelopathy or meningopathy is suspected, myelography is not indicated (Ticer and Brown, 1974; Bailey and Holliday [in press]). Cerebrospinal fluid analysis must be performed prior to myelography if these disseminated disorders are suggested clinically (Ticer and Brown, 1974; Bailey and Holliday [in press]). Myelography is also contraindicated unless the neurologic deficit appears reversible and unless decompressive surgery is planned should the myelographic findings suggest it (Bailey and Holliday [in press]).

Technique

Patient Preparation. The patient is anesthetized and a survey radiographic examination is performed. If the differential diagnosis includes disseminated myelopathies or meningopathies, a cerebrospinal fluid analysis should be performed to rule out the presence of infectious myelitis, since the injection of a positive contrast medium into the subarachnoid space may disseminate the infection and the medium may further damage the spinal cord (Bailey and Holliday [in press]). The caudal lumbar region is clipped, scrubbed, and draped.

Materials. All myelographic contrast materials have technical drawbacks and postmyelographic complications. However, 20 per cent sodium methiodal (Skiodan, 40%, Winthrop Laboratories) has been found to produce the most diagnostic myelograms, especially in chondrodystrophoid breeds (Morgan, 1972). Skiodan is diluted to 20 per

cent by adding 0.5 ml of 2 per cent Xylocaine (Xylocaine HC1, 2%, Astra Pharmaceutical Products, Inc.) and 4.5 ml bacteriostatic water to 5 ml of 40 per cent sodium methiodal.

A 3 inch, 20 gauge, short beveled needle with stylet ("Pitkin" needle, catalogue #1161, Becton-Dickinson) is used to make the injection. The short beveled needle decreases epidural spill of contrast medium (Ticer and Brown, 1974). A 2 or 3 ml syringe is needed to aspirate cerebrospinal fluid, and a suitable-sized syringe is needed to inject the contrast medium. A fluoroscope with image intensification is necessary to perform cervical myelography accurately and safely from a lumbar puncture site (Ticer and Brown, 1974).

Dosage of Contrast Material. A volume of 0.3 ml of 20 per cent Skiodan per kilogram of body weight is used to delineate thoracolumbar lesions from a lumbar puncture site (Bullock and Zook, 1967; Funquist, 1962). The volume of contrast medium required to fill the subarachnoid space of the cervical spinal cord from a lumbar puncture site is extremely variable and requires fluoroscopic monitoring. The total volume required may exceed 0.5 ml per kilogram of body weight. In some patients, this dose may be sufficient to fill the subarachnoid space of the brain stem and may result in respiratory arrest.

Procedure. The patient is placed in lateral recumbency and the spinal needle is inserted through the dorsal intervertebral space between L5 and L6. This procedure is facilitated by passing the needle lateral to the dorsal spinous process of L6 and directing the needle point medioventrally to enter the spinal canal. This increases the angulation of the needle and simplifies spinal canal entry (Ticer and Brown, 1974). Moderate flexion of the patient's trunk will aid in opening the dorsal intervertebral space, making spinal canal entry easier. The beveled edge of the spinal needle is directed cranially.

If fluoroscopic monitoring is available to confirm spinal canal entry, an attempt should be made to enter the dorsal subarachnoid space. After visualization of spinal canal entry, the needle is advanced slowly until a slight contraction of the rear limb musculature is detected. The stylet is then removed and the needle hub is observed for signs of cerebrospinal fluid. The needle may be slightly advanced or retracted until CSF flow is obtained. The calculated dose of contrast medium is then injected slowly (over a period of approximately one minute) to prevent epidural spill.

If fluoroscopic control of spinal canal entry is not available, the needle is advanced through the spinal cord to the ventral floor of the spinal canal. The stylet is then removed and the needle hub is checked for cerebrospinal fluid. In chondrodystrophoid breeds, the lumen of the needle is usually located in the subarachnoid space when the needle tip is on the ventral floor of the spinal canal. In other breeds, the needle may need to be retracted slightly from the ventral canal floor before CSF flow is obtained.

If CSF flow is not readily obtainable, excessive needle manipulation is not indicated. In the absence of CSF flow, to confirm the location of the needle lumen, a small dose (0.25 ml) of contrast medium may be injected and the characteristic rear limb muscle contraction observed as an indication of subarachnoid space injection. The total dose of contrast medium should not be injected unless either CSF flow or positive muscle contraction is obtained, since epidural injections are generally not of diagnostic quality and intraparenchymal injections are disas-

trous. After proper needle placement is attained, the calculated dose of contrast medium is injected slowly. The needle is then removed.

Radiographs are made in the following sequence (Morgan et al., 1972): (1) lateral recumbent view of the thoracolumbar region immediately after the injection; (2) ventrodorsal view of the T-L region; (3) opposite lateral recumbent view of the T-L region; (4) coned-down view of the region of the suspected lesion; (5) lateral view of the cervicothoracic region.

Care should be taken not to allow flexion of the trunk during lateral recumbent radiography since this may cause an artifactual narrowing of the ventral subarachnoid space at the thoracolumbar region (Ticer and Brown, 1974).

Aftercare. Recovery from anesthesia is usually uncomplicated; however, postmyelographic convulsions are a problem in some patients. Elevation of the head may decrease this problem. Convulsive activity may be satisfactorily controlled by small intravenous doses of diazepam (Valium, Roch Laboratories) given as indicated (Hoerlein, 1965; Ticer and Brown, 1974).

Interpretation. The myelographic outline should approximate the normal subarachnoid space (Figs. 10–27 to 10–31). The

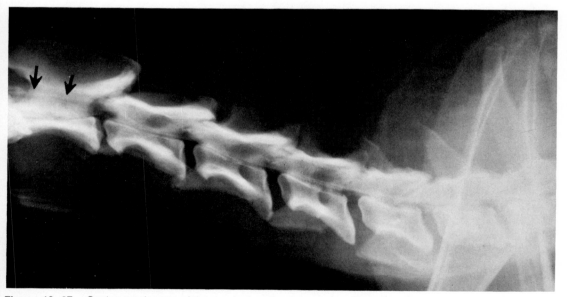

Figure 10–27. Canine myelogram of the cervical region, lateral view. Note the relatively increased width of the subarachnoid space in the dorsal aspect of the C_2 cord (arrows).

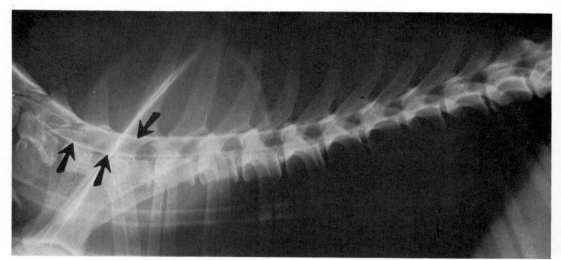

Figure 10—28. Canine myelogram of the thoracic region, lateral view. Note the relatively increased width of the subarachnoid space in the caudal cervical and cranial thoracic region (arrows).

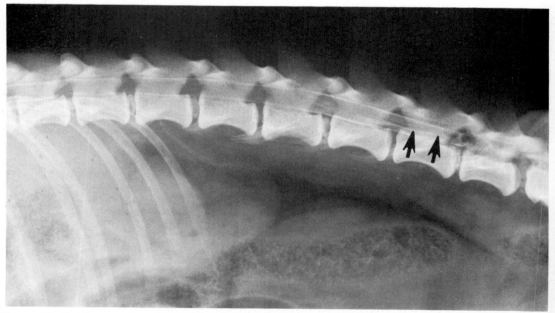

Figure 10—29. Canine myelogram of the lumbar region, lateral view. Note the radiopaque longitudinal striations of the cauda equina (arrows).

width of the radiopaque column should be of uniform magnitude over most of its course. A slight narrowing of the ventral subarachnoid space may occur over the intervertebral spaces, especially in chrondro-dystrophoid breeds. The lateral view of the cranial cervical (Fig. 10–27) and caudal cervical and cranial thoracic (Fig. 10–28)

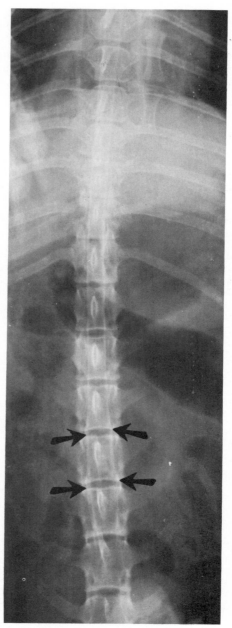

Figure 10–31. Canine myelogram of the caudal thoracic and lumbar region, VD view. Note the relatively increased diameter of the spinal cord in the region of L_{4-5} (arrows).

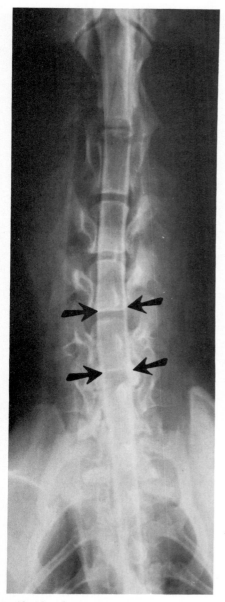

Figure 10–30. Canine myelogram of the cervical region, VD view. Note the relatively increased diameter of the spinal cord in the caudal cervical region (arrows).

regions usually shows an increased width of the subarachnoid space. The radiopaque medium delineates the longitudinal striations of the cauda equina (Fig. 10–29). The spinal cord usually shows an increased diameter in caudal cervical regions (Fig. 10–

30) and the area of the fourth and fifth lumbar vertebrae (Fig. 10–31), especially when viewed in VD projection. Generally, the diameter of the spinal cord is disproportionately smaller than the spinal canal in large breeds of dogs.

REFERENCES

Bailey, C. S., and Holliday, T. A.: Diseases of the Spinal Cord. *In* Ettinger, S. J. (Ed.): Textbook of Veterinary Internal Medicine: Diseases of the Dog and Cat. Philadelphia, W. B. Saunders Co. (in press).

Bullock, L. P., and Zook, B. C.: Myelography in dogs using water-soluble contrast mediums. J.A.V.M.A., *151*:321, 1967.

Funkquist, B.: Thoraco-lumbar myelography with water-soluble contrast medium in dogs. I. Technique of myelography; side effects and complications. J. Sm. An. Pract., *3*:53, 1962.

Hoerlein, B. F.: Canine Neurology: Diagnosis and Treatment. 2nd ed. Philadelphia, W. B. Saunders Co., 1965.

Morgan, J. P.: Radiology in Veterinary Orthopedics. Philadelphia, Lea & Febiger, 1972.

Morgan, J. P., Suter, P. F., and Holliday, T. A.: Myelography with water-soluble contrast medium: Radiographic interpretation of disc herniation in dogs. Acta Radiol. Suppl., *319*:217, 1972.

Olsson, S. E.: *In* Pettit, G. D. (Ed.): Intervertebral Disc Protrusion in the Dog. New York, Appleton-Century-Crofts, 1966.

Suter, P. F., Morgan, J. P., Holliday, T. A., and O'Brien, T. R.: Myelography in the dog: Diagnosis of tumors of the spinal cord and vertebrae. J. Amer. Vet. Radiol. Soc., *12*:29, 1971.

Ticer, J. W., and Brown, S. G.: Water-soluble myelography in canine intervertebral disc protrusion. J. Amer. Vet. Radiol. Soc., *15*:3, 1974.

Wortman, J. A.: Radiographic diagnosis of intervertebral disc disease in the dog: A comparison of non-contrast and myelographic studies. Scientific Presentations and Seminar Synopses of the 41st Meeting, American Animal Hospital Association, 1974, p. 689.

11
HEAD AND CERVICAL REGION

SKULL

Anatomical variations among species and breeds of animals often necessitate comparison of skull radiographs for disturbances in the bilateral symmetrical relationships. Radiographic examination of the skull, therefore, requires accurate positioning. This can be accomplished in most patients only with the aid of chemical restraint, preferably general anesthesia.

Pathologic processes, such as those resulting from trauma, may contraindicate anesthesia, but in most cases restraint assistance may be obtained by some form of sedation.

Exposure factors for skull radiography are generally determined by measuring the widest part of the cranium, since underexposure of this area usually results in a nondiagnostic radiograph. Regional measurements are made when anatomic features such as the nasal, maxillary or mandibular structures are specifically examined.

Some patients, such as brachycephalic canines, possess increased bone content per unit thickness compared to the average density composition of other anatomic regions and therefore require increased exposure. Generally, the addition of 7 to 10 KV or doubling the mas will produce satisfactory radiographic density for these patients.

Lateral View. The patient is placed in lateral recumbency and the rostral aspect of the skull is elevated with dry sponges to create a parallel relationship between the sagittal plane of the skull and the film, and to prevent obliquity (Fig. 11–1).

If the base of the skull is of primary interest, the mandibles may be opened to avoid overlay of the mandibular coronoid processes.

TABLE 11–1

SUGGESTED VIEWS FOR DEMONSTRATION OF VARIOUS REGIONS OF THE SKULL

Regions	View
1. Routine survey	Lateral, VD, frontal and frontal of the cranium.
2. Base of skull	Open mouth lateral, both lateral obliques, VD and open mouth frontal.
3. Frontal sinus and ethmoid regions	Both lateral obliques, frontal and open mouth VD.
4. Middle and inner ear	Both lateral obliques, VD and open mouth frontal.
5. Mandibular rami	Both lateral obliques and VD.
6. Temporomandibular joints	Both lateral obliques, sagittal oblique temporomandibular view, VD and open mouth frontal.
7. Zygomatic and orbital	Both lateral obliques, VD open mouth and frontal.
8. Maxillary teeth	Lateral oblique open mouth and VD open mouth.
9. Mandibular teeth	Lateral oblique open mouth and VD of the mandible.
10. Maxillary incisor teeth	Lateral and DV with intraoral film.
11. Mandibular incisor teeth	Lateral and VD with intraoral film.

Figure 11–2 illustrates the normal radiographic anatomy of an oligocephalic canine skull in lateral view.

Lateral Oblique View. Oblique views are utilized to examine the dorsal or ventral aspects of the skull in lateral projection without the interference created by the overlying contralateral side.

By elevating the ventral aspect of the skull so that the sagittal plane is rotated laterally approximately 20 degrees to the film, adequate visualization of the lower tympanic bulla and temporomandibular joint regions may be obtained (Fig. 11–3). The contralateral frontal sinus is also projected in a manner that will allow visualization.

Figure 11–4 illustrates the normal radiographic anatomy of the canine os bulla and temporomandibular joint regions in lateral oblique view.

If examination of the frontal sinus region is the primary objective, the dorsal aspect of the skull should be elevated (Fig. 11–5). This will profile the lower frontal sinus region.

Figure 11–6 illustrates the normal radiographic anatomy of the canine frontal sinus region in lateral oblique view.

Sagittal Oblique View of the Temporomandibular Joint. The lateral oblique view of the skull for visualization of the temporomandibular joint may be supplemented by a sagittal oblique view. The patient is placed in lateral recumbency, the rostral aspect of the skull is elevated so that the sagittal plane of the skull is rotated rostrocaudally approximately 30 degrees to the film and the mouth is opened with a dry sponge (Fig. 11–7). The joint to be examined should be placed down.

The central x-ray beam is directed at the joint being examined. This position aligns the long axis of the mandibular condyle perpendicular to the film and allows better evaluation of the intra-articular space (Douglas and Williamson, 1972).

Figure 11–8 illustrates the normal radiographic anatomy of the canine temporomandibular joint in sagittal oblique view.

Lateral Oblique Open Mouth View of the Maxillary Dental Arcades. The patient is placed in lateral recumbency and the mouth is opened maximally, with a dry sponge used as a gag. The dental arcade to be examined is placed down. Views of the maxillary arcade are produced by elevating

(*Text continued on page 234.*)

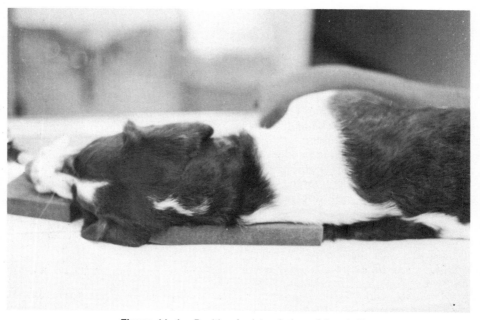

Figure 11–1. Position for lateral view of the skull.

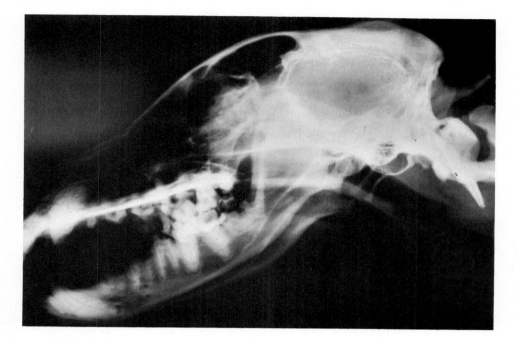

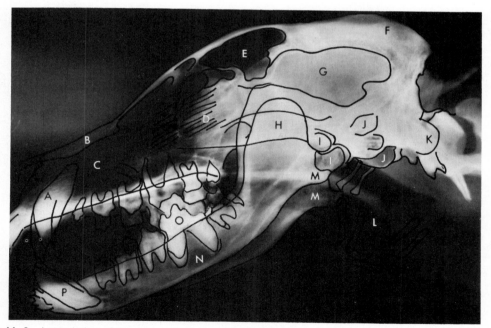

Figure 11–2. Lateral view of the canine skull. In some small canine breeds the frontal sinuses are diminished in size or absent.

A. Maxillary canine teeth superimposed
B. Nasal bone
C. Nasal passage
D. Ethmoid turbinates
E. Frontal sinuses
F. External sagittal protuberance
G. Cranium
H. Coronoid processes of the mandibles superimposed

I. Mandibular condyles
J. Tympanic bullae
K. Occipital condyles
L. Hyoid bones
M. Angular process of the mandible
N. Ramus of the mandible
O. 1st molar
P. Mandibular canine teeth superimposed

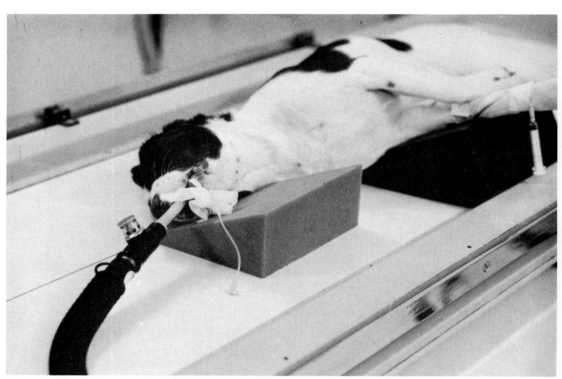

Figure 11–3. Position for the lateral oblique view of the canine skull for demonstration of the tympanic bulla, temporomandibular joint, and mandibular ramus.

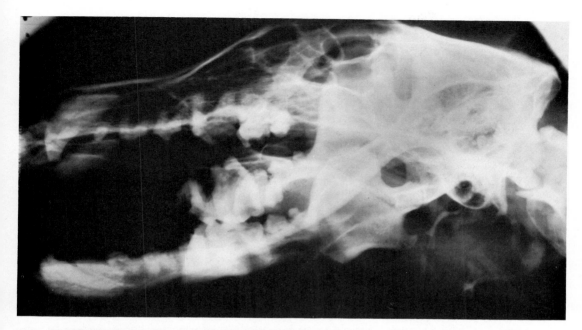

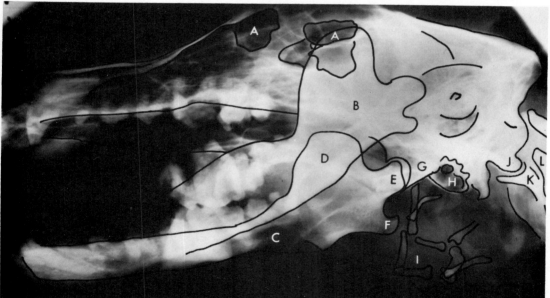

Figure 11–4. Lateral oblique view of the canine skull for demonstration of the tympanic bulla, temporomandibular joints, and mandibular ramus.

A. Frontal sinuses
B. Upper mandibular ramus
C. Lower mandibular ramus
D. Coronoid process of lower mandible
E. Mandibular condyle
F. Angular process of the mandible

G. Retroglenoid process
H. Tympanic bulla
I. Hyoid bones
J. Occipital condyle
K. Atlas (C_1)
I. Dens

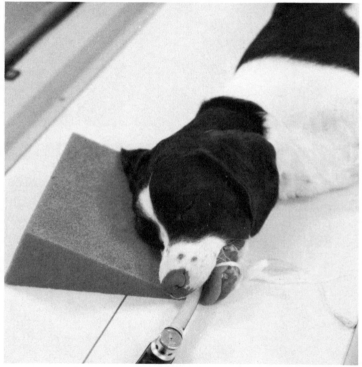

Figure 11–5. Position for the lateral oblique view of the canine skull for demonstration of the frontal sinus region.

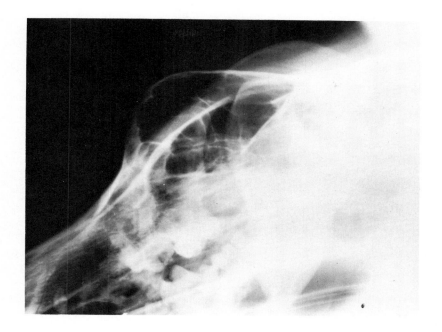

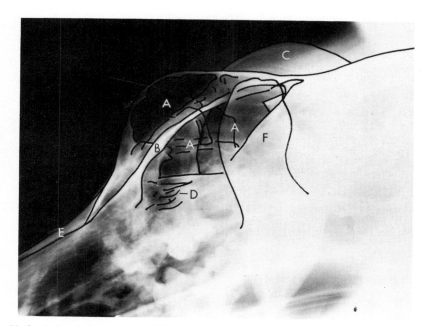

Figure 11–6. Lateral oblique view of the canine skull for demonstration of the frontal sinus region.

A. Frontal sinus
B. Frontal bone
C. Zygomatic arch

D. Ethmoid region
E. Nasal bone
F. Coronoid process of the mandible

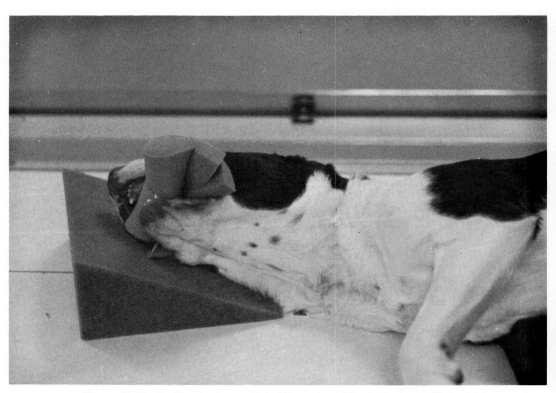

Figure 11–7. Position for the sagittal oblique view of the temporomandibular joint.

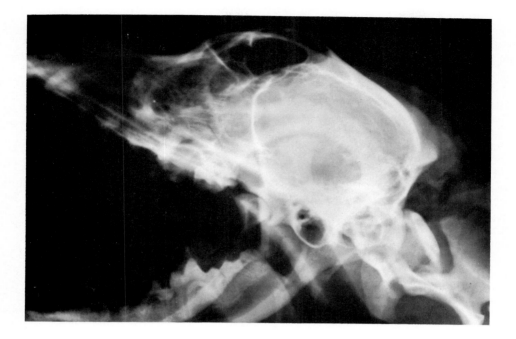

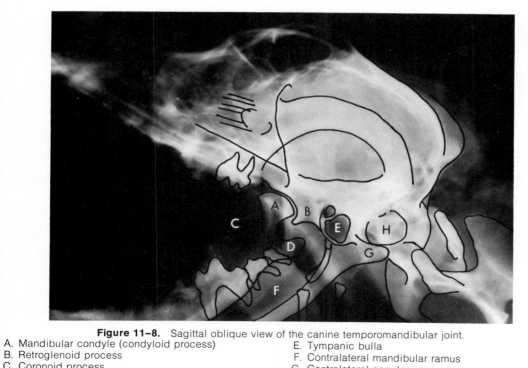

Figure 11–8. Sagittal oblique view of the canine temporomandibular joint.

A. Mandibular condyle (condyloid process)
B. Retroglenoid process
C. Coronoid process
D. Angular process

E. Tympanic bulla
F. Contralateral mandibular ramus
G. Contralateral angular process
H. Contralateral tympanic bulla

the ventral aspect of the skull so that the sagittal plane is rotated laterally approximately 45 degrees to the film (Fig. 11–9). The use of nonscreen film or detail screens provides increased detail for dental radiography.

Figure 11–10 illustrates the normal radiographic anatomy of the canine maxillary dental arcade in lateral oblique view.

Lateral Oblique Open Mouth View of the Mandibular Dental Arcade. The mandibular arcade is examined by elevating the dorsal aspect of the skull approximately 45 degrees (Fig. 11–11).

Figure 11–12 illustrates the normal radiographic anatomy of the canine mandibular arcade in lateral oblique view.

VD View. The patient is placed in dorsal recumbency and the occipital-atlantal articulation is extended so that the hard palate is parallel to the film (Fig. 11–13). The tracheal tube should be removed just prior to exposure.

Figure 11–14 illustrates the normal radio-

graphic anatomy of the canine skull in VD view.

VD Open Mouth View of the Nasal and Ethmoid Regions. The patient is placed in dorsal recumbency, and the mouth is opened maximally by a positioning device (Fig. 11–15), gauze bandages or tape. The hard palate is positioned parallel to the film. The central x-ray beam is angled into the mouth 20 degrees toward the caudal aspect of the trunk and is placed at the level of the upper third premolar.

This position allows visualization of the entire nasal passage and maxillary and frontal sinuses without overlying mandibular shadows. This complete VD view should replace the limited DV view of the nasal passage produced with the film or cassette located intraorally.

Figure 11–16 illustrates the normal radiographic anatomy of the canine nasal cavity in VD open mouth view.

DV View of the Maxillary Incisor Teeth. The patient is placed in ventral recumbency
(*Text continued on page 242.*)

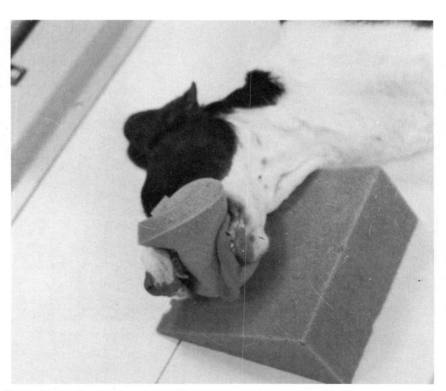

Figure 11–9. Position for lateral oblique open mouth view of the maxillary dental arcade.

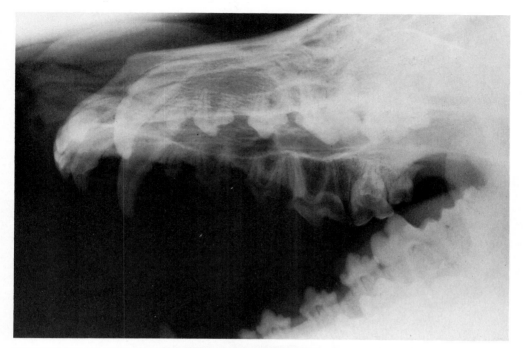

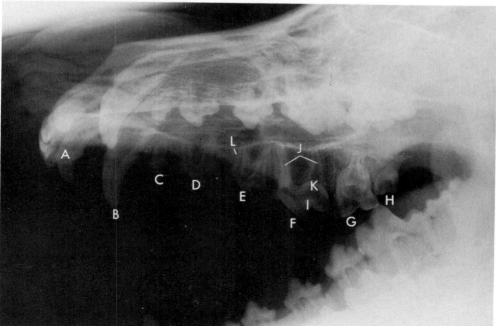

Figure 11-10. Lateral oblique open mouth view of the canine maxillary dental arcade.

A. Incisor teeth
B. Canine tooth
C. 1st premolar tooth
D. 2nd premolar tooth
E. 3rd premolar tooth
F. 4th premolar tooth (carnasial tooth)

G. 1st molar tooth
H. 2nd molar tooth
I. Crown
J. Roots
K. Pulp cavity
L. Lamina dura

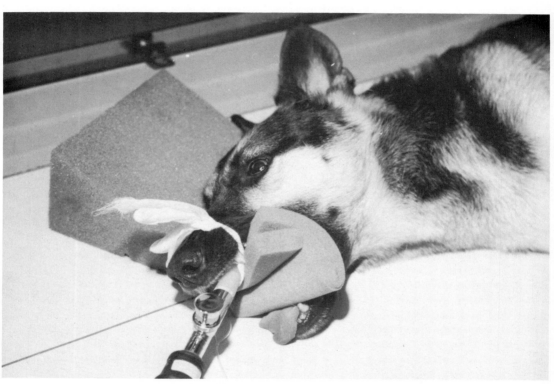

Figure 11–11. Position for lateral oblique open mouth view of the mandibular dental arcade.

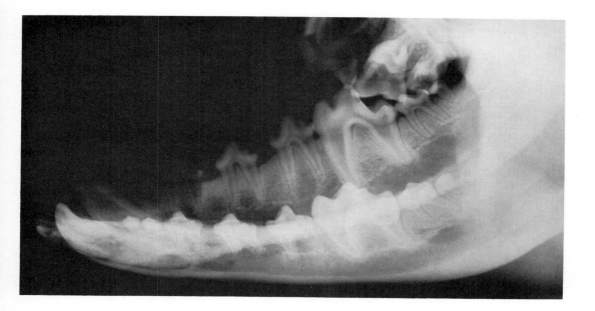

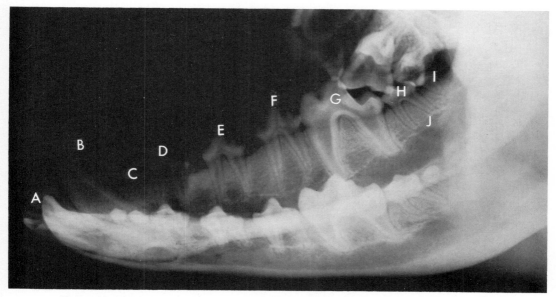

Figure 11–12. Lateral oblique open mouth view of the canine mandibular dental arcade.

A. Incisor teeth
B. Canine tooth
C. 1st premolar tooth
D. 2nd premolar tooth
E. 3rd premolar tooth

F. 4th premolar tooth
G. 1st molar (carnasial tooth)
H. 2nd molar tooth
I. 3rd molar tooth
J. Lamina dura

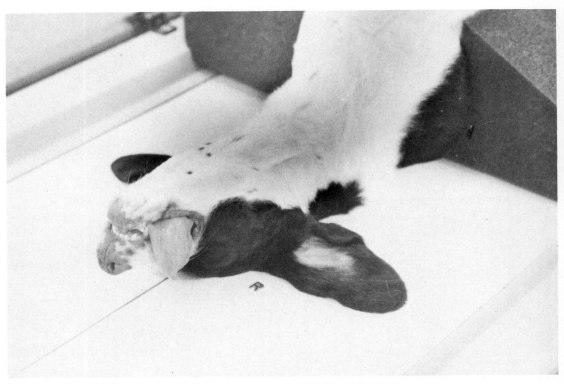

Figure 11–13. Position for VD view of the skull.

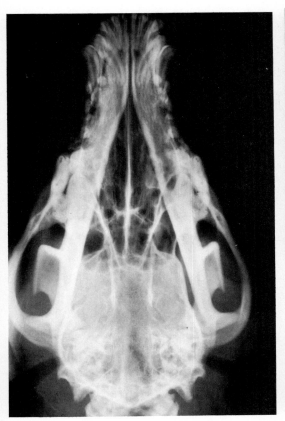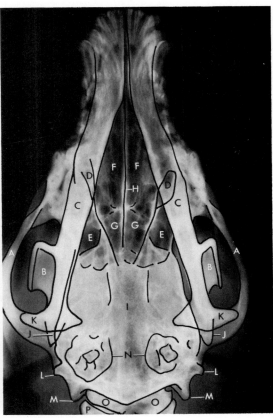

Figure 11–14. VD view of the canine skull.

A. Zygomatic arch
B. Coronoid process of the mandible
C. Ramus of the mandible
D. Maxillary sinus
E. Frontal sinus
F. Nasal passage
G. Ethmoid turbinates
H. Nasal septum (palatine suture)

I. Cranium
J. Angular process of the mandible
K. Mandibular condyle (condyloid process)
L. Mastoid process
M. Jugular process
N. Tympanic bullae
O. Occipital condyles
P. Atlas (C$_1$)

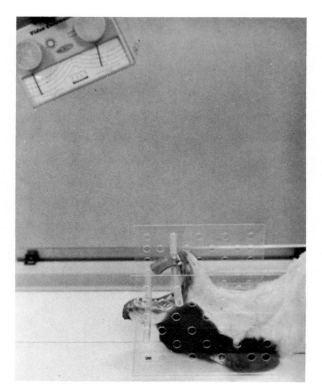

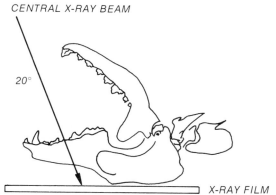

Figure 11–15. Position for VD open mouth view of the nasal and ethmoid regions.

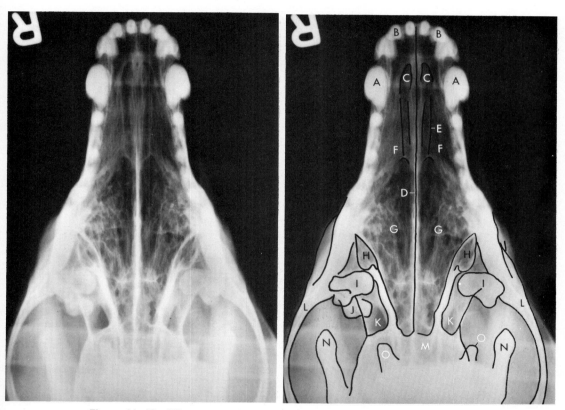

Figure 11–16. VD open mouth view of the canine nasal and ethmoid regions.

A. Maxillary canine teeth
B. Maxillary incisor teeth
C. Palatine fissure
D. Nasal septum (palatine suture)
E. Base of vomer bone
F. Maxilloturbinates
G. Ethmoturbinates
H. Maxillary sinus

I. 1st molar
J. 2nd molar
K. Frontal sinus
L. Zygomatic arch
M. Cranium
N. Coronoid process of mandible
O. Mandibular canine teeth

and a nonscreen film in a cardboard holder is placed intraorally (Fig. 11–17). The x-ray beam is angled caudally approximately 20 degrees so that it bisects the longitudinal axis of the incisor teeth.

Figure 11–18 illustrates the normal radiographic anatomy of the canine maxillary incisor teeth in DV view.

VD View of the Mandibular Incisor Teeth. The patient is placed in dorsal recumbency

and a nonscreen film in a cardboard holder is placed intraorally (Fig. 11–19). The x-ray beam is angled caudally approximately 20 degrees so that it bisects the longitudinal axis of the incisor teeth.

Figure 11–20 illustrates the normal radiographic anatomy of the canine mandibular incisor teeth in VD view.

VD View of the Mandible. The patient is placed in dorsal recumbency and a non-

(*Text continued on page 246.*)

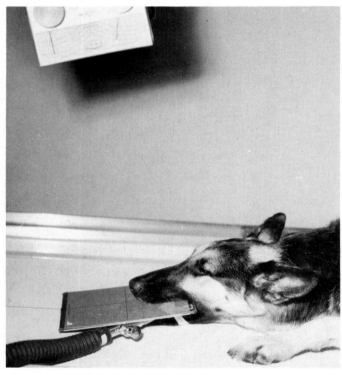

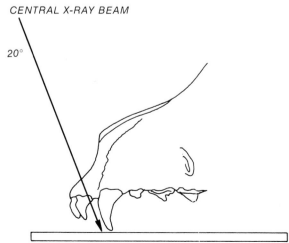

Figure 1–17. Position for DV view of the maxillary incisor teeth.

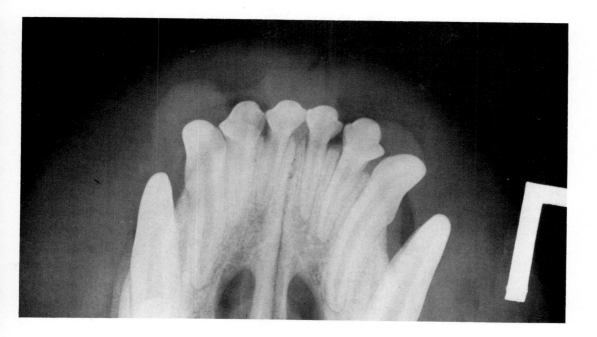

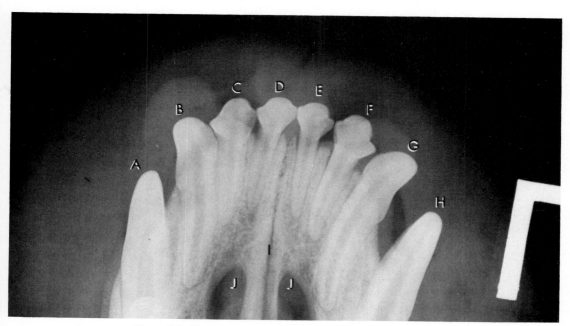

Figure 11–18. DV view of the canine maxillary incisor teeth.

A. Canine tooth, right side
B. 3rd incisor tooth, right side
C. 2nd incisor tooth, right side
D. 1st incisor tooth, right side
E. 1st incisor tooth, left side

F. 2nd incisor tooth, left side
G. 3rd incisor tooth, left side
H. Canine tooth, left side
I. Palatine suture
J. Palatine fissure

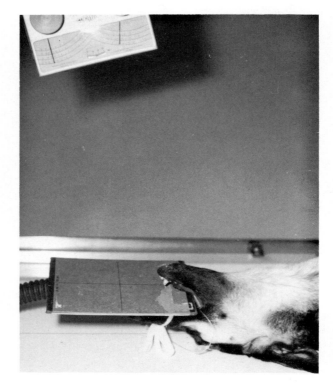

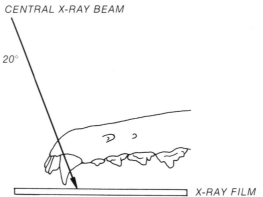

Figure 11–19. Position for VD view of the mandibular incisor teeth.

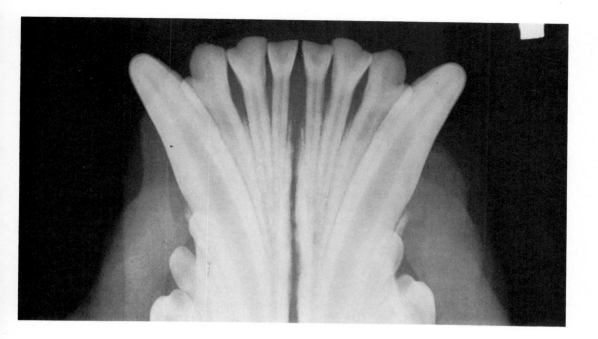

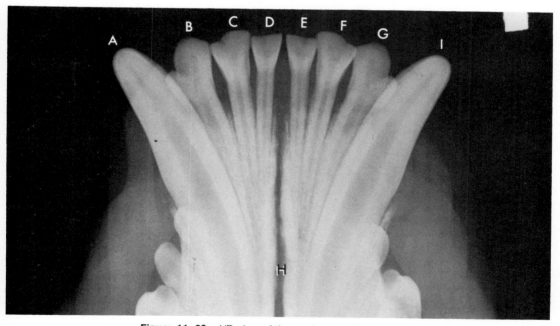

Figure 11-20. VD view of the canine mandibular teeth.

A. Canine tooth, right side
B. 3rd incisor tooth, right side
C. 2nd incisor tooth, right side
D. 1st incisor tooth, right side
E. 1st incisor tooth, left side

F. 2nd incisor tooth, left side
G. 3rd incisor tooth, left side
H. Canine tooth, left side
I. Mandibular symphysis

screen film in a cardboard holder is placed intraorally to the commissure of the mouth. The central x-ray beam is placed midmandibularly at a 90 degree angle to the rami (Fig. 11–21).

Figure 11–22 illustrates the normal radiographic anatomy of the canine mandible in VD view.

Frontal View of the Skull. The patient is placed in dorsal recumbency and the occipital-atlantal articulation is flexed approximately 90 degrees so that the hard palate is perpendicular to the film and parallel to the central x-ray beam (Fig. 11–23). Measurement to determine exposure is made from the occipital protuberance to approximately one half the distance from the intrapupillar line to the tip of the nose.

This examination is indicated when a frontal view of the nasal passages and frontal sinuses is desired.

Figure 11–24 illustrates the normal radiographic anatomy of the canine skull in frontal view.

Frontal View of the Cranium. The patient is placed in dorsal recumbency and the occipital-atlantal articulation is flexed 110 to 120 degrees so that the frontal sinuses are superimposed over the ventral skull in a manner that profiles the middle and caudal cranium (Fig. 11–25).

Measurement to determine exposure is made from the occipital protuberance to the intrapupillary line.

This examination is indicated when a frontal view of the cranium is desired without superimposition of the frontal sinuses and nasal passages.

Figure 11–26 illustrates the normal radiographic anatomy of the canine cranium in frontal view.

Open Mouth Frontal View. The patient is placed in dorsal recumbency and the occipital-atlantal articulation is flexed approximately 55 degrees. The mouth is opened in such a manner that the central x-ray beam (which is 90 degrees to the film) bisects the angle of the opened temporomandibular

(*Text continued on page 252.*)

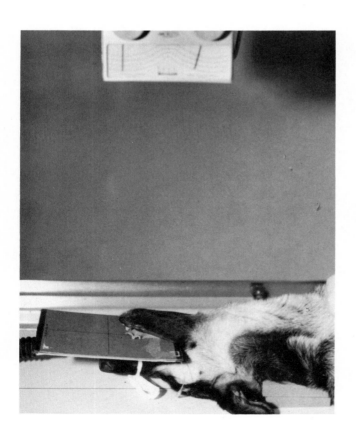

Figure 11–21. Position for VD view of the mandible.

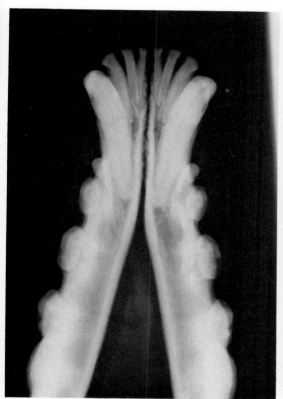 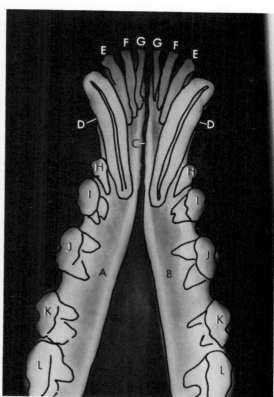

Figure 11–22. VD view of the canine mandible.

A. Right ramus of the mandible
B. Left ramus of the mandible
C. Mandibular symphysis
D. Canine teeth
E. 3rd incisor teeth
F. 2nd incisor teeth

G. 1st incisor teeth
H. 1st premolar teeth
I. 2nd premolar teeth
J. 3rd premolar teeth
K. 4th premolar teeth
L. 1st molar

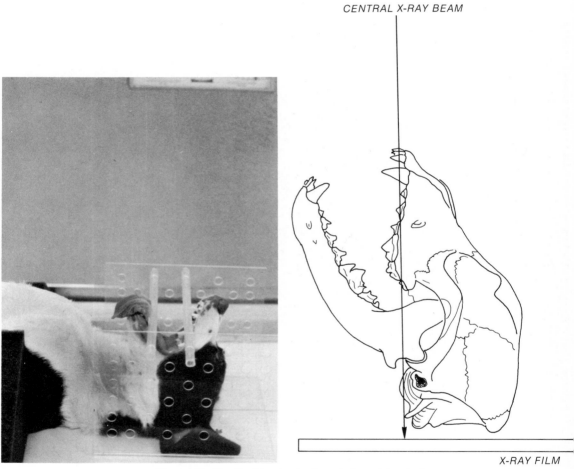

Figure 11–23. Position for the frontal view of the skull.

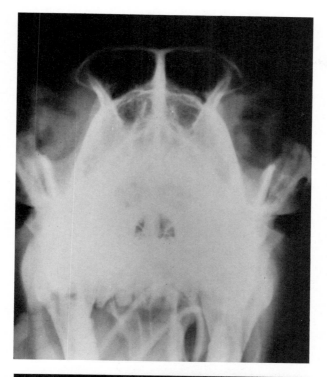

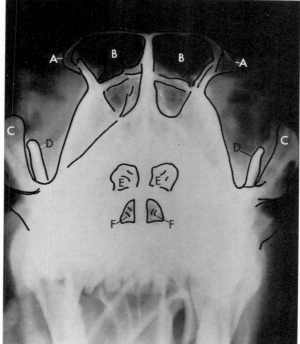

Figure 11–24. Frontal view of the canine skull. In some small canine breeds the frontal sinuses are diminished in size or absent.

A. Zygomatic processes of the frontal bones
B. Frontal sinuses
C. Zygomatic arch

D. Coronoid process of the mandible
E. Nasal passages
F. Nasopharynx

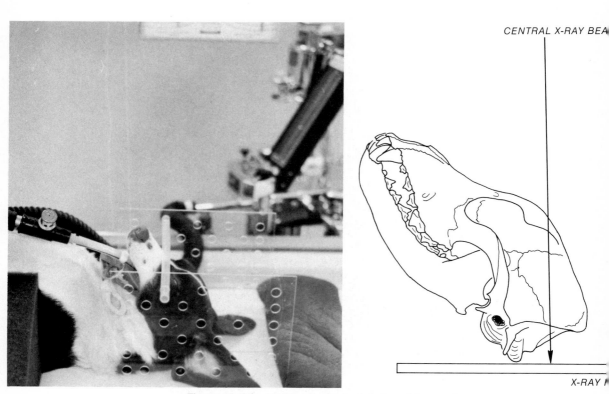

CENTRAL X-RAY BEAM

X-RAY

Figure 11–25. Position for the frontal view of the cranium.

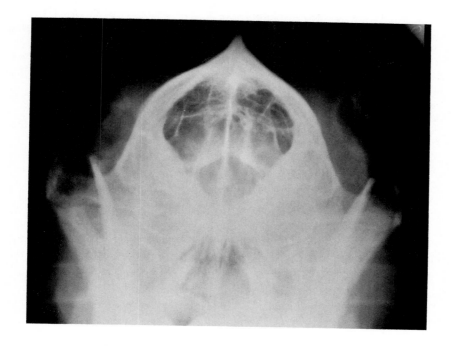

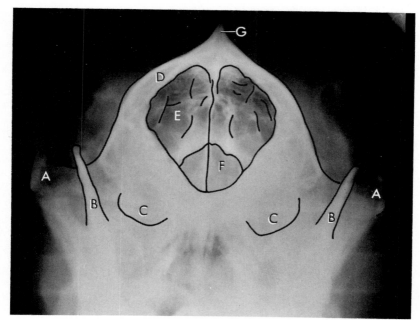

Figure 11–26. Frontal view of the canine cranium.

    A. Zygomatic arch
    B. Coronoid process of the mandible
    C. Tympanic bulla
    D. Calvarium
    E. Cranial cavity
    F. Foramen magnum
    G. Sagittal crest

articulation (Fig. 11–27). The hard palate and the mandible are angled approximately 35 degrees to the film in opposite directions. Measurement to determine exposure is made from the occipital protuberance to the commissure of the mouth.

This examination is indicated when a frontal view of the middle (os bullae) or inner ear regions and the temporomandibular joints is needed.

Figure 11–28 illustrates the normal radiographic anatomy of the canine skull in open mouth frontal view.

CERVICAL REGION

Lateral View. The patient is placed in lateral recumbency and the forelimbs are re-tracted over the cranial thorax (Fig. 11–29). The vertebrae are elevated from the x-ray table with a dry sponge pad so that the cervical and thoracic vertebrae are on the same level. The occipital-atlantal articulation is moderately flexed (45 degrees to the vertebral column).

The x-ray beam is centered mid-cervically. The beam is collimated to include the caudal aspect of the skull and the thoracic inlet.

Figure 11–30 illustrates the normal radiographic anatomy of the canine cervical region.

A marked variation in the position of the laryngeal structures may occur and is related to function (O'Brien et al., 1969). Mineralization of the larynx may occur in all dogs, particularly large breeds, in which the cricoid cartilage may mineralize at an

(Text continued on page 256.)

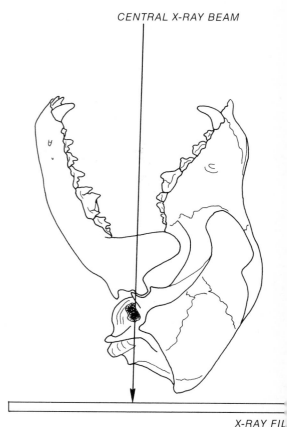

CENTRAL X-RAY BEAM

X-RAY FIL

Figure 11–27. Position for the open mouth frontal view of the skull.

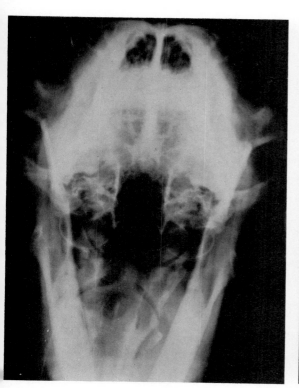 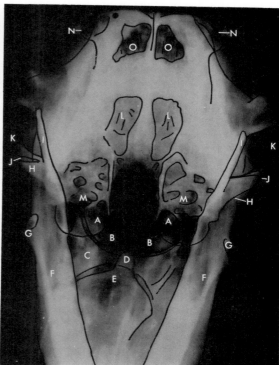

Figure 11–28. Open mouth frontal view of the canine skull.

A. Tympanic bullae
B. Occipital condyles
C. Atlas (C₁)
D. Dens
E. Axis (C₂)
F. Mandibular ramus
G. Angular process of the mandible
H. Mandibular condyle
I. Coronoid process of the mandible
J. Temporomandibular joint
K. Zygomatic arch
L. Nasal passages
M. Inner ear region of petrous temporal bone
N. Zygomatic process of the frontal bone
O. Frontal sinuses

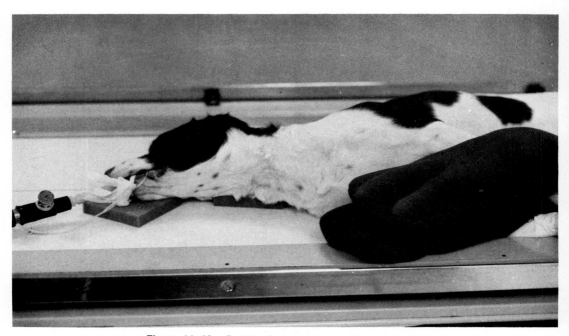

Figure 11–29. Position for lateral view of the cervical region.

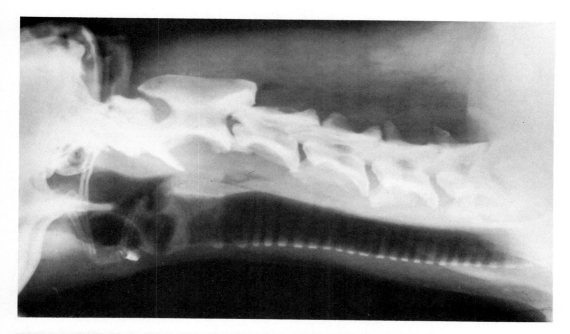

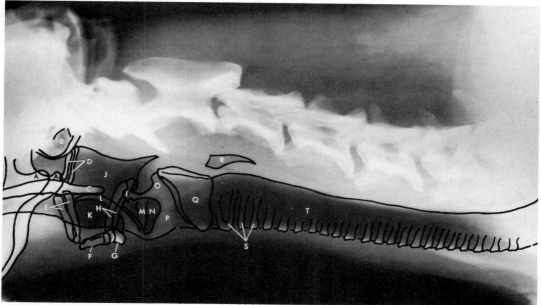

Figure 11–30. Lateral view of the canine cervical region.

A. Angular processes of the mandibles
B. Tympanic bullae
C. Soft palate
D. Stylohyoid bones
E. Epihyoid bones
F. Keratohyoid bones
G. Basihyoid bone
H. Thyrohyoid bones
I. Cranial cornu of the thyroid cartilage
J. Nasopharynx

K. Oropharynx
L. Epiglottis
M. Vocal cord
N. Lateral ventricular saccules
O. Corniculate process of arytenoid cartilage
P. Thyroid cartilage
Q. Cricoid cartilage
R. Air in esophagus
S. Tracheal cartilaginous rings
T. Tracheal lumen

TABLE 11-2

THE RELATIONSHIPS BETWEEN AGE AND MINERALIZATION OF LARYNGEAL CARTILAGES IN DOGS (FROM GASKELL, 1974)

Age	No. of Dogs Examined	Percentage of Dogs Showing Radiographic Evidence of Mineralization			
		Cricoid	Thyroid	Arytenoid	Epiglottis
0–6 mo	18	0	0	0	0
6 mo–1 yr	23	78	65	0	30
1–4 yr	39	97	64	15	28
5–8 yr	46	93	68	30	48
8+ yr	14	100	71	64	57

early age. Table 11–2 lists the relationships between age and mineralization of laryngeal cartilages in dogs.

The basihyoid bone normally appears mineralized in the lateral view in all dogs. Tracheal rings may also appear mineralized, especially in large dogs.

VD View. The patient is placed in dorsal recumbency with the forelimbs secured laterally to the thoracic walls (Fig. 11–31).

The x-ray beam is centered mid-cervically and is collimated to include the caudal aspect of the skull and the thoracic inlet.

Figure 11–32 illustrates the normal radiographic anatomy of the canine cervical region in VD view.

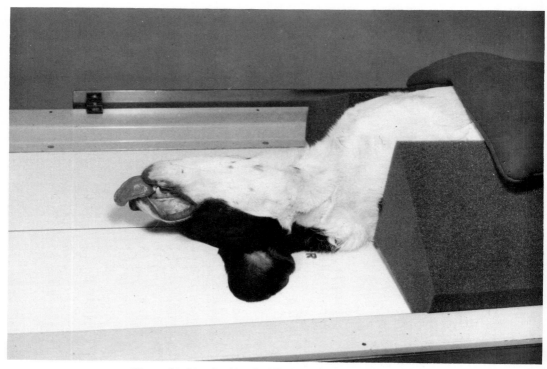

Figure 11–31. Position for VD view of the cervical region.

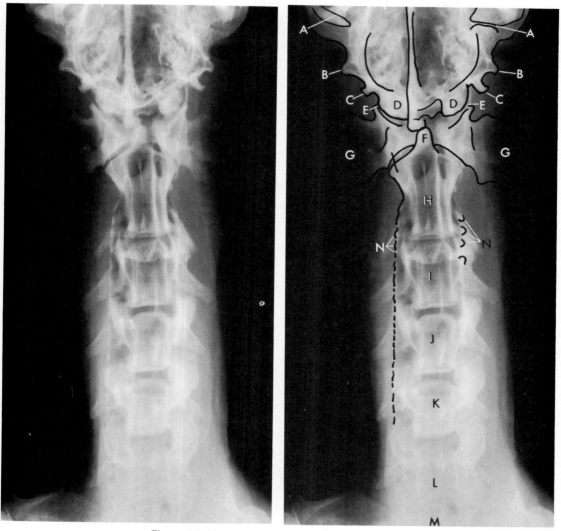

Figure 11–32. VD view of the canine cervical region.

A. Temporomandibular joints
B. Mastoid processes
C. Jugular processes
D. Occipital condyles
E. Atlanto-occipital joint
F. Dens
G. Wings of the atlas (C_1)
H. Axis (C_2)
 I. C_3
J. C_4
K. C_5
L. C_6
M. C_7
N. Tracheal rings

Orbital Angiography

Orbital angiography may be accomplished by simple retrograde injection of contrast medium through the infraorbital artery.

INDICATIONS

Orbital angiography may assist in diagnosing neoplasms (Glatt et al., 1970) and vascular abnormalities (Rubin and Patterson, 1965). Visualization of deviation of the large orbital vessels and increased vascularity (tumor blush) caused by certain neoplasms can aid in surgical planning (Glatt et al., 1970). Exact radiographic location of the eye within the orbit is made possible by angiographic outline of the choroid.

CONTRAINDICATIONS

No specific contraindications for orbital angiography in the dog have been reported; however, orbital pain, ocular hemorrhage, and transient to permanent blindness have been reported in man (Lombardi, 1967).

TECHNIQUE

Patient Preparation

Patient preparation consists of routine pre-anesthetic procedures. General anesthesia is required.

Materials

A 21-gauge vein infusion set (Butterfly 21 Infusion Set, Abbott Laboratories) and a 5 or 10 ml syringe are used to make the injection of contrast medium. Heparinized physiologic saline solution is needed to flush the infusion set. A 50 to 60 per cent iodine-based, water soluble contrast medium is used (Hypaque 50%, Winthrop Laboratories; Renografin-60, Squibb & Sons). Surgical instrumentation for simple arteriotomy is used to isolate the artery.

Dosage

Five to 10 ml of contrast medium is used for each injection.

Procedure

The patient is anesthetized and the region of the infraorbital foramen is prepared for surgery. The skin is incised over the foramen, and the superficial facial muscles are bluntly separated to expose the infraorbital artery, nerve and vein. The infraorbital artery is usually located medial or ventral to the nerve but may occasionally be found in the infraorbital nerve bundle (Glatt et al., 1970). A segment of the artery approximately 1 cm long is isolated and elevated with two lengths of nonabsorbable suture material. The artery is then cannulated in a proximal direction with a 21-gauge vein infusion set, and the needle is tied into place with the previously placed ligature. Heparinized physiologic saline solution is used to flush the needle and tubing periodically to maintain patency.

After the patient has been placed with the

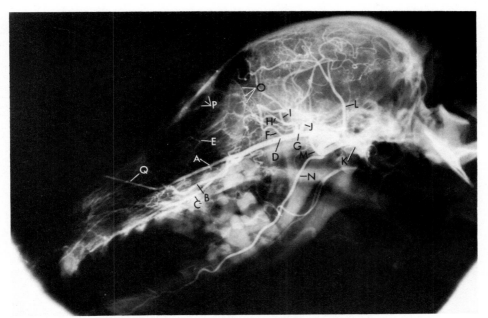

Figure 11–33. Orbital angiogram, canine, lateral view. Radiograph was produced after a retrograde injection of contrast medium into the infraorbital artery.

A. Infraorbital artery
B. Sphenopalatine artery
C. Major palatine artery
D. Maxillary artery
E. Malar artery
F. Anterior deep temporal artery
G. Orbital artery
H. Ventral muscular branch
 I. External ethmoid artery
J. External ophthalmic artery
K. External carotid artery
L. Superficial temporal artery
M. Posterior deep temporal artery
N. Mandibular alveolar artery
O. Choroid
P. Ciliary body
Q. Cannula

side to be examined next to the film, 5 to 10 ml of contrast medium is injected with moderate pressure to produce retrograde flow into the infraorbital artery. A lateral radiograph is produced near the end of the injection period. The injection and radiographic procedure are repeated in the VD open mouth projection. Radiographic exposure technique should be increased from 5 to 7 KV above the normal factors.

The cannula is then removed and moderate digital pressure is applied to the artery for a short time. If hemorrhage persists, the vessel may be ligated without adverse effects (Glatt et al., 1970). The skin incision is closed in the routine manner.

Interpretation

The number of arteries visualized will vary with the amount of contrast medium injected. A large-volume injection results in radiographic visualization of the arteries arising from the external carotid and internal maxillary arteries. The superficial facial, auricular, mandibular and glossal vessels are usually demonstrated (Figs. 11–33 and 11–34). Arteries of the orbital floor and choroid are also seen (Figs. 11–33 and 11–34).

The detection of displacement of the large vessels and abnormal vascularization may be diagnostically useful in defining masses in the orbital region.

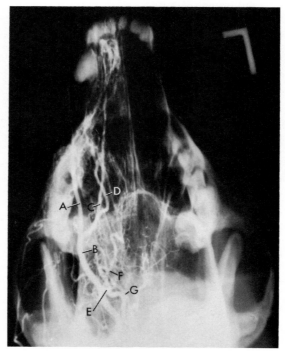

Figure 11–34. Orbital angiogram, canine, VD open mouth view. Radiograph was produced after a retrograde injection of contrast medium into the infraorbital artery.

A. Infraorbital artery
B. Maxillary artery
C. Major palatine artery
D. Sphenopalatine artery
E. Orbital artery
F. External ethmoid artery
G. External ophthalmic artery

Sialography

Sialography is the radiographic examination of the salivary ducts and glands after the introduction of a radiopaque medium.

INDICATIONS

Sialography is useful in the diagnosis of disease involving the salivary ducts and glands. In the dog, sialography has helped to definitively locate salivary mucoceles and to elucidate their mechanism of formation (Harvey, 1969). In any fluid-containing swelling that is suspected of being congenital, sialography is useful in eliminating lesions of the salivary gland and ducts. Parotid sialography should be a routine part of the diagnostic investigation of recurrent swellings of the cheek (Harvey, 1969). In addition, confirmation of diagnoses of neoplasia, abscess, sialolithiasis, sialoangiectasis and sialadenitis has been an indication for sialography in humans (Hettwer and Folsom, 1968; Schulz and Weisberger, 1948).

CONTRAINDICATIONS

No specific contraindications for sialography have been reported. Probably, however, a contraindication for general anesthesia would also constitute a contraindication for sialography.

TECHNIQUE

Patient Preparation

Patient preparation consists of routine pre-anesthetic procedures. General anesthesia is usually required.

Materials

Blunt cannulas made from shortened (1 cm long) 22-, 25-, and 26-gauge hypodermic needles or lacrimal cannulas are used for opaque medium injection. A pair of fine tissue forceps, syringes and a mouth gag are also needed. A 60 per cent suspension of propyliodone in peanut oil (Dionosil Oily, Glaxo Laboratories, Ltd., distributed by Picker Corp.) is used as the medium.

Dosage

A contrast medium dose of 0.1 to 0.3 ml. is used for retrograde injection into the salivary ducts.

Procedure

Parotid Duct. Scout radiographs of the skull in the lateral and VD projections are produced. The parotid salivary duct opens into the mouth on a papilla located on the labial oral mucosa opposite the upper fourth premolar (carnassial) tooth (Fig. 11–35). The parotid duct enters the mouth perpendicularly to the oral mucosa and bends caudally 90 degrees immediately beneath the duct papilla (Miller et al., 1964). Cannulation of the duct may be simplified by straightening the distal portion of the duct by grasping the oral mucosa caudal to the duct papilla with a fine tissue forceps and retracting it rostromedially (Harvey, 1969). A 22-gauge needle (smaller for small dogs) is then directed into the duct opening and gently pushed caudally. This procedure should require very little force. The cannula is then inserted to the hub and the contrast medium injected. Lateral and VD radiographs are then produced. Generally, the lateral view possesses the most diagnostic information and should be produced first.

Zygomatic Duct. Scout radiographs of the skull are made in the lateral and VD open mouth projection. The zygomatic salivary gland has one major duct and two to four minor ducts. The major duct opens into the mouth approximately 1 cm caudal and slightly dorsal to the parotid duct papilla (Fig. 11–36). It lies on a mucosal ridge that runs lateral to the last upper molar tooth. The duct is approximately one half the size of the parotid duct. Fine tissue forceps are used to steady the oral mucosa next to the major duct opening, and a 25- to 26-gauge cannula is directed into the duct opening and passed gently dorsally and slightly caudally.

The methods of injection of contrast medium and radiography are the same as those used for parotid duct sialography. Radiographs in the lateral and VD open mouth projections are produced.

Mandibular and Sublingual Ducts. Scout radiographs of the skull in lateral and VD views are produced. The mandibular salivary duct opens on the lateral surface of the lingual caruncles (Fig. 11–37). The duct opening is a slit-like orifice approximately 1 mm long. The sublingual duct enters the mouth 1 to 2 mm caudal to the mandibular duct opening and appears as a small red dot in approximately two thirds of dogs (Fig. 11–38). In approximately one third of dogs, the sublingual and submandibular ducts join and enter the mouth at a common opening (Miller et al., 1964). This variation may be bilateral or unilateral. Careful inspection of the lateral surfaces of the caruncles should be performed prior to excessive manipulation or application of forceps since marks left on the oral mucosa may resemble a duct opening (Harvey, 1969).

A 22- or 25-gauge cannula may be used to enter the mandibular duct. A 26-gauge cannula is used for the sublingual duct. Forceps are utilized to retract the lingual caruncle rostrally. The mandibular duct is entered by placing the cannula tip just rostral to the opening and sliding the cannula caudally.

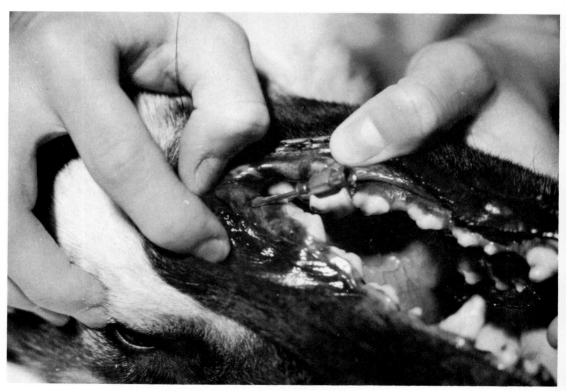

Figure 11–35. Cannula in the parotid salivary duct.

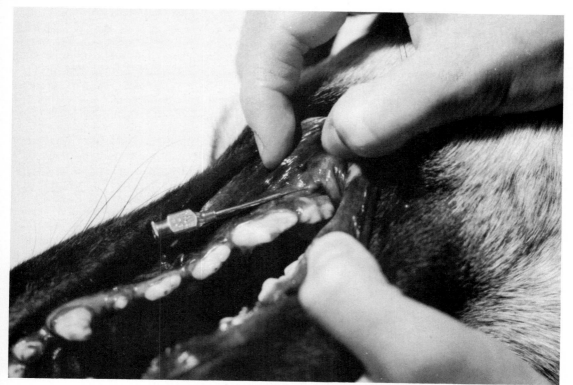

Figure 11–36. Cannula in the zygomatic salivary duct.

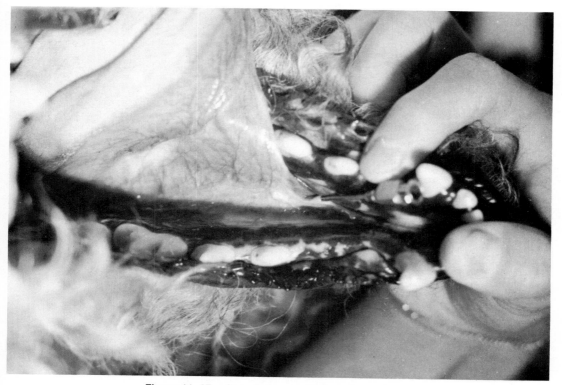

Figure 11–37. Cannula in mandibular salivary duct.

Cannulation should be to the cannula hub. If both ducts open into the mouth at a single orifice, the mandibular duct may be entered by sliding the cannula directly caudal from the common opening. A 26-gauge cannula is then inserted at the dorsomedial edge of the opening, and an attempt is made to locate the sublingual duct by gently probing in a medial and dorsal direction from the mandibular duct (Harvey, 1969).

This method of injection of contrast medium and radiography is the same as that used for parotid duct sialography.

Figures 11–39 and 11–40 illustrate the normal radiographic anatomy of a canine mandibular sialogram, showing the normal appearance of the salivary duct and salivary gland ductules.

Interpretation

Parotid Duct and Gland. The parotid duct course varies with the degree of mouth opening. Decreased mouth opening causes the duct to arc slightly ventrally (Harvey, 1969). The duct should be smooth in outline and course to the angle of the jaw, where it divides into several small ductules before entering the gland. The intraglandular ductules show progressive bifurcation, producing a tree-branch pattern. The parotid gland is an irregular, lobulated structure that lies lateroventrally to the external auditory meatus.

Zygomatic Duct and Gland. The main zygomatic duct is short and courses in a dorsocaudal direction. The intraglandular ductules show progressive bifurcation, producing a tree-branch pattern. The gland is a large, single-lobed structure located ventral to the rostral end of the zygomatic arch.

Mandibular Duct and Gland. The mandibular duct courses caudally and parallel to the ramus of the mandible to the angle of the jaw and twists slightly before coursing ventrally to the gland. The intraglandular ductules show progressive bifurcation, producing a tree-branch pattern. The mandibular gland is smooth, single-lobed and located immediately ventral to the angle of the jaw. The hyoid bones may be superimposed in

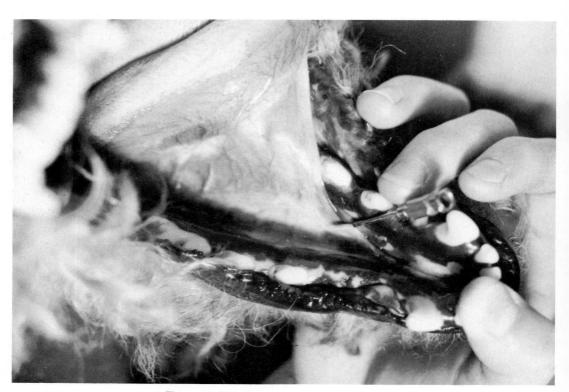

Figure 11–38. Cannula in sublingual salivary duct.

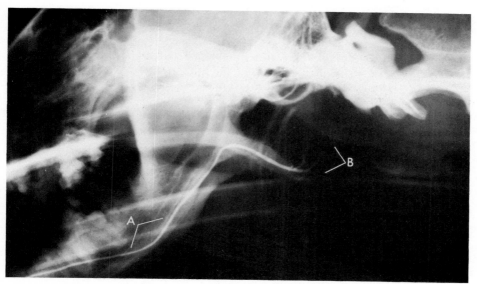

Figure 11–39. Mandibular sialogram, canine, lateral view. Radiograph produced after retrograde injection of contrast medium into the mandibular duct.

A. Mandibular salivary duct
B. Ductules of the mandibular salivary gland

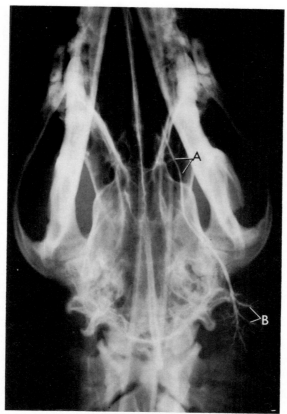

Figure 11–40. Mandibular sialogram, Canine, VD view. Radiograph produced after retrograde injection of contrast medium into the mandibular duct.

A. Mandibular salivary duct
B. Ductules of the mandibular salivary gland

the region of the gland on the lateral view and should not be mistaken for extravasation of dye from the duct or gland.

Sublingual Duct and Gland. The sublingual duct courses caudally in a manner similar to that of the mandibular duct. Superimposed upon the duct are several lobules, which vary in size and position. A small, isolated lobule is located cranial to the first lower molar tooth, and a collection of small lobules is located at the level of or caudal to this tooth. The main part of the gland is located at the level of the second molar tooth and courses caudoventrally. The main part of the gland consists of two parts: a bilobed cranial part, and a caudal part, which is located caudoventral to the cranial part. The intraglandular ductules show progressive bifurcation, producing a tree-branch pattern.

Dacryocystorhinography

Dacryocystorhinography is a radiographic examination of the nasolacrimal duct after the introduction of a positive contrast agent into the puncta lacrimalia.

INDICATIONS

Contrast examination of the lacrimal drainage system is indicated in cases of chronic recurring or intractable conjunctivitis, dacryocystitis (Yakely and Alexander, 1971) and neoplasia of the lacrimal duct or periductal tissue (Glatt et al., 1970).

CONTRAINDICATIONS

Contraindications for dacryocystorhinography are limited to those that might prevent the administration of anesthesia or profound sedation.

TECHNIQUE

Dacryocystorhinography is best performed on anesthetized patients. Survey radiographs of the rostral aspect of the skull are then produced in the lateral and open mouth views. The patient is placed in lateral recumbency with the diseased side up. The superior puncta is then cannulated with a 17- to 22-gauge beveled polyethylene intravenous catheter (I.V. Catheter Placement Unit, Jelco Laboratories), which is then taped to the side of the head to prevent dislodging during subsequent positioning maneuvers (Fig. 11–41). The inferior puncta is occluded with fixation forceps (Graeff Fixation Forceps, Milten Instrument Co.) and the system is flushed with physiologic saline solution. A 50 to 60 per cent solution of water-soluble iodine-based contrast medium (Hypaque 50%, Winthrop Labora-

tories, or Renographin-60, Squibb & Sons) or an oily medium (Dionosil Oily, Glaxo Laboratories, Ltd., distributed by Picker Corp.) is then injected continuously until several drops are emitted from the nose. Moderate digital pressure applied to the medial canthus will prevent spillage of medium into the conjunctival sac. Placing the nose close to the table during injection and lateral recumbent radiography will prevent excessive retrograde flow of the medium into the nasal ·turbinates, where it may overlie the course of the lacrimal duct and obscure adequate visualization.

After the injection, the patient is placed with the side to be examined closest to the film, and a lateral recumbent radiograph is produced, using a slightly increased exposure than for the scout radiographic technique (add 5 to 7 KV). A moderately oblique open mouth view is then produced.

Interpretation

The lacrimal drainage system in the dog is devoid of a distinct lacrimal sac (Miller et al., 1964). The duct is seen as a smooth, well-delineated structure joining the second canaliculus and continuing rostroventrally and slightly medially through the lacrimal bone into the maxilla, where it opens ventrally to the maxilloturbinate crest (approximately 2 cm caudal to the external nares on the lateral floor of the nasal cavity) (Figs. 11–42 and 11–43). The medial wall of the canal may be thin and incomplete in the maxilla and may protrude into the maxillary sinus (Miller et al., 1964).

There should be no alterations in luminal size nor in the course of the duct. The periductal osseous structures should not show changes in the normal trabecular pattern.

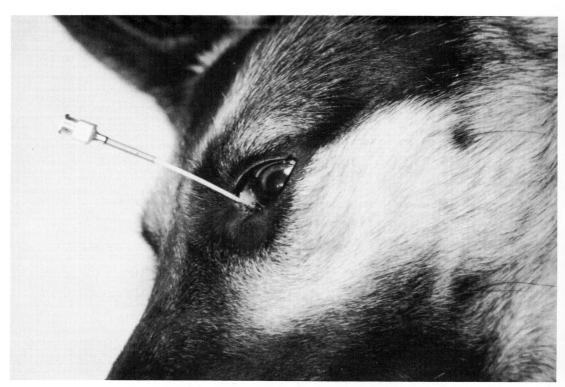

Figure 11–41. Catheter placed in the superior puncta for dacryocystorhinography.

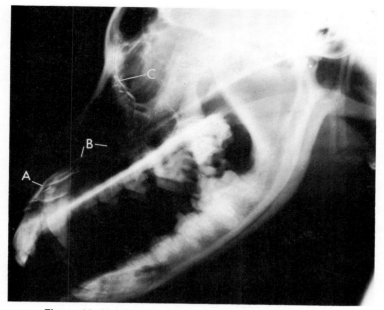

Figure 11–42. Dacryocystorhinography, canine, lateral view.

    A. Contrast medium in nasal passage
    B. Nasolacrimal duct
    C. Superior and inferior canaliculi

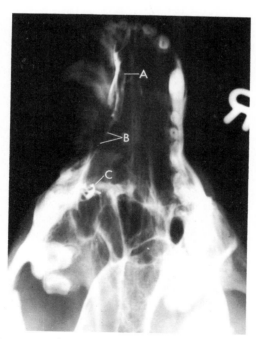

Figure 11–43. Dacryocystorhinography, canine, moderately oblique open mouth view.

    A. Contrast medium in nasal passage
    B. Nasolacrimal duct
    C. Superior and inferior canaliculi

REFERENCES

Carlson, W. D.: Veterinary Radiology. 2nd ed. Philadelphia, Lea & Febiger, 1967.

Douglas, S. W., and Williamson, H. D.: Principles of Veterinary Radiography. 2nd ed. Baltimore, Williams & Wilkins Co., 1972.

Gaskell, C. J.: The radiographic anatomy of the pharynx and larynx of the dog. J. Sm. Anim. Pract., 14:89, 1974.

Glatt, K. N., Guffy, M. M., and Boggess, T. S.: Radiographic contrast techniques for detecting orbital and nasolacrimal tumors in dogs. J.A.V.M.A., 156:741, 1970.

Harvey, C. E.: Sialography in the dog. Am. J. Vet. Radiol. Soc., 10:18, 1969.

Hettwer, K. J., and Folsom, T. C.: The normal sialogram. Oral Surg., Oral Med. and Oral Path., 26:790, 1968.

Lombardi, G.: Radiology in Neuro-ophthalmology. Baltimore, Williams & Wilkins Co., 1967.

Miller, M. E., Christensen, G. C., and Evans, H. E.: Anatomy of the Dog. Philadelphia, W. B. Saunders Co., 1964.

O'Brien, J. A., Harvey, C. E., and Tucker, J. A.: The larynx of the dog: Its normal radiographic anatomy. Am. J. Vet. Radiol. Soc., 10:38, 1969.

Rubin, L. F., and Patterson, D. F.: Arteriovenous fistula of the orbit in a dog. Cornell Vet., 55:471, 1965.

Schebitz, H., and Wilkins, H.: Atlas of Radiographic Anatomy of Dog and Horse. Berlin, Paul Parley, 1968.

Schulz, M. D., and Weisberger, D.: Sialography, its value in diagnosis of swelling about the salivary glands. Oral. Surg., Oral Med. and Oral Path., 1:233, 1948.

Spreull, J. S. A., and Archibald, J.: Glands of the head and neck. In Archibald, J. (Ed.): Canine Surgery, First Archibald Edition. Santa Barbara, Calif., American Veterinary Publications, Inc., 1965.

Yakeley, W. L., and Alexander, J. E.: Dacryocystorhinography in the dog. J.A.V.M.A., 159:1417, 1971.

Cerebral Ventriculography

J. E. OLIVER, JR.,
AND C. R. CONRAD

Ventriculography is the radiographic process in which a contrast material is injected into the cerebral ventricular system in order to visualize the size and shape of the ventricles of the brain (Hoerlein, 1971).

INDICATIONS

The contents of the cranial vault — nervous tissue, cerebrospinal fluid and vascular structures — all have the same radiographic density. Radiographs of the cranium demonstrate the structures of the skull, but not its contents. Since most pathologic processes (such as tumors, hematomas and hydrocephalus) are of the same radiographic density as the other structures within the skull, special techniques are required to demonstrate most brain lesions.

Ventriculography is the method of choice for evaluating the size of the ventricles, as is necessary in cases of suspected hydrocephalus. Intracranial mass lesions may be detected by lateral shift in the position of the ventricles or by deviations in their contours.

CONTRAINDICATIONS

Ventriculography requires general anesthesia and the placement of needles through the cerebral cortex into the lateral ventricles. There are no specific contraindications, but each animal must be evaluated in view of its physical condition and the information to be derived from the procedure.

NORMAL ANATOMY

The cerebral ventricular system consists of paired lateral ventricles, a midline third ventricle, the mesencephalic aqueduct and a fourth ventricle.

The lateral ventricles are located in each cerebral hemisphere. They are separated by the septum pellucidum and communicate with the third ventricle by the interventricular foramina. The lateral ventricles are divided into three parts: the body, the rostral horn, with an extension into the olfactory bulb, and a caudal or temporal horn, which curves around the caudal margin of the thalamus in the temporal lobe of the cerebrum (Fitzgerald, 1961).

Each lateral ventricle is bounded by the cerebral white matter dorsally and laterally, the septum pellucidum medially and the caudate nucleus and hippocampus ventrally (Miller et al., 1964).

The third ventricle is a median, unpaired cavity surrounding the interthalamic adhesion, between the two sides of the thalamus. The dorsal margin of the third ventricle is formed by ependyma and tela choroidea. The ventral boundaries are primarily the structures of the hypothalamus, but include an invagination into the hypophysis. The third ventricle communicates with the lateral ventricles through the paired interventricular foramina and with the fourth ventricle by way of the mesencephalic aqueduct.

The mesencephalic aqueduct extends from the caudal end of the third ventricle to the rostral end of the fourth ventricle. It lies entirely within the midbrain.

The fourth ventricle lies above the pons and medulla oblongata. The roof of the fourth ventricle is composed of the cerebellum, the choroid plexus and the rostral and caudal medullary vela. Laterally it is bounded by the rostral and caudal cerebellar

271

peduncles. The fourth ventricle communicates rostrally with the third ventricle through the mesencephalic aqueduct, laterally with the subarachnoid space through lateral apertures (foramina of Luschka), and caudally with the central canal of the spinal cord. Most authors agree that there is no caudal aperture to the subarachnoid space (foramen of Magendie), although it has been described (Fitzgerald, 1961; Jenkins, 1972).

PROCEDURE

Patient Preparation

The patient should be prepared for general anesthesia. If there are no specific contraindications, corticosteroids should be administered for 24 to 48 hours prior to the procedure in order to reduce the chances of cerebral edema which may result from trauma to the brain.

Anesthesia

Inhalation anesthesia should be administered through an endotracheal tube. It is extremely important that respiration be monitored, since some animals may become apneic during the procedure. A moderate degree of hyperventilation is recommended to help prevent cerebral edema.

Positioning

If possible, the animal should be positioned with a head holder (Oliver, 1966). Such a device allows the animal to be manipulated easily, provides easy access to the cranium, and avoids compression of the jugular veins and trachea. Radiographs can be made using a horizontal beam, which best demonstrates the contours of the ventricles when air is used as the contrast medium.

Contrast Media

Air is the safest and most frequently used contrast material for ventriculography. Good visualization of the lateral and third ventricles can be obtained with air. However, it is difficult to manipulate the animal properly to move air through the mesen-

cephalic aqueduct into the fourth ventricle. Even when this can be accomplished, contrast is usually insufficient to truly evaluate these structures.

Iophendylate (Pantopaque, Lafayette Pharmaceuticals) has been used in ventriculography (Hoerlein, 1971). Good contrast is obtained and patency of the mesencephalic aqueduct is readily demonstrated. Residual iophendylate has been shown to produce a granulomatous reaction in the meninges. Such a reaction may reduce absorption of cerebrospinal fluid (CSF) sufficiently to produce hydrocephalus.

Water-soluble positive contrast media have also been used for ventriculography. Excellent visualization of the entire ventricular system is produced, Unfortunately, some animals have convulsions following the use of these materials (Albert, 1967).

Air is the contrast medium of choice for most procedures. If the mesencephalic aqueduct or fourth ventricle must be visualized, one of the aqueous contrast media should be used, with precautions to control possible convulsions.

Technique

A 22-gauge 1- to 2-inch short bevel spinal needle with a stylette is inserted into each lateral ventricle (Fig. 11–44). The injection site is 0.5 to 1.0 cm from the midline, midway between a line drawn through the lateral canthus of the eyes and a line through the external occipital protuberance (Fig. 11–45). In most dogs and cats, this will place the needles just caudal to the coronal suture and dorsal cerebral veins in the parietal lobe of the brain. The injection must be lateral to the midline to avoid the dorsal sagittal sinus. Depth of needle insertion depends on the thickness of the calvarium and temporal muscles and can be estimated on lateral radiographs of the skull.

The injection must be performed using aseptic techniques. The site can be exposed by a midline skin incision and lateral reflection of the temporal muscles. A stab incision through the skin and temporal muscles with a No. 11 surgical blade is a simpler technique, however. The needle may be inserted directly into the brain through the lateral margin of the large open fontanelles of animals with hydrocephalus. A Steinman pin in a hand chuck, or a twist drill, can be

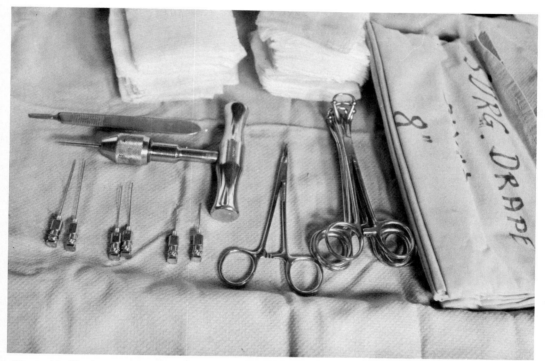

Figure 11–44. Instruments needed for ventriculography include knife, pin and chuck, and spinal needles.

used to penetrate the skull in other animals (Fig. 11–46). If possible, the last portion of the inner table of the skull should not be penetrated, so that the needle can be pushed through for a tight fit. This prevents lateral motion of the needle during the procedure.

Both needles are inserted to the estimated depth; the stylette is removed from one needle; jugular veins are compressed to increase CSF pressure slightly; and the needle is slowly withdrawn until fluid appears in the hub (Fig. 11–47). When fluid is obtained from both needles, a sample of CSF is obtained for analysis, and the veins are released. Approximately 3 cc of air is in-jected first into one ventricle, then into the other, with both needles open to prevent sudden increases in the pressure. It is *imperative* that the pulse be monitored constantly throughout the procedure for alterations in rate or strength. The injection should be stopped if any changes are noted and completed only when the pulse returns to normal.

The objective of the procedure is to place a bubble of air in each ventricle, which can be manipulated to various portions of the system. Complete filling of the ventricular system is neither necessary nor desirable (Fig. 11–48).

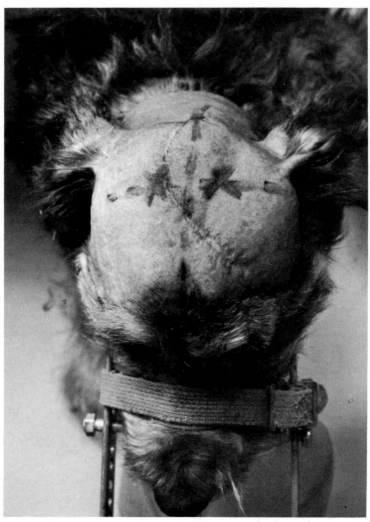

Figure 11–45. The injection site is approximately 1 cm off the midline, midway between the lateral canthus of the eyes and the external occipital protuberance.

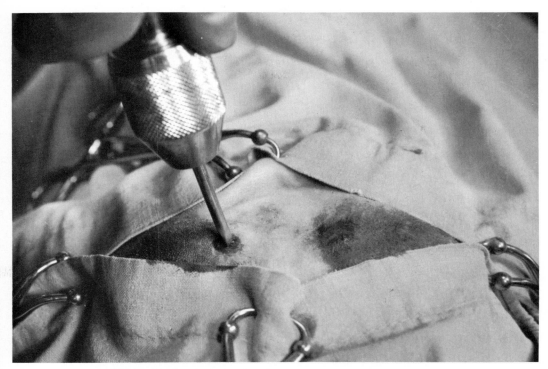

Figure 11–46. A pin in a hand chuck is used to penetrate the skull.

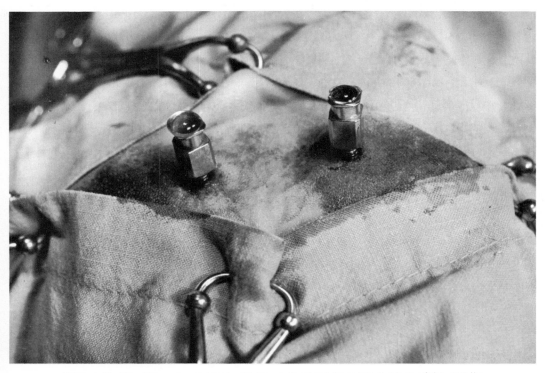

Figure 11–47. When the stylet is withdrawn, fluid will flow into the hub of the needle.

Interpretation

Enlarged ventricles may be the result of increased pressure, as in obstructive hydrocephalus, or of cerebral atrophy. The ventricles normally enlarge slightly with age, because of senile atrophy. Occlusion of the ventricular pathways (especially the mesencephalic aqueduct) is difficult to demonstrate using air, but may be seen when positive contrast media are used.

Displacement of the lateral ventricle away from cerebral mass lesions (tumor, subdural hematoma) can be seen best on the frontal view of the cranium. Masses may also encroach directly on the ventricular system (choroid plexus papilloma) and can be visualized by ventriculography.

Ventriculography is primarily beneficial in determining alterations in size of the ventricular system (hydrocephalus) and in locating mass lesions of the cerebral hemispheres which displace the lateral ventricles.

Precautions

Table 11–3 lists the major complications of ventriculography with recommended procedures to prevent their occurrence.

Morbidity is very low if this technique is performed properly. Animals with increased intracranial pressure may even improve following ventriculography because of the reduction in pressure.

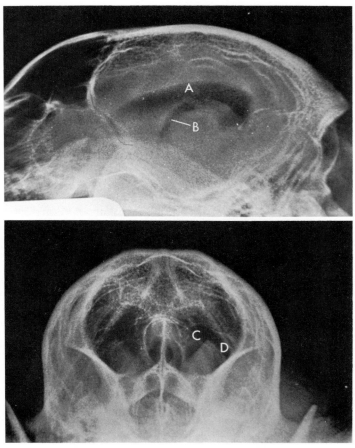

Figure 11–48. Pneumoventriculogram of normal dog.

Above, Lateral view	*Below,* Frontal view of the cranium
A. Lateral ventricle	C. Body of lateral ventricle
B. Third ventricle	D. Temporal horn of lateral ventricle.

TABLE 11-3

PREVENTION OF COMPLICATIONS OF VENTRICULOGRAPHY

Complications	Problem	Prevention
1. Laceration of vein or sinus	Improper injection site	Proper placement of needles (see text)
2. Cardiac or respiratory difficulty	Sudden changes in intracranial pressure	Monitor pulse constantly. Inject slowly, be sure both needles are patent
3. Collapse of ventricles, subdural hematoma	Removal of too much fluid, especially in hydrocephalic animal	Remove no more than 2 ml of fluid initially. Allow fluid to escape during injection of opposite ventricle. Use only 2 to 4 cc of air in each ventricle
4. Laceration of brain	Movement of needles during procedure	Penetrate inner table of skull with needle to insure stability. Keep needles absolutely still throughout procedure

REFERENCES

Albert, R. A.: Canine ventriculography and encephalography. Master of Science Thesis. Auburn, Alabama, Auburn University, 1967.

Fitzgerald, T. C.: Anatomy of the cerebral ventricles of domestic animals. Vet. Med., 56:38, 1961.

Hoerlein, B. F.: Canine Neurology. 2nd ed. Philadelphia, W. B. Saunders Co., 1971.

Jenkins, T. W.: Functional Mammalian Neuroanatomy. Philadelphia, Lea & Febiger, 1972.

Miller, M. E., Christensen, G. C., and Evans, H. E.: Anatomy of the Dog. Philadelphia, W. B. Saunders Co., 1964.

Oliver, J. E., Jr.: Principles of canine brain surgery. An. Hosp., 2:73, 1966.

Cerebral Arteriography

C. R. Conrad and J. E. Oliver, Jr.

Cerebral arteriography is the radiographic procedure in which a contrast medium is injected into the arterial system of the brain in order to visualize the course and distribution of the cerebral vessels. By appropriate timing of radiographs, the capillaries and veins may also be demonstrated following an arterial injection (Rosen, 1965).

Indications

The contents of the cranial vault (nervous tissue, cerebrospinal fluid, and vascular structures) all have the same radiographic density. Radiographs of the cranium demonstrate the bony structures of the skull, while its contents appear as a homogeneous mass. Most pathologic processes, such as tumors and hematomas, produce structures of the same density as the normal components of the skull. Therefore, special radiographic procedures are required to demonstrate most brain lesions.

Cerebral arteriography is the procedure of choice for demonstrating abnormalities involving the blood supply to the brain and for visualizing mass lesions of the brain stem. In some cases arteriography will localize mass lesions of the cerebral hemispheres more accurately than ventriculography.

Contraindications

Cerebral arteriography requires general anesthesia and catheterization of a major artery for placement of contrast material. There are no specific contraindications, but each animal must be evaluated in view of its physical condition and the information to be derived from the procedure. Toxic or ana-phylactic reactions to organic iodine base contrast media have not been reported in the dog. Cerebral anoxia and anesthesia-related deaths have been described (James and Hoerlein, 1960; Dorn, 1972) but have not been a problem in our experience.

Normal Anatomy

The arterial supply to the brain arises from four major sources: the left and right internal carotid arteries and the left and right vertebral arteries. These four arteries are interconnected by anastomotic branches, both internal and external to the cranial vault, that do not directly supply the brain (de la Torre et al., 1959). The common carotid artery terminates as two branches, the external and internal carotid arteries caudoventral to the angle of the mandibles. The internal carotid artery enters the cranial vault through the carotid canal.

The left vertebral artery is a branch of the left subclavian artery, arising at the level of the cranial margin of the first rib. The right vertebral artery is a branch of the brachiocephalic trunk and arises just caudal to the origin of the costocervical trunk. The paired vertebral arteries course dorsocraniad to the transverse foramen of the sixth cervical vertebra and then continue craniad in the transverse foramina of the remaining cervical vertebrae. As the arteries course craniad, they give rise to the segmental arteries of the cervical spinal cord. The vertebral arteries terminate after passing through the intervertebral foramen of the atlas and anastomosing to form the basilar artery. The basilar artery courses rostrad on the floor of the brain stem, giving rise to the caudal cerebellar arteries just cranial to the roots of the hypoglossal nerves. The paired acoustic arteries arise just caudal to the abducens nerve. Rostral to the abducens nerve are the pontine arteries, which supply the pons of the brain stem. The basilar artery terminates in the bifurcation which contributes to the arterial circle of the base of the brain.

The internal carotid artery, upon entering the cranial vault, runs dorsorostrad and inside the lumen of the cavernous sinus to the level of the optic chiasm. At this level, it perforates the dura to the subarachnoid space and terminates in three major branches: the rostral and middle cerebral arteries and the caudal communicating artery. The rostral and middle cerebral arteries supply the cerebral hemispheres (Miller et al., 1964). The caudal communicating arteries contribute to the arterial circle of the brain. The caudal intercarotid artery is a small branch of the internal carotid artery which leaves the internal carotid artery just before it perforates the inner layer of the dura. The paired caudal intercarotid arteries join just cranial to the hypophysis and they give off branches which supply the caudal lobe of the hypophysis.

The arterial circle of the brain is formed caudally and caudolaterally by the terminal bifurcation of the basilar artery, laterally by the caudal communicating artery, craniolaterally by the internal carotid artery, and cranially by the terminal communicating branches of the internal carotid arteries. The other major and constant branches of the arterial circle of the brain, beginning caudally, are paired rostral cerebellar arteries which arise just caudal to the oculomotor nerve and the paired caudal cerebral arteries which arise just rostral to the oculomotor nerve. The arterial circle may have other small and quite variable branches.

The major arterial supply to the meninges of the brain arises from the external carotid artery or its branches. It includes the rostral, middle and caudal meningeal arteries.

Procedure

Patient Preparation

The patient should be prepared for general anesthesia. Unless contraindicated, corticosteroids should be administered for 24 to 48 hours prior to the procedure to help prevent cerebral edema.

Anesthesia

The patient should be given atropine 15 to 30 minutes before induction of anesthesia. Inhalation anesthesia should be administered through an endotracheal tube fitted with an inflatable cuff. It is important that respiration and depth of anesthesia be monitored throughout the procedure. A surgical plane of anesthesia is required.

Materials

Cerebral arteriography requires specialized radiographic equipment. Fluoroscopy is necessary for catheter placement for vertebral artery cannulation. Rapid, sequential, short duration exposures are necessary for complete evaluation. This is accomplished with a rapid cassette changer. Injection must be made with a power syringe to insure adequate filling of the cerebral vessels. A No. 5 or No. 8 French catheter is needed for internal carotid arteriography. A long end-hole catheter is needed for vertebral arteriography.

Positioning

Internal Carotid Artery Injection. The animal should be restrained in dorsal recumbency for cannulation of the internal carotid artery.

Vertebral Artery Injection. The animal should be restrained in lateral recumbency with the uppermost hind limb flexed and retracted, exposing the medial surface of the other hind limb for cannulation of the femoral artery.

Positioning of the head for radiographs is the same for both procedures. A ventrodorsal (VD) view is obtained with the hard palate parallel to the table top. The central x-ray beam should be centered on the midline at the level of the temporomandibular articulation. A lateral view is taken with the sagittal plane of the head parallel to the table top. The x-ray beam should be centered on the temporomandibular articulation. The frontal view of the cranium may be useful in some cases; this is taken with the animal in dorsal recumbency. The hard palate is brought perpendicular to the table top and then the neck is flexed further, creating a 10 degree to 20 degree angle between the hard palate and the perpendicular axis. The central x-ray beam is then centered between the eyes on the midline, using a vertical beam.

Precise positioning is essential for adequate interpretation.

Contrast Media

Numerous contrast materials have been used for cerebral arteriography (Hoerlein, 1971). The present medium of choice of these authors is meglumine iothalamate (Conray, Mallinckrodt Chemical Works) in a 60 per cent solution, at a dosage rate of approximately 1 ml per 3 kg of body weight. Sodium salts of organic iodine often cause severe reactions at the time of injection, manifested as spastic muscular contractions.

They also produce vascular spasm, which alters the distribution of the contrast medium. These reactions are transient and have not caused post-procedural deterioration of the patient.

Technique

Internal Carotid Artery

The ventral cervical region is prepared for aseptic surgery. A ventral midline skin incision is made centered at the level of the atlas. The common carotid artery is isolated and traced rostrally to its division into the internal and external carotid arteries. The

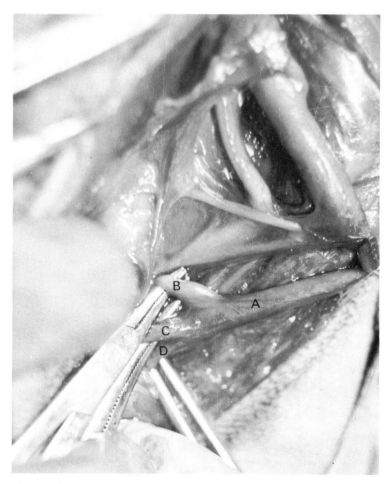

Figure 11–49. Termination of common carotid artery (*A*) into internal carotid (*B*) occipital (*C*) and external carotid arteries (*D*).

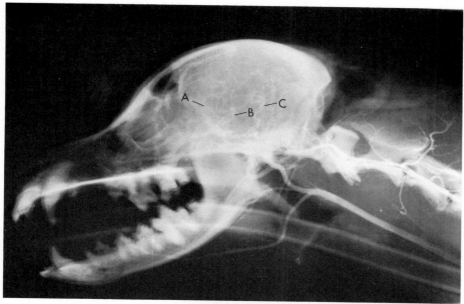

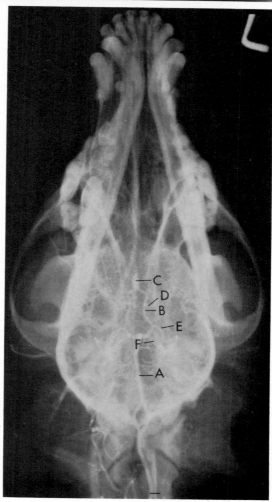

Figure 11–50. Arterial phase of vertebral arteriogram

Above, Lateral view
　　A. Rostral cerebral artery
　　B. Middle cerebral artery
　　C. Caudal cerebral artery
Below, Ventrodorsal view
　　A. Basilar artery
　　B. Arterial circle of brain
　　C. Rostral cerebral artery
　　D. Middle cerebral artery
　　E. Caudal cerebral artery
　　F. Rostral cerebellar artery

internal carotid artery may be distinguished from the occipital artery by the carotid bulb at its origin (Fig. 11–49). The external and common carotid arteries are ligated or occluded with bulldog clamps. A No. 5 or No. 8 French catheter is inserted into the common carotid artery and threaded up so that the lumen opening is adjacent to the origin of the internal carotid artery. The catheter is tied securely in place. The catheter is flushed frequently with heparinized saline while it is in place. The opening in the common carotid artery is sutured, or the artery is ligated when the procedure is completed.

Vertebral Artery

The medial aspect of the thigh is surgically prepared and the femoral artery is exposed as close to its origin as possible. The artery is cannulated using an end-hole catheter. The catheter is advanced proximally through the external iliac artery and into the aortic trunk. Using fluoroscopic examination, the catheter is advanced craniad to the arch of the aorta. As the arch of the aorta is approached, the curved end of the catheter is directed dorsad into the brachiocephalic trunk. Further advancement of the catheter places it in the vertebral artery. The tip of the catheter should be advanced as far as possible since it is desirable to have it at the level of the second cervical vertebra. During the placement of the catheter, it should be continuously flushed with heparinized saline by a slow drip. Upon completion of the procedure, the catheter is withdrawn, the femoral artery is sutured, and the skin incision is closed.

With the catheter in place and the patient properly positioned over a rapid cassette changer, injection is made using a power syringe. The pressure at the catheter tip should not exceed 750 psi. The catheter diameter should be such that injection of the required amount of contrast media can be completed in 2 seconds or less. Exposures following injection should be made at a minimum of two per second, but preferably four per second. The first exposure is made just prior to the beginning of the injection phase. Filming is continued at the pre-set rate for a minimum of 4 seconds to visualize the capillary phase and for 6 seconds to visualize the venous phase. If the film changer allows for a change in filming rate, there is no need to exceed two films per second after the capillary phase.

Once filming is complete and films are processed, they should be placed on multiple view boxes in the order in which they were exposed (Figs. 11–50 and 11–51). This permits the radiologist to visually and mentally reconstruct the flow pattern of the contrast media through the cerebral vasculature. To more easily visualize the vascular outline, "subtraction" can be used (Fig. 11–52). This procedure is discussed in Chapter 15. In order for this to be accomplished there can be no patient movement during the filming cycle. The enhancement of the vascular pattern by subtraction reveals more minute changes than those which can be evaluated on the original sequential radiographs.

Interpretation

Failure of vessels to fill must be interpreted very cautiously. Thrombi, emboli, or vascular spasm could prevent filling by contrast media (vascular spasm is minimized using non-sodium containing contrast media). However, the failure of opacification of all vessels is commonly encountered in normal dogs. The rostral cerebral artery is frequently not filled in vertebral arteriography, and the caudal cerebral and the cerebellar arteries are frequently not filled by carotid injections. Carotid injection may result in one side of the brain being more opacified than the other.

Alterations in vascular patterns may be the result of avascular structures displacing normal vessels (hematoma, abscess) or increased vascularity in an area (tumor).

Enlargement of the lateral ventricles will cause dorsal deviation of the rostral cerebral artery (callosal branch) (Fig. 11–51).

Arteriovenous fistulae or other vascular malformations can also be visualized by arteriography.

The carotid arteriogram is especially useful for visualizing structures in the supratentorial fossa, which are supplied by the rostral or middle cerebral arteries. The vertebral arteriogram is useful for visualization of the structures supplied by the caudal cerebral artery, and the branches of the basilar artery. The rostral and middle cerebral arteries will usually, but not always, be

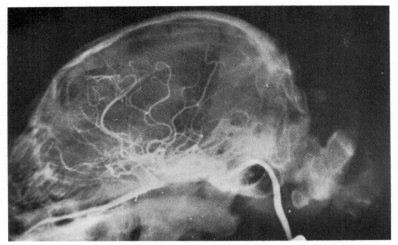

Figure 11–51. Arterial phase of carotid arteriogram, lateral view. Notice that rostral cerebral artery is slightly elevated as compared to Figure 11–50. This dog had slightly enlarged ventricles elevating this vessel which courses along the dorsal surface of the corpus callosum.

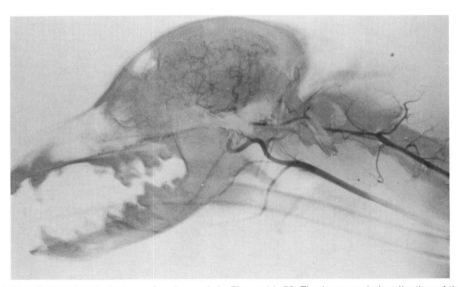

Figure 11–52. Subtraction technique of radiograph in Figure 11–50. The increased visualization of the vessels, especially the smaller branches, is of considerable benefit in interpretation of arteriograms.

filled by vertebral artery injection. The basilar artery and its branches may be filled by the carotid injection, but it is not as reliable as the vertebral injection. The course of the basilar artery may be tortuous.

Clinical diagnosis should be used as the guide for selection of the appropriate technique.

Precautions

Some contrast agents have caused muscle spasms during injection. These have created problems with regard to radiographic technique, but have not caused residual defects in the patients.

Any procedure requiring arterial catheterization is a potential hazard of arterial thrombi or emboli, or of sepsis. Meticulous attention to detail during the technique will prevent these complications. Catheteriza-

tion procedures and injection pressure must be monitored carefully to prevent rupture of an arterial wall.

REFERENCES

de la Torre, E., Netsky, M. G., and Meschan, I.: Intracranial and extracranial circulations in the dog: Anatomic and angiographic studies. Am. J. Anat., *105*:3, 1959.

Dorn, A. S.: A standard technique for canine cerebral angiography. J.A.V.M.A., *161*:12, 1972.

Hoerlein, B. F.: *Canine Neurology,* 2nd ed. Philadelphia, W. B. Saunders Co., 1971.

James, C. W., and Hoerlein, B. F.: Cerebral angiography in the dog. Vet. Med., *55*:12, 1960.

Miller, M. E., Christensen, G. C., and Evans, H. E.: *Anatomy of the Dog.* Philadelphia, W. B. Saunders Co., 1964.

Rising, J. L., and Lewis, R. E.: Femoro-vertebral cerebral angiography in the dog. Am. J. Vet. Res., *33*:665, 1970.

Rosen, L., Weidner, W., and Hanafee, W.: Angiographic visualization of the subarachnoid cisterns. Radiology, *85*:1, 1965.

Thoracic radiography provides an opportunity to examine a body cavity that is relatively inaccessible by other methods. When properly produced, thoracic radiographs can provide valuable diagnostic information, but when inadequately produced, they may be misleading. Exact positioning and exposure factors must be observed to prevent the introduction of multiple misleading artifacts.

Generally, exposure times must be less than 1/20 second to ensure that imperceptible respiratory movements do not result in a loss of radiographic detail. This requires x-ray equipment with milliamperage capabilities of 100 or more for most canine patients (see Chap. 4).

A grid should be used to reduce fog-producing scatter radiation in normal patients with thoracic thicknesses of 15 cm or greater. Patients with thoracic contents that have densities similar to the abdomen (patients with extensive pleural or pulmonary parenchymal fluid) require the use of a grid when the thoracic measurement exceeds 9 cm.

Thoracic radiographs are usually produced during maximum inhalation to enhance the contrast between radiolucent and radiodense structures. An exception to this procedure is made when patients are examined for signs of minimal or moderate pneumothorax, in which case increased density of the visceral pleural surface may be accomplished by producing the radiograph at maximum expiration (Fraser and Paré, 1970). This results in a relative collapse of the pulmonary parenchyma and pleura without changing the pleural air density, thereby increasing the contrast between these regions and aiding the diagnostic quality of the radiographs.

The thorax is examined with a minimum of two views. Survey radiographs should include the right lateral and DV views. Standing lateral and erect views using a horizontal x-ray beam and the VD view may be useful in demonstrating pleural fluid in some patients.

The x-ray beam should be collimated to include the entire thorax from 2 cm cranial to the first rib to a point just caudal to the first lumbar vertebra (Ettinger and Suter, 1970). In patients with serious cough, the the caudal cervical trachea should be included on the lateral view. A separate lateral view of the cervical trachea should be produced if clinical signs suggest tracheal disorders (Ettinger and Ticer [in press]).

PROCEDURE

Right Lateral View. The patient is positioned in right lateral recumbency and the forelegs are pulled cranially so that most of the triceps musculature is displaced from the cranial aspect of the thorax (Fig. 12–1). The sternum is elevated to a level above the x-ray table equal to that of the thoracic vertebrae to prevent rotation. The neck is extended and the occipital-atlantal joint is allowed to flex approximately 45 degrees to avoid displacement of the trachea. The x-ray beam is centered at the fifth intercostal space. The radiograph is produced at maximum inspiration.

Figure 12–2 illustrates the normal radiographic anatomy of the canine thorax in right lateral view.

Left Lateral View. The patient is positioned in left lateral recumbency and the forelegs are pulled cranially so that most of the triceps musculature is displaced from

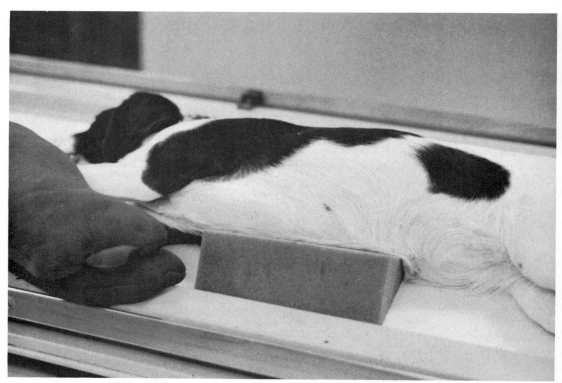

Figure 12–1. Position for right lateral view of the thorax.

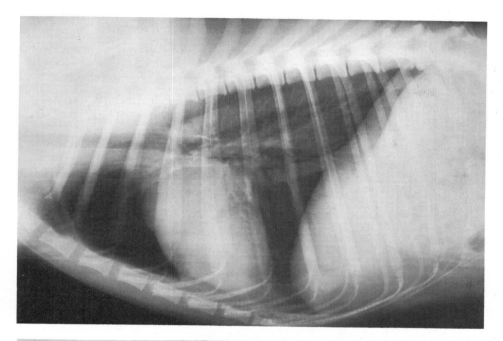

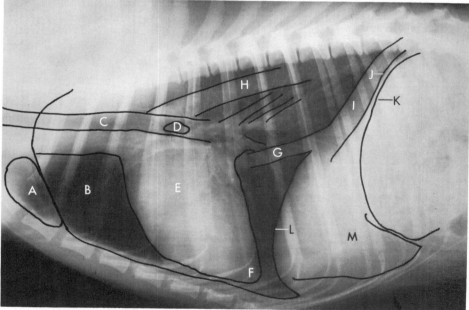

Figure 12–2. Right lateral view of the canine thorax. Note that the apex of the heart (*F*) is more conically shaped than in the left lateral view (Fig. 12–4) because the cardiophrenic ligament prevents it from moving to the dependent portion of the pleural cavity. The dependent (right) crus is cranially displaced (*I*).

A. Cranial aspect of the left cranial lung lobe viewed end on
B. Cranial lung lobes superimposed
C. Trachea
D. Common origin of the left cranial and middle lobar bronchi viewed end on
E. Cardiac silhouette
F. Cardiac apex

G. Caudal vena cava
H. Descending aorta
I. Right diaphragmatic crus
J. Left diaphragmatic crus
K. Stomach wall
L. Diaphragmatic cupula
M. Liver

the cranial aspect of the thorax (Fig. 12–3). The sternum is elevated to a level above the x-ray table equal to that of the thoracic vertebrae to prevent rotation. The neck is extended and the occipital-atlantal joint is allowed to flex approximately 45 degrees to avoid displacement of the trachea. The x-ray beam is centered at the fifth intercostal space. The radiograph is produced at maximum inspiration.

Figure 12–4 illustrates the normal radiographic anatomy of the canine thorax in left lateral view.

Dorsoventral View. The patient is placed in ventral recumbency with the thoracic vertebrae superimposed over the sternum. The forelegs are pulled slightly forward and the elbows are rotated outward (abducted), so that the shoulders are displaced craniomedially and the scapulae are shifted laterally away from the cranial lung field (Fig. 12–5). The rear limbs are allowed to flex in a crouching position, and the head is lowered between the forelimbs to decrease the thickness of the caudal cervical musculature over the cranial lung fields.

The x-ray beam is centered over the fifth intercostal space, which is usually located at the level of the caudal aspect of the scapulae. The radiograph is produced at maximum inspiration.

Figure 12–6 illustrates the normal radiographic anatomy of the canine thorax in DV view.

Ventrodorsal View. The patient is placed in dorsal recumbency and the forelimbs are pulled forward (Fig. 12–7). The sternum should be superimposed over the thoracic vertebrae to avoid rotation in the sagittal plane.

The x-ray beam is centered over the fifth intercostal space, which is usually located at the junction of the cranial two thirds to the caudal one third of the sternum. The radiograph is produced at maximum inspiration.

Figure 12–8 illustrates the normal radiographic anatomy of the canine thorax in VD view.

Horizontal X-ray Beam Radiographs. Radiographs using a horizontal x-ray beam may be indicated when the diagnosis of pleural fluid is equivocal on survey radio-

(*Text continued on page 294.*)

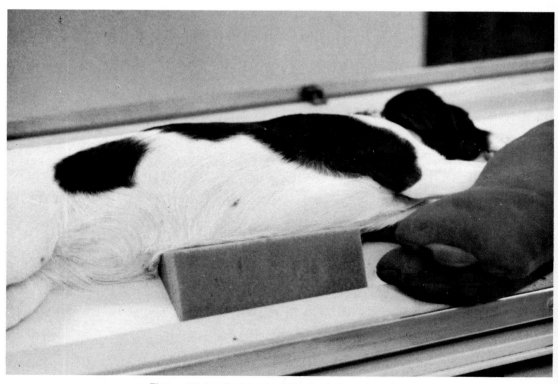

Figure 12–3. Position for left lateral view of the thorax.

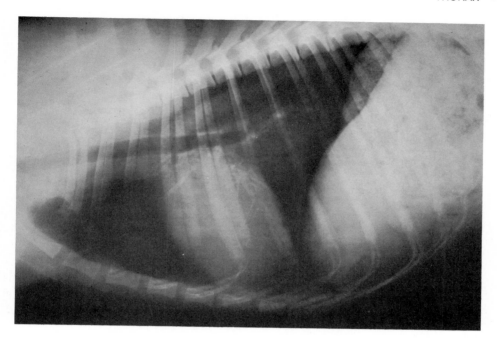

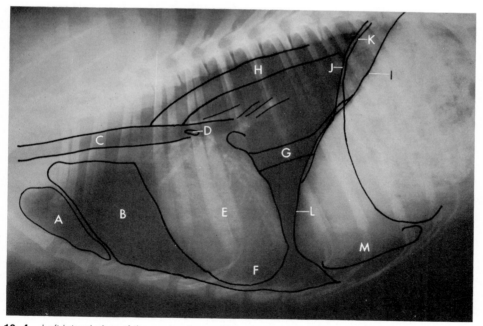

Figure 12–4. Left lateral view of the canine thorax. Note that the apex of the heart (F) is allowed to change position when compared to the right lateral view (Fig. 12–2), giving a rounded appearance. The left diaphragmatic crus, which is in direct contact with the fundus of the stomach, is displaced cranially (J).

A. Cranial aspect of the left cranial lung lobe viewed end on
B. Cranial lung lobes superimposed
C. Trachea
D. Common origin of the left cranial and middle lobar bronchi viewed end on
E. Cardiac silhouette
F. Cardiac apex

G. Caudal vena cava
H. Descending aorta
I. Right diaphragmatic crus
J. Left diaphragmatic crus
K. Stomach wall
L. Diaphragmatic cupula
M. Liver

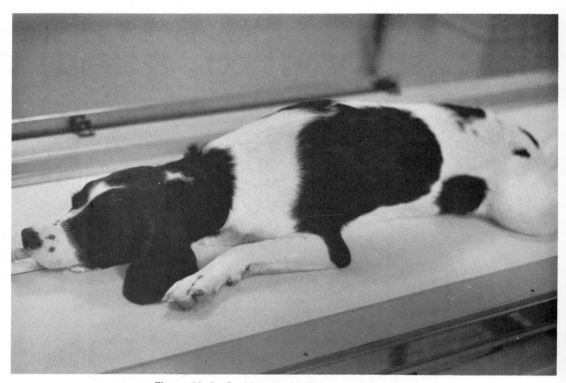

Figure 12–5   Position for the DV view of the thorax.

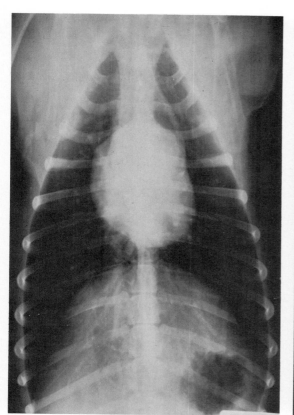 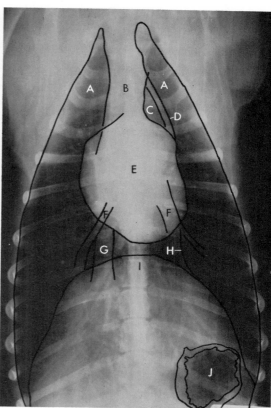

Figure 12–6 DV view of the canine thorax.

A. Cranial lung lobes
B. Cranial mediastinum
C. Ventral aspect of the right cranial
   lung lobe
D. Ventral mediastinum displaced to
   the left
E. Cardiac silhouette
F. Caudal lobar pulmonary arteries
G. Caudal vena cava
H. Cardiophrenic ligament
 I. Diaphragmatic cupula
J. Air-filled fundus of the stomach

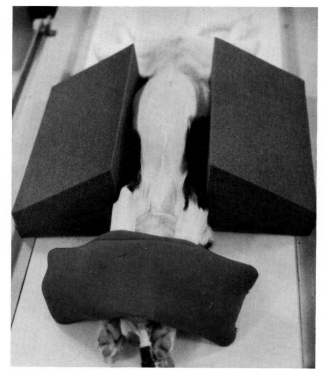

Figure 12–7 Position for VD view of the thorax.

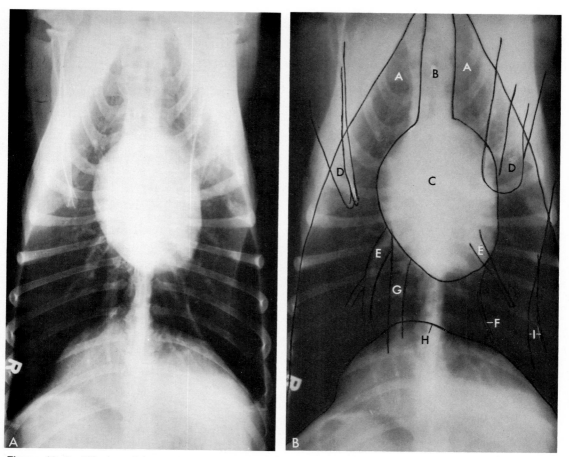

Figure 12–8. VD view of the canine thorax. Note the scapular overlay of the cranial thorax and the increased prominence of the axillary skin folds (I) compared to the DV view (Fig. 12–6).

A. Cranial lung lobes
B. Cranial mediastinum
C. Cardiac silhouette
D. Scapulae
E. Caudal lobar pulmonary arteries
F. Cardiophrenic ligament
G. Caudal vena cava
H. Diaphragmatic cupula
I. Axillary skin folds

graphs. The standing lateral or erect (patient suspended by forelimbs) positions may cause gravitation of fluid to the dependent portions of the pleural space and enhance visualization. Usually, however, clinically significant quantities of pleural fluid may be detected on radiographs produced in the VD view using a routine vertical x-ray beam. The VD view is also useful in allowing the postural drainage of pleural fluid to the dorsolateral aspects of the pleural space, thus allowing better visualization of the mediastinal structure, cardiac silhouette, lung margins and pulmonary parenchyma than with the DV view in patients with moderate to large amounts of pleural fluid (Fig. 12–9).

INTERPRETATION

The position and appearance of the normal thoracic viscera vary, depending on postural relationships, phases of the respiratory cycle, physiologic states, body types and x-ray beam geometry. Generally the most variable appearance is observed in the shape of the cardiac silhouette and diaphragm and in the appearance of the pulmonary parenchyma.

Heart

Postural changes in the thorax result in changes in the cardiac silhouette. Since the apex of the heart is not attached to the sternum, changes in posture result in apical displacement. In the VD view, the cardiac apex may shift to the left laterally and dorsally in spite of absolute sagittal plane alignment. This displacement will result in increased cardiac elongation with a moderate left lateral shift in most dogs and cats, compared to the DV view. The DV view, therefore, becomes the position of choice when radiographing the thorax in this plane (Ettinger and Suter, 1970).

The cardiophrenic ligament tends to prevent the cardiac apex from shifting in the dependent direction in right lateral recum-

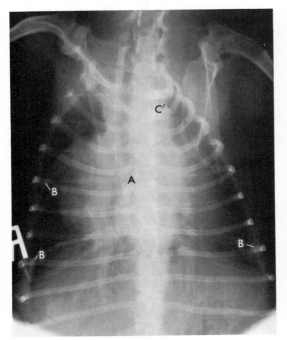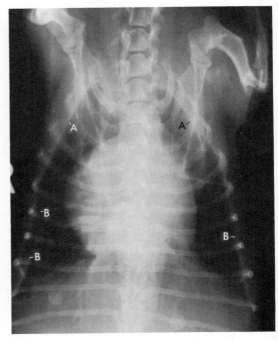

Figure 12–9. *Left,* DV view of a canine thorax with pleural effusion, showing collection of the fluid ventrally around the cardiac silhouette (*A*). Fluid may also be seen in the interlobar fissures (*B*) and around the cranial mediastinum (*C*), causing an artifactual widening. *Right,* VD view of a canine thorax with pleural effusion (same patient as on the right), showing redistribution of fluid away from the heart and cranial mediastinum. Moderate cranial lobe atelectasis with fluid between the visceral and parietal pleural (*A*) and interlobar fissure fluid (*B*) may be seen as evidence of the pleural fluid.

bency, thus producing an apical silhouette that is more conical in shape (Fig. 12–2) when compared to the cardiac apex on the left lateral view (Fig. 12–4). It is therefore preferable to radiograph the lateral view of the thorax in right recumbency for routine survey examination of the thorax.

There is considerable variation in the cardiac silhouette among the different breeds of dogs. Dogs with a deep thorax, such as setters, sight hounds and collies, have a cardiac silhouette that is more upright than that of dogs with a wide, shallow thorax, such as beagles and Boston terriers (Ettinger and Suter, 1970). In dogs with a deep thorax, the heart occupies a relatively smaller proportion of the thoracic cavity compared to the relatively greater volume and wider appearance of the heart in dogs with a wide, shallow thorax. Animals approximately three months of age or younger have a relatively rounder heart than adult animals (Ettinger and Suter, 1970). In some breeds of dogs, such as the borzoi, Irish wolfhound and Irish setter, the cardiac apex may not reach the sternum in the lateral view, and this sign should not be mistaken for pneumothorax.

DV radiographs produced during deep inspiration show the apex of the heart nearer the midline than when radiographs are produced during expiration. Exposures of 1/20 sec or less may demonstrate differences between systole and diastole on the shape and position of the heart (Ettinger and Suter, 1970). The left border may look straighter and the pulmonary artery larger, and the heart may appear slightly smaller and more sharply delineated at the end of systole than during diastole. Exposures of 1/10 sec or longer usually show the heart in diastole because the slightly enlarged diastolic heart effectively absorbs the x-ray beam, preventing visualization of the smaller cardiac silhouette of systole. The change in cardiac size during exposure accounts for the relative loss of radiographic detail on radiographs produced with long exposures.

A cranial displacement of the central x-ray beam will result in a shortening of the cardiac silhouette in the DV view.

Lateral View. In the lateral thoracic view, most normal dogs have a cranial cardiac border that is located near the third rib, and the caudal border extends to about the eighth rib. The cranial border consists of the right ventricular wall and right auricle. The dorsal portion of the cranial border joins the ventral outline of the cranial vena cava. In some patients, the dorsal aspect of the cranial border is composed of the aortic arch and the conus arteriosus of the main pulmonary artery. Where the cranial vena cava joins the atrium, there may be a slight indentation, which is called the cranial waist. The angle of the cranial waist varies with the inclination of the heart. This angle is more acute in dogs with upright hearts and more obtuse in dogs with greater inclination of the heart.

The curve of the cranial border usually runs parallel to the sternum for various distances, depending upon the cardiac axis inclination. Increased sternal contact is normal in dogs with a wide thorax. Retrosternal fat accumulates around the cardiac apex and may obscure the junction of the cranial border and apex, especially in left lateral recumbency, during which the apex shifts in the dependent direction.

The caudal cardiac border is formed by the left ventricle and atrium. The caudal border may merge with or overlie the diaphragmatic cupula, especially in dogs with a wide and short thorax. The distance between the cardiac apex and the diaphragmatic cupula varies with the respiratory cycle. The left ventricular border usually curves inward at the base of the heart to form the caudal waist as it meets the left atrium. The caudal waist corresponds to the atrioventricular groove. The angle of the caudal waist is most acute in hearts with increased inclination. The left atrial border extends caudodorsally to join the pulmonary veins. The caudal vena cava joins the cardiac silhouette just ventral to the atrioventricular groove.

In the lateral view, the dorsal aspect of the cardiac silhouette is composed of the densities of the right and left atria and the main pulmonary arteries and veins.

The main pulmonary artery contributes to the cranial border of the heart only rarely (Ettinger and Suter, 1970) and usually becomes visible only after it bifurcates into the right and left branches immediately cranial to the carina. The left caudal lobar artery passes over the radiographically lucent oval structure of the common origin of the left cranial and middle lobar bronchi and may be seen for a variable distance into the pulmonary parenchyma. The right pulmonary artery crosses from left to right under the carina and may be seen end on as a dense, round structure at the cardiac base. This normal structure is sometimes mistaken for an enlarged hilar lymph node. The right caudal lobar artery is superimposed on the left atrium toward the periphery, making it difficult to distinguish this artery from the pulmonary veins. The pulmonary veins are normally less dense than the arteries, as they converge before joining the left atrium.

The aorta may be seen leaving the cardiac silhouette in a variety of positions, depending on the thoracic conformation. In dogs with a deep thorax, the aortic arch extends farther cranially and emerges more ventrally from the area of the right auricle. The aorta is well delineated only after it crosses the trachea and courses dorsocaudally between the trachea and the thoracic vertebrae.

Dorsoventral View. Moderate rotation of the thorax about the sagittal plane can cause marked change in the shape and size of the lateral borders of the cardiac silhouette (Ettinger and Suter, 1970). If the thorax is rotated clockwise, the diaphragmatic cupula and the left cardiac border and apex appear closer to the left thoracic wall than normal. The pulmonary artery is moved in the direction of the apex, and the left side of the heart appears rounder. This should not be mistaken for left ventricular enlargement. If the thorax is rotated counterclockwise, the diaphragmatic cupula appears closer to the right thoracic wall. The right cardiac border appears rounder and closer to the right thoracic wall than normal and should not be mistaken for right ventricular enlargement. The left auricle appears enlarged and the left ventricular border appears straighter than normal. The pulmonary artery becomes superimposed under the vertebral column.

In the true DV view, the cardiac silhouette has been described as a "lopsided egg" (Wyburn and Lawson, 1967). The cranial and right borders are rounded and the left border almost straight, which makes its appearance lopsided.

The cardiac silhouette usually extends from the third to about the eighth rib in the DV view but may vary greatly, depending upon the thoracic conformation. In dogs with a deep thorax, the distance is decreased because of the more nearly upright position of the heart as it is suspended in the thoracic cavity. The base of the heart lies on the midline, and the apex is directed toward the left side. In breeds with a wide thorax, the apex is directed more toward the left side than in breeds with a narrow thorax, in which the longitudinal axis of the heart almost parallels the midsagittal plane of the thorax. In some brachycephalic breeds, the cardiac apex may lie on the right side.

The DV view is characterized by superimposition of the cardiac silhouette, great vessels, trachea and esophagus.

The right cranial quadrant of the cardiac silhouette is formed by the right atrium. Caudally, the atrial border merges with the right ventricle and right pulmonary artery. The vena cava interrupts the right ventricular border as it courses caudomedially. The right ventricle usually ends immediately to the right of the cardiac apex and may be demarcated by a notch at the interventricular septum.

The cardiophrenic ligament extends as a thin band of tissue from the cardiac apex to the diaphragm. The entire apex and most of the left cardiac border are formed by the left ventricle. Cranial to the fourth intercostal space, the left cardiac border is created by the pulmonary artery and the right ventricular outflow tract. The left auricle, which lies between the pulmonary artery and the left ventricle, seldom extends beyond the left cranial cardiac border in normal dogs. The medial portion of the pulmonary artery merges medially with the aortic arch.

Mediastinum

In lateral views, the cranial mediastinal structures are demarcated ventrally by the ventral border of the cranial vena cava. The tracheal lumen is usually the only structure visualized within the cranial mediastinum except when air or ingesta are present in the esophageal lumen. Usually the esophageal lumen is air-filled only during anesthesia or during severely depressing disease states.

In the DV view, the right mediastinal border is formed by the cranial vena cava. The left subclavian artery forms the left mediastinal border.

The trachea enters the thoracic cavity at the midline or slightly to the right and courses caudally with a slight right lateral curve. The trachea ends by bifurcating to form the main bronchi, which is referred to as the carina.

The width of the mediastinum varies greatly and tends to be increased in brachycephalic breeds.

Lungs

The vascular markings are the most prominent structures of the lungs. The air-filled alveoli provide an excellent contrast medium against the dense pulmonary vasculature. The degree of contrast between these structures varies greatly with the respiratory cycle, position, age of the patient and radiographic technique (Ettinger and Suter, 1970). Older patients usually have denser pulmonary structures caused by nodular or linear markings of interstitial origin (Reif and Rhodes, 1966). Overexposure of lung fields tends to simulate decreased density compared to radiographs of properly exposed lungs produced during the same phase of the respiratory cycle (Fig. 12–10).

The intrapulmonary vasculature may be divided into three zones for purposes of description (Ettinger and Suter, 1970): (1) the central or hilar zone; (2) the middle zone, which contains the large bronchial and vascular branches; and (3) the peripheral zone, which is composed of pulmonary parenchyma. The pulmonary vasculature is best evaluated in the middle zone. The peripheral zone usually contains relatively few visible vascular or bronchial markings.

On the lateral view, the pulmonary vasculature is best evaluated in the cranial lobar vessels. The dorsal pair of vessels are the left cranial lobar artery and veins, from dorsal to ventral, respectively; and the ventral pair of vessels are the right cranial lobar artery and vein.

In the DV projection, the caudal lobar pulmonary arteries are usually visible lateral to the caudal lobar bronchus, and the vein is located medially.

The lateral view may show the cranial aspect of the left cranial lobe end on as it courses medially in front of the right cranial lobe.

The retrosternal fat pad may appear as a moderately dense structure that may elevate the lung lobes and cardiac silhouette dorsally from the sternum in obese patients. The magnitude of this elevation decreases on inhalation and increases on expiration (Fig. 12–11). The normal retrosternal fat pad should not be mistaken for pleural fluid.

Most survey radiographs of the thorax should be produced in the DV view, but when pleural fluid is suggested on clinical examination or on survey radiographs, the VD view is useful in defining the presence and distribution of the fluids. Figure 12–9 illustrates the effect of this positional variation on the radiographic appearance of a moderate amount of pleural fluid. The DV view shows that the ventral collection of fluid obscures the normal lucency of the lung fields and the delineation of the cardiac borders. By placing the patient in dorsal recumbency, the fluid distribution is changed, allowing improved visualization of these structures and confirmation of the presence of pleural fluid in the interlobar fissures.

Some patients, especially dogs with a deep thorax, show extensive visualization of the axillary skin folds in the DV and VD positions (Fig. 12–12). These shadows should not be considered pathologic.

Diaphragm

The radiographic appearance of the diaphragm varies markedly with body conformation and phase of the respiratory cycle. In patients with a deep thorax, the DV view shows the distinct outline of the left and right crus and the medially located cupula. This is particularly evident on the VD view of the thorax (Grandage, 1974).

Patients with a wide, shallow thorax have a single-lobed diaphragmatic outline with a slightly right lateral cranial location. The cupula may have contact with the cardiac apex and show a slight depression at the point of contact.

In the lateral view, the dependent crus is located cranial to the contralateral crus (Grandage, 1974).

The crus normally intersects the ventral border of the vertebral column between T_{11} and T_{13}, although it may attach as far forward as T_9 and as far back as L_1 in normal dogs. The position of the diaphragm may vary as much as two vertebral body lengths. Quietly breathing dogs may show a

(*Text continued on page 301.*)

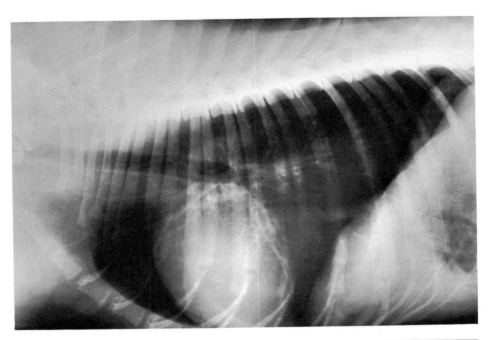

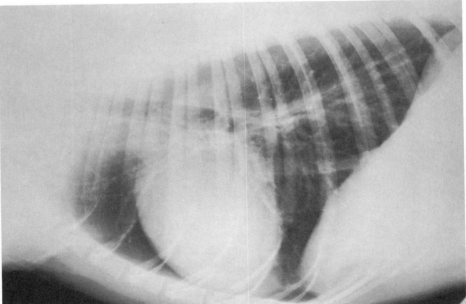

Figure 12–10. *Top,* Lateral view of a canine thorax produced with moderate overexposure, resulting in a relatively decreased density of the lung fields. *Bottom,* Lateral view of a canine thorax (same patient as in top) produced with proper exposure. Notice the visualization of the bronchovascular markings throughout the entire lung field.

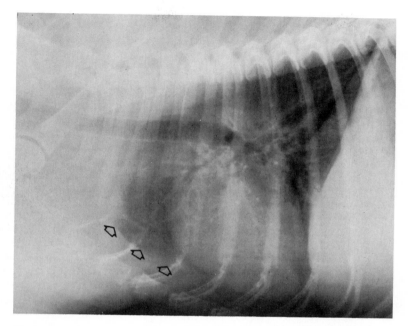

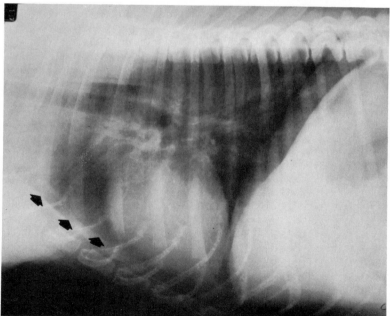

Figure 12–11. *Top*, Lateral view of a canine thorax produced during expiration (note the position of the diaphragm), illustrating the relative increased thickness of the retrosternal fat pad (arrows) when compared to an inhalation radiograph of the same patient (*bottom*). *Bottom*, Lateral view of a canine thorax produced during inspiration (note the position of the diaphragm), illustrating the relative decreased thickness of the retrosternal fat pad when compared to an exhalation radiograph of the same patient (*top*).

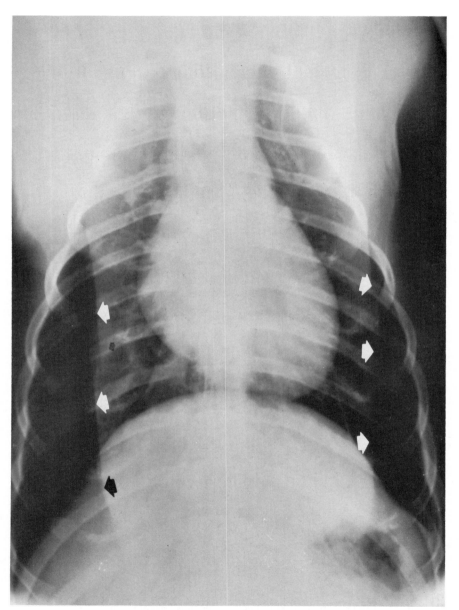

Figure 12–12. DV view of a two year old female boxer, showing the appearance of the axillary skin folds (arrows) that are seen in some dogs with a deep thorax.

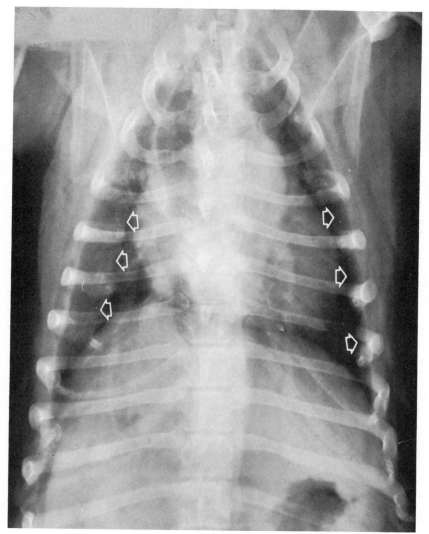

Figure 12–13. DV view of a 15 year old male dachshund, showing the appearance of undulating longitudinal density produced by an invagination of the ribs and pleura at the costochondral junctions (arrows). This structure should not be mistaken for pleural fluid or thickened pleural margins.

diaphragmatic excursion of less than one vertebral length.

Ribs and Sternum

The ribs usually arch laterally from the vertebral column, then course medially to the costochondral junction. In some breeds of dogs, such as the basset hound and some dachshunds, the ribs may invaginate at the costochondral junction, producing a longitudinal indentation on the sides of the thorax in apparently normal animals. The DV or VD view shows this invagination as an undulating longitudinal density on the lateral aspect of the thoracic cavity (Fig. 12–13). This structure should not be mistaken for pleural fluid or thickened pleural margins.

The costal cartilages may become mineralized at a relatively young age in some apparently normal dogs. Early in the stages of mineralization, the densities may appear mottled.

The caudal aspect of the sternum may show rather a bizarre structure in the lateral view in apparently normal animals. These deformities should not be mistaken for pathologic processes.

Pneumopericardiography

J. W. TICER AND S. J. ETTINGER

Pneumopericardiography is a negative contrast radiographic examination of the pericardial sac.

INDICATIONS

Pneumopericardiography is indicated when a complete evaluation of the etiology of pericardial fluid cannot be determined from conventional methods of examination.

CONTRAINDICATIONS

When a diagnosis of pericardial fluid has been positively established on the basis of available clinical data, the only contraindication for pneumopericardiography is congestive heart failure (Ettinger, 1974). In patients with congestive heart failure, the stress of lateral recumbent posture may be an indication to modify the procedure to allow a ventral recumbent posture. Patients with pericardial effusion secondary to congestive heart failure usually respond well to digitalization and diuretic therapy. These animals should generally not be subjected to the procedure unless the usual therapeutic agents fail to resolve the problem. In the latter case, pericardiocentesis is in order and pneumopericardiography may then be performed.

TECHNIQUE

Patient Preparation

Prior to performing pericardiocentesis, a clinical diagnosis of pericardial fluid must be made. Clinical, radiographic, electrocardiographic and clinical pathologic evidence must strongly indicate a diagnosis of pericardial fluid accumulation (Ettinger and Suter, 1970; Ettinger, 1974). Patients with severe congestive heart failure, signs of pulmonary edema, cyanosis and respiratory distress are poor candidates for pneumopericardiography. Rapid digitalization and administration of diuretic and narcotic sedatives may be indicated prior to performing the procedure. In apprehensive patients, tranquilizers aid in restraint during the relatively long procedure of fluid drainage.

The left ventral thorax is clipped and scrubbed.

Materials

A large syringe, 16-gauge Venocath set (Venocath, Abbott Laboratories), three-way stopcock and lidocaine for local anesthesia are needed to perform the pericardiocentesis, fluid drainage and air injection. Fluid collection and sterile culture tubes are required for pericardial fluid analysis.

Procedure

The site for pericardiocentesis is determined from the survey radiographs. Usually the left fourth to sixth intercostal spaces near the junction of the lower and middle thirds of the thorax provide the most convenient site. The patient is placed in right lateral recumbency and electrocardiographic leads are attached in a normal manner. Lidocaine is used to infiltrate the skin and intercostal musculature at the site of the needle entry.

A sample of venous blood should be withdrawn to compare with the pericardial fluid. Its color and clotting time are noted prior to the procedure. The needle from the Venocath unit is attached to a large syringe. The needle and syringe are held at an angle of approximately 45 degrees to the intercostal space, and the needle is inserted through the thoracic wall in a mediodorsal direction. As the needle touches the pericardium, it is thrust into the pericardial sac.

Electrocardiographic monitoring will show no disturbance in cardiac rhythm if the needle is scratching the pericardial sac or has passed through it. If the needle touches the epicardium or enters the myocardium, one or more premature contractions will be noted (Ettinger, 1974). This suggests that pericardial fluid is not present or that the needle is within the sac and is touching and irritating the epicardial surface. Epicardial contact through the needle and syringe has a scratching-like sensation, Since coronary vessels could be lacerated, the needle should immediately be pulled back.

Twenty-five to 30 ml of fluid are then withdrawn for comparison with the previously drawn peripheral venous blood and for laboratory samples. No additional fluid is withdrawn until a comparison with clotting time has been made. If clotting occurs readily, it is assumed that the sample is whole blood, which indicates that the procedure should be stopped. This usually requires a waiting period of from 5 to 10 minutes. The Venocath catheter and wire guide are inserted into the pericardial sac through the needle. The catheter is advanced, while the wire guide is held in place just within the pericardial sac. The needle is then retracted from the thorax and the plastic guards around it are folded into place. A three-way stopcock and syringe are then attached to the catheter. If the sample is not whole blood, the withdrawal of fluid is then started. Since the catheter lumen is small, the entire procedure may require 30 to 60 minutes or more. The patient is rotated about the sagittal plane of the thorax to assist in complete drainage. After fluid collec-

tion is completed, the total volume of fluid is noted and a like amount of air is injected into the pericardial sac.

Dorsoventral and lateral radiographs are then produced. At times, a standing lateral view using a horizontal x-ray beam is produced to visualize the dorsal aspect of the pericardial sac when a residual amount of fluid makes delineation of these structures difficult.

Upon completion of fluid removal and special radiographic procedures, the catheter is withdrawn. The patient may require antibiotic therapy for several days. Digitalis and diuretics may also be necessary to assist in mobilization of other body fluids and to improve cardiac function if failure has been evident (Ettinger, 1974).

The air in the pericardium will be resorbed in a period of 24 to 96 hours. The patient should be reradiographed 48 hours following the procedure to determine the degree of recurrence of pericardial fluid.

Figure 12–14 is a thoracic radiograph of a seven year old male German shorthaired pointer with benign pericardial effusion. Figure 12–15 shows this same patient after pericardial drainage and the production of a pneumopericardiogram. This pneumopericardiogram shows normal cardiac conformation. The cranioventral aspect of the cardiac silhouette is composed of a smoothly marginated right auricular appendage, which is not visualized to this degree in a normal heart that is covered by pericardium. Figure 12–16 shows a nine year old female springer spaniel with a heart-base tumor that is visualized with a pneumopericardiogram. The right auricular appendage is displaced caudoventrally by the mass, which shows a roughened marginal outline.

COMPLICATIONS

Rupture of a coronary vessel may lead to fatal hemorrhage. Excessive irritation of the epicardium may result in ventricular premature contractions which may develop into life-threatening arrhythmia. Neither of these complications is common and therefore should not present a contraindication for the procedure if it is performed correctly.

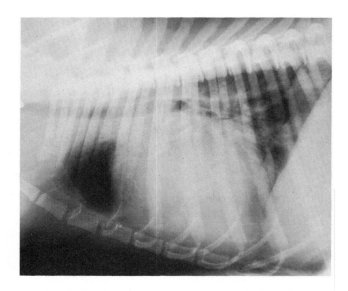

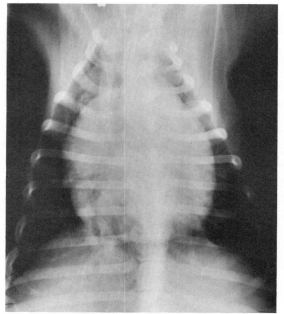

Figure 12–14.   *Top*, Lateral view of a seven year old male German shorthaired pointer with a markedly enlarged cardiac silhouette due to pericardial fluid that was secondary to benign pericardial effusion. *Bottom*, DV view of the same patient.

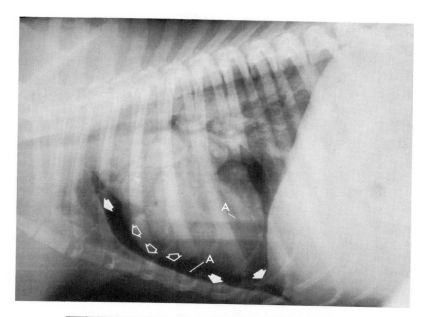

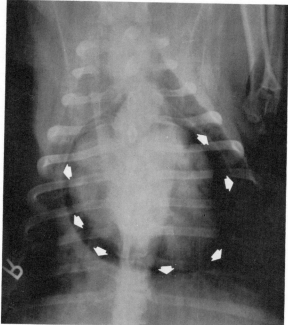

Figure 12–15. Lateral and DV views of a pneumopericardiogram of a seven year old male German shorthaired pointer with a markedly enlarged pericardium due to pericardial fluid that was secondary to benign pericardial effusion (same patient as in Fig. 12–14). Note the outline of the parietal pericardium as it is contrasted with the pericardial air (arrows). The radiopaque catheter may be seen within the pericardial sac (*A*). The normal right auricular appendage is seen on the cranioventral aspect of the cardiac silhouette (open arrows).

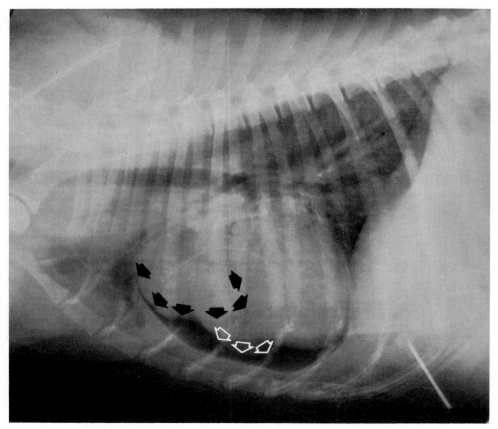

Figure 12–16. Lateral view of a pneumopericardiogram of a nine year old female springer spaniel showing the outline of heart-based tumor (arrows). The right auricular appendage (open arrows) is partially hidden by the tumor mass. Note the lack of smooth margination shown by the tumor silhouette.

REFERENCES

Carlson, W. D.: Veterinary Radiology. 2nd ed. Philadelphia, Lea & Febiger, 1967.

Douglas, S. W., and Williamson, H. D.: Principles of Veterinary Radiography. 2nd ed. Baltimore, Williams & Wilkins Co., 1972.

Ettinger, S. J., and Suter, P. F.: Canine Cardiology. Philadelphia, W. B. Saunders Co., 1970.

Ettinger, S. J.: Pericardiocentesis. Vet. Clin. N. Amer., 4:403, 1974.

Ettinger, S. J., and Ticer, J. W.: Tracheal Diseases. In Ettinger, S. J. (Ed.): A Textbook of Veterinary Internal Medicine: Diseases of Dog and Cat. Philadelphia, W. B. Saunders Co., (in press).

Fraser, R. G., and Paré, J. A. P.: Diagnosis of Diseases of the Chest. Vol. II. Philadelphia, W. B. Saunders Co., 1970.

Grandage, J.: The radiology of the dog's diaphragm. J. Small Anim. Pract., 15:1, 1974.

Miller, M. E., Christensen, G. C., and Evans, H. E.: Anatomy of the Dog. Philadelphia, W. B. Saunders Co., 1964.

Reif, J. S., and Rhodes, W. H.: The lungs of aged dogs: A radiographic-morphologic correlation. J. Amer. Vet. Radiol. Soc., 7:5, 1966.

Schebitz, H., and Wilkens, H.: Atlas of Radiographic Anatomy of Dog and Horse. Berlin, Paul Parey, 1968.

Suter, P. F., and Chan, K. F.: Disseminated pulmonary disease in small animals: A radiographic approach to diagnosis. J. Amer. Vet. Radiol. Soc., 9:67, 1968.

Wyburn, R. S., and Lawson, D. D.: Simple radiography as an aid to the diagnosis of heart disease in the dog. J. Small Anim. Pract., 8:163, 1967.

Contrast Pleurography

James K. Burt

Radiographic demonstration of pleural disease and the differentiation of pleural and pulmonary lesions are a matter of concern to all who interpret thoracic radiographs. Lesions may be masked by the density of vascular structures in the mediastinum, may involve the pleura in several areas of the chest, or may become obliterated in varying amounts of pleural fluid. Many times, pleural lesions are unrecognized until they become extensive in size or are widespread. Because the healthy pleura is a thin layer of fibrous tissue, it cannot be visualized radiographically until disease increases the thickness sufficiently for it to be contrasted by the air-filled lungs or the ribs. At times, increased amounts of pleural fluid will collect between the lung lobes and separate the pleural surfaces, yet these surfaces cannot be visualized and evaluated because of their contact with fluid that has the same radiographic density.

Contrast pleurography provides good visualization of pleural surfaces (Rudy et al., 1968). Pleurography is the coating of parietal and visceral pleura with an aqueous contrast material containing iodide. Pleural reflections are then seen as opaque lines and deposits of contrast material, which have a predictable and characteristic pattern. As with any contrast procedure, the definition or detail depends upon a clearly demonstrated difference in adjacent densities. The objective in pleurography is to opacify spaces between pleural surfaces and to note any filling defects along the margins of the contrast material or abnormal deposits (pooling). Properly executed, pleurography can be extremely beneficial in delineating mass lesions in the mediastinum and pleura, as well as pleural adhesions. Often, differentiation of pleural and pulmonary lesions is possible only with contrast pleurography.

If more than a few milliliters of pleural fluid is present, the contrast material is diluted and detail is markedly diminished. Dilution of the contrast material is not as critical a problem in the evaluation of mass lesions as it is in the defining of less obvious pleural defects, such as chronic pleuritis, pleural adhesions or miliary carcinomatosis. Pleurography should not be attempted, therefore, in the presence of pleural effusion. In these cases, pleuracentesis for the removal of most of the pleural fluid should be done prior to pleurography.

PREPARATION OF THE PATIENT

Fasting for 24 hours prior to the pleurographic examination is desirable, particularly when general anesthesia will be needed. Although contrast pleurography is a percutaneous technique, general anesthesia facilitates the procedures by preventing any movement while placing the needle. In the debilitated or critically ill patient, the procedure can be done by local anesthesia of the skin, intercostal muscles, and parietal pleura.

Routine radiographs of the thorax should be made on the day of the pleurographic examination. Correlation of the contrast study and the plain radiographs is an important facet of this examination. The plain radiographs should be made with a short exposure time in order to eliminate motion of the lungs. The exposure for the pleurogram should be increased by 6 to 10 kilovolts over that of the noncontrast (scout) radiographs.

The catheterization site on the right side of the thorax (approximately 3 inches lateral to the dorsal spinous processes of the sixth

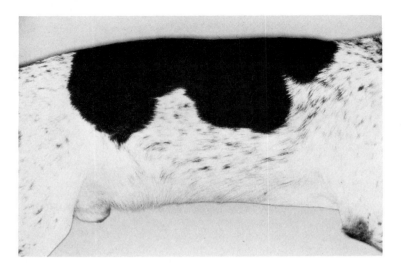

Figure 12–17. Dog in left lateral recumbency, positioned for contrast pleurography.

to the ninth thoracic vertebrae) is clipped and scrubbed, using routine techniques of surgical preparation (Figs. 12–17 and 12–18). The animal is then draped in a routine manner to minimize contamination of equipment by the hair coat.

MATERIALS

A 15-gauge catheter with a 14-gauge needle is satisfactory for large dogs. An 18-gauge catheter with a 17-gauge needle is better for medium and small-sized dogs. An Intrafusor, which combines these items, is an easily handled instrument. (Intrafusor, McGaw Laboratories and Sorenson Research Co.).

Good pleurographic contrast agents are the aqueous iodide compounds, methylglucamine diatrizoate and combination of sodium and methylglucamine diatrizoate (Renograffin, Renovist; Squibb & Sons). Other aqueous iodides possess good contrast qualities; however, the rate of absorption and rapidity of diffusion through the mediastinum make them less desirable pleurographic contrast media.

Because of the pleural irritation caused by all aqueous contrast materials, lidocaine hydrochloride (Spinal Xylocaine) is added to the solution before injection. Muscle fascic-

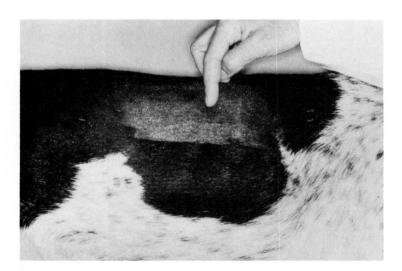

Figure 12–18. Site of percutaneous injection of contrast material. Local anesthesia of skin, muscle, and pleura is necessary at this site if a general anesthetic is not used.

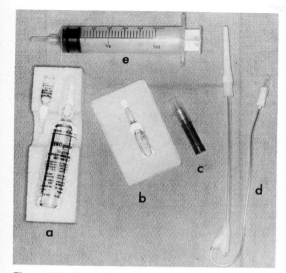

Figure 12–19. Materials used in contrast pleurography. *a*, Aqueous iodide (urographic contrast material); *b*, 2 cc. ampule of lidocaine hydrochloride; *c*, hypodermic needle; *d*, Intrafusor; *e*, syringe.

TECHNIQUE

The animal is prepared and draped as previously described. Contrast material is measured in amounts of 0.3 to 0.5 ml per pound of body weight. Lidocaine hydrochloride is then added to obtain a final concentration of 0.1% (0.1 ml lidocaine per milliliter of contrast material). After thorough mixing, the Intrafusor is attached to the syringe and filled. Filling the Intrafusor minimizes iatrogenic pneumothorax or bubbles in the pooled areas.

The Intrafusor needle is removed from the needle cover (Fig. 12–20) and inserted in one of the intercostal spaces between the sixth and ninth ribs, approximately 3 inches lateral to the dorsal spinous processes (in a 40 to 60 lb dog). This area is high on the chest wall and the exact location will vary with the size of the dog. The needle is inserted at a 5 to 10 degree angle, directed toward the sternum. The bevel of the needle should be flat against the skin when inserted, so that when the needle reaches the pleura, the bevel will be parallel to the pleural surface.

With the lateral surface of the palm resting on the chest wall, the needle is slowly advanced until a snap is felt, which identifies penetration of the parietal pleura. The catheter is then advanced through the needle into the pleural space between parietal and visceral pleura. The needle is withdrawn, leaving the catheter in place (Fig. 12–21). A test injection of 0.5 ml is made to

ulations are seen when a local anesthetic is not added to the contrast material, even with a light plane of general anesthesia. Spinal Xylocaine is available in 2 ml ampules or in multiple dose vials. The product containing epinephrine should not be used.

A syringe and hypodermic needle (Fig. 12–19) are used to measure and mix the contrast solutions. Sterile surgical gloves should also be used for this procedure.

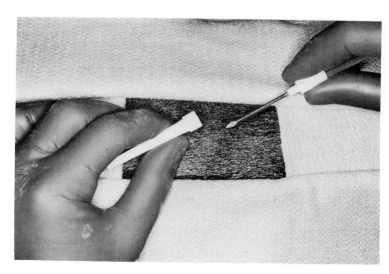

Figure 12–20. Draped patient, prepared for pleurography. The needle cover has been removed from the Intrafusor. The Intrafusor should be filled with the contrast material.

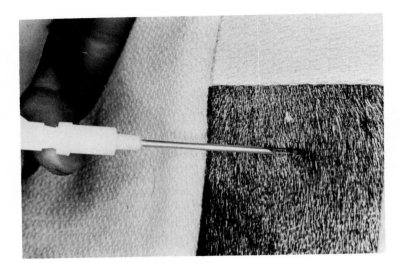

Figure 12-21. Withdrawn needle after the catheter has been advanced in the pleural space.

determine the ease of injection and any adverse reaction to the contrast material, such as coughing from inadvertent pulmonary parenchymal injection. A slight increase in respiratory rate is expected, but the plane of anesthesia can effect this response. After one minute, the remaining contrast material is injected (Fig. 12-22). The Intrafusor catheter is removed and the animal is rolled from side to side, onto its sternum and back, and then tipped cranially and caudally to distribute the contrast material throughout the pleural cavity. Leaving the animal in one position for several minutes will cause pooling of contrast material in the various recesses of the dependent hemithorax.

Lateral and ventrodorsal radiographs are made immediately after positional distribution. Although not always necessary, four views (both left and right laterals, a ventrodorsal and dorsoventral) are beneficial. The results should show an even, smooth distribution of contrast material over pleural surfaces, with minor pooling in the pleural recesses (Figs. 12-23 to 12-26).

The contrast material is absorbed rapidly from the thorax and excreted by the kidneys within 30 minutes. This rapid absorption necessitates immediate exposures following injection and positional distribution. If sterile conditions are maintained, no aftercare is needed.

(*Text continued on page 314.*)

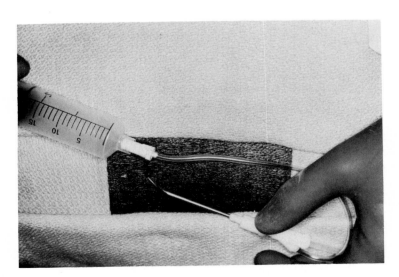

Figure 12-22. Injection of contrast material into the pleural space.

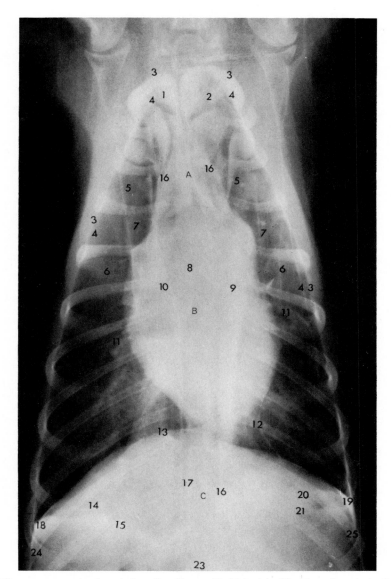

Figure 12–23. Pleurogram, ventrodorsal view. See Figure 12–24 for identification of symbols. Reprinted by permission of the Journal of the American Veterinary Radiology Society.

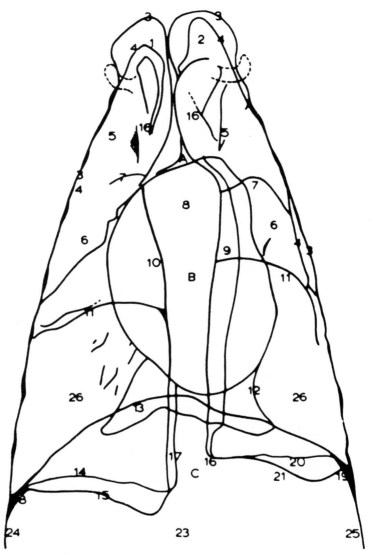

Figure 12–24. Line drawing of contrasted pleura, ventrodorsal positioning. *1,* right pleural cupula; *2,* left pleural cupula; *3,* parietal pleura; *4,* pulmonary pleura; *5,* cranial lobe of lung; *6,* middle lobe of lung; *7,* interlobular reflection of pleura between cranial and middle lobes of lungs; *8,* pleural reflection over pericardium; *9,* left mediastinal border; *10,* right mediastinal border; *11,* interlobular reflection of pleura between middle and caudal lobes of lung; *12,* pleural reflection on the accessory lobe of the lung; *13,* caudal pleura; *14,* ventral caudal end of the right lung; *15,* dorsal caudal border of the right lung; *16,* dorsal mediastinal line; *17,* caudal border of accessory lobe of the lung; *18,* right costophrenic angle; *19,* left costophrenic angle; *20,* ventral caudal end of left lung; *21,* dorsal caudal end of the left lung; *22,* diaphragm; *23,* extension of pleura caudal to right costodiaphragmatic angle; *24,* extension of pleura caudal to left costodiaphragmatic angle; *25,* caudal lobe of lung; *A,* cranial mediastinal pleura; *B,* middle mediastinal pleura; *C,* caudal mediastinal pleura. Reprinted by permission of the Journal of the American Veterinary Radiology Society.

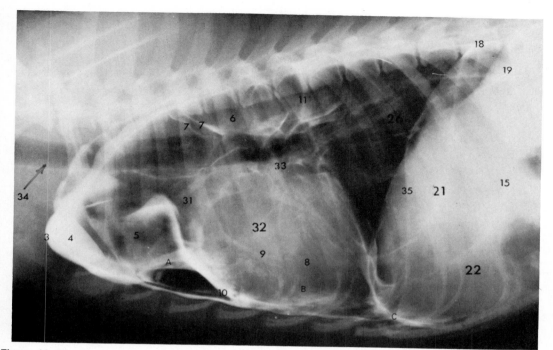

Figure 12–25. Pleurogram, right lateral view. See Figure 12–26 for identification of symbols. Reprinted by permission of the Journal of the American Veterinary Radiology Society.

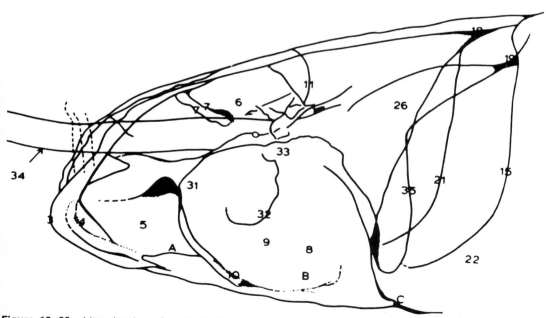

Figure 12–26. Line drawing of contrasted pleura, right lateral positioning. *3,* parietal pleura; *4,* pulmonary pleura; *5,* cranial lobe of lung; *6,* middle lobe of lung; *7,* interlobular fissure between cranial and middle lobe; *8,* pleural reflection over pericardium; *9,* heart; *10,* ventral mediastinal pleura; *11,* interlobar fissure between middle and caudal lobe of the lung; *15,* caudal margin of right lung; *18,* costophrenic angle of the left side; *19,* costophrenic angle of the right side; *21,* caudal margin of the left lung; *22,* diaphragmatic pleura; *31,* cranial vena cava; *32,* caudal margin of left auricle; *33,* contrast material trapped in folds of pulmonary pleura; *34,* thoracic inlet; *35,* caudal margin of accessory lobe; *A,* cranial mediastinal pleura; *B,* middle mediastinal pleura; *C,* caudal mediastinal pleura; *arrow,* trachea. Reprinted by permission of the Journal of the American Veterinary Radiology Society.

COMPLICATIONS

Complications may arise due to faulty catheterization technique. Extending the needle beyond the pleural space will result in the penetration of the lung and intrapulmonary injection of the contrast material. Coughing after an injection in the awake patient indicates an intrapulmonary injection. The contrast material is absorbed from the lung without permanent parenchymal changes and the procedure can be repeated in a few hours or delayed 24 hours.

Lung laceration, with subsequent pneumothorax, is more common if the needle bevel is not parallel to the pleural surface. In such circumstances, the procedure should not be repeated until pleural air is absent on thoracic radiographs.

Laceration of an intercostal vessel can result in a hematoma at the injection site, but this is not a common problem if care is taken to select an injection site in the center of the intercostal space. Palpation of the ribs before needle placement is important in obese dogs, since the ribs are not easily seen.

Failure to penetrate the parietal pleura results in an injection in the intercostal muscles. Pleurography should be delayed until absorption of this contrast material is complete. When the contrast material contains a local anesthetic, ectopic intramuscular injections are seldom painful.

REFERENCES

Bhargava, A. K., Rudy, R. L., and Diesem, C. D.: Radiographic anatomy of the pleura in dogs visualized by contrast pleurography. J. Amer. Vet. Radiol. Soc., *10*:61, 1969.

Bhargava, A. K., Burt, J. K., Rudy, R. L., and Wilson, G. P.: Diagnosis of mediastinal heart base tumors in dogs using contrast pleurography. J. Amer. Vet. Radiol. Soc., *11*:56, 1970a.

Bhargava, A. K., Kentner, D. C., Rudy, R. L., and Burt, J. K.: Contrast pleurography in rhesus monkeys *(Macaca mulatta)*. Brit. Vet. J., *126*:57, 1970b.

Rudy, R. L., and Bhargava, A. K.: The diagnosis of pleuropulmonary lesions utilizing contrast pleurography. Acta Radiol. Suppl., *319*:215, 1972.

Rudy, R. L., Bhargava, A. K., and Roenigk, W. J.: Contrast pleurography. A new technic for the radiographic visualization of the pleura and its various reflections in dogs. Radiology, *91*:1034, 1968.

Bronchography in the Dog

WILLIAM J. ZONTINE

Bronchography is a specialized radiologic procedure in which radiopaque medium is introduced into the lumen of the bronchial tree in order to visualize the anatomical details fluoroscopically or radiographically. It is a method of establishing anatomical and topographical diagnoses of bronchial lesions.

INDICATIONS

There are a number of indications for this type of study in veterinary medicine. It is the only accurate method of determining the extent of bronchiectasis. This disease results in definite changes on the plain radiograph, but requires either tomography or bronchography to delineate the findings more efficiently. Bronchography is particularly useful in assessing partial or complete airway obstruction from such sources as tumors, foreign bodies or strictures. Bronchograms will show the displacement and compression produced by extrabronchial lesions. Tracheal or bronchial fistulas can be confirmed or localized, as can abscesses, cysts and cavities. Bronchography has also been used to demonstrate the persistence of a residual cavity, following therapy for a lung abscess (Cracovaner, 1957). It can be used to identify both normal structures, such as a lung lobe, and anomalies such as a bronchial dilatation. It is a valuable aid to the surgeon in properly planning his surgical technique.

CONTRAINDICATIONS

Bronchography should always be used with caution as the introduction of any foreign material into the lungs will compromise respiratory function. Patients should be carefully selected after a thorough clinical evaluation and assessment of the plain radiographs. The main contraindication is poor general health of the patient. Since general anesthesia must usually be employed, any contraindication to anesthesia is likewise a contraindication to bronchography. It should not be used where there is acute pulmonary disease (Whitehouse, 1971), acute bronchitis, or severe emphysema (Nelson et al., 1959). Another contraindication is any known idiosyncrasy to the contrast material.

ANATOMY

The evaluation of the radiographs obtained requires knowledge of normal bronchial tree anatomy. The criterion for naming the lung lobes is the division of the bronchi rather than the external fissures of the lungs (Fig. 12–27). In the dog, both lungs have a cranial (apical), middle (cardiac) and caudal (diaphragmatic) lobe. The right lung has an additional lobe, the accessory (intermediate or azygos) (Nomina Anatomica Veterinaria, 1968). Each lung lobe has its own main bronchus which then continues to branch dichotomously into smaller bronchioles terminating in alveoli. The epithelium of the bronchi is ciliated columnar as far as the final branching.

The trachea terminates by dividing into the left and right main stem bronchi. All of the bronchi to the 4 right lobes arise separately from the right main stem bronchus. However, on the left, the cranial and middle lobe bronchi arise from a common branch from which the cranial lobe bronchus

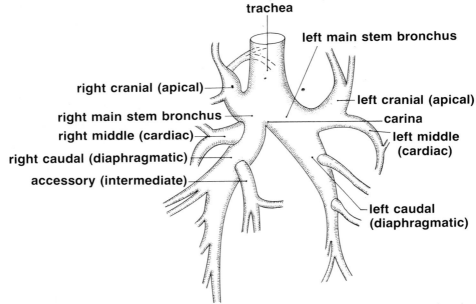

Figure 12–27. Sketch of normal anatomy of the canine bronchial tree seen in the ventrodorsal projection.

courses cranially after an acute bend. This anatomical feature accounts for the difficulty experienced in filling the entire left lung during bronchography.

The cranial lobes bronchi lie in a plane parallel to the trachea, directed in a cranial direction. The middle lobes bronchi are directed ventrally and slightly caudally. The caudal lobes bronchi are directed primarily caudally and dorsally, while the accessory lobe bronchus courses ventrally and caudally with a medial branch which curves ventrally around the right side of the heart across the midline.

A knowledge of the anatomic arrangement and direction of the bronchi is important in performing bronchography, as proper positioning of the patient must be accomplished in order to permit the contrast material to flow into the appropriate bronchus by gravity.

TECHNIQUE

Patient Preparation and Anesthesia

Food should be withheld for 12 to 24 hours prior to the procedure. General anesthesia is necessary in order to introduce the contrast material and to suppress coughing which will interfere with the procedure. Gas anesthesia (halothane or methoxyflurane) is the ideal anesthetic agent since rapid recovery is essential in order for the patient to regain cough reflexes and remove the contrast material as quickly as possible.

Following induction with a general anesthetic, the patient is intubated with as large an endotracheal tube as feasible in order to provide maximum ventilation. As much of the bronchial secretions as possible should be removed by postural drainage and suction. The use of atropine sulfate to dry secretions is not recommended in diseased animals since it interferes with mucociliary action, which prevents clearing of the contrast material and may cause secretions to become tenacious and form plugs (Hersman et al., 1972). The contrast material may then be introduced through the endotracheal tube via a catheter attached to a syringe.

Catheter

The catheter must be of soft material in order not to tear or scratch the delicate lining of the tracheobronchial tree. Many types of polyethylene arterial catheters or disposable intravenous tubing can be utilized for this purpose. The tip of the catheter should be cut at a slight bevel and then carefully smoothed to remove all sharp edges. If the catheter material is too flexible, an inserted wire stylet can be used to improve its rigidity and to render the catheter radiopaque.

The catheter must be long enough to permit placement of the contrast medium in the bronchial tree well beyond the tracheal bifurcation. A means of roughly estimating adequate length is to measure from the proximal end of the endotracheal tube to the caudal edge of the rib cage. Once the catheter is positioned, the stylet is withdrawn and the contrast-filled syringe attached. If a stylet is not used, the non-radiopaque catheter should be filled with contrast medium in order to visualize it fluoroscopically or radiographically.

Fluoroscopy is necessary in order to properly position the catheter in the bronchus under study. The trachea and main stem bronchi may be visualized by blind introduction of the contrast material. However, this is not recommended as good technique.

Bronchographic Contrast Materials

The ideal contrast medium should have high radiopacity and the ability to coat bronchial walls uniformly and rapidly. In addition, it must be of a viscosity which will prevent entry into the alveoli (alveolization). It should be able to be quickly and completely expelled from the lungs and be physiologically and pharmacologically inert (Johnson et al., 1960). There is no agent presently available which meets all of these criteria. Several materials are presently used both clinically and experimentally in animals: organically bound iodine in an oily or aqueous base (Bishop et al., 1955; Bjork and Lodin, 1957; Douglas and Hall, 1959; Dyce, 1955; Nelson et al., 1968), powdered tantalum (Nadel et al., 1968; Upham et al., 1971), and barium sulfate as a powder or in suspension (Johnson and Howland, 1968; Nelson et al., 1968; Shook and Felson, 1970; Willson et al., 1959).

Any foreign material, including sterile saline, introduced into the lungs will cause a tissue reaction (Hellstrom and Holmgren, 1949). Alveolization of the contrast material impairs ventilation, may cause atelectasis and predispose to secondary infection

(Farinas and Zaldivar, 1958) and interferes with good visualization of the bronchi. For these reasons, alveolization should be avoided whenever possible by not overfilling the lungs and by using a material of sufficient viscosity to reduce the probability.

The contrast material which is most useful in animals is a 50 to 60% w/v suspension of barium sulfate in a carboxymethylcellulose base.* The desired 50 to 60% suspension is obtained by dilution with sterile saline.

Barium sulfate is relatively inert and results in only a mild reaction in the lungs (Huston et al., 1952). This is a nonspecific foreign body reaction which is seen with all other bronchographic media (Nelson et al., 1959) except tantalum (Nadel et al., 1968). It has the advantage of greater radiopacity than iodine since it has a higher atomic number (56 vs. 53). It can produce a foreign body granuloma as do other nonabsorbable contrast media and vehicles (Nelson et al., 1964). Even when barium is accidentally aspirated into the lungs, it is usually completely eliminated in a year or less in most patients. Deposits which remain longer apparently do not cause any ill effects (Nelson et al., 1964) and will collect in the regional lymph nodes.

The largest volume of the foreign material introduced into the lungs in bronchography is not the radiopaque substance but, rather, the vehicle. With the vehicles presently in use, the acute tissue reaction appears to readily subside. When the concentration of the iodine-containing media is high, tissue changes are more intense because of the additional iodine-tissue chemical reaction. Barium does not produce this additional reaction because it is inert (Christoforidis et al., 1967).

Procedure

It is advisable to study one lung at a time (Figs. 12–28 and 12–29). Also, the lateral view of a completely filled bronchial tree is quite confusing due to superimposition (Figs. 12–30 and 12–31). The trachea and

---

*The material is commercially available in a sterile form for gastrointestinal use under the trade name Redi-Flow, 100% w/v (Flow Pharmaceuticals, Inc. Palo Alto, CA 94303).

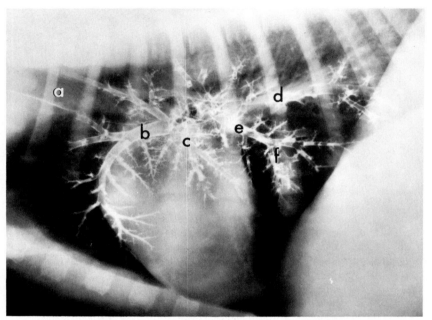

Figure 12–28. Bronchogram of the left lung, lateral view. *a,* Trachea; *b,* left cranial lobe bronchus; *c,* left middle lobe bronchus; *d,* left caudal lobe bronchus; *e,* right caudal lobe bronchus; *f,* accessory lobe bronchus.

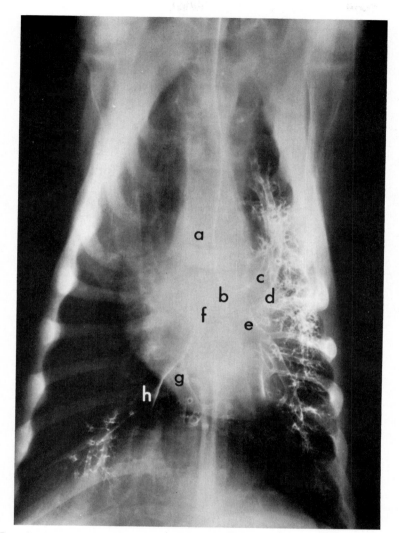

Figure 12–29. Bronchogram of the left lung, ventrodorsal projection. Note a small amount of contrast material in the right lung. This cannot be appreciated when seen on the lateral projection. *a*, Trachea; *b*, left main stem bronchus; *c*, left cranial lobe bronchus; *d*, left middle lobe bronchus; *e*, left caudal lobe bronchus; *f*, carina; *g*, accessory lobe bronchus; *h*, right caudal lobe bronchus.

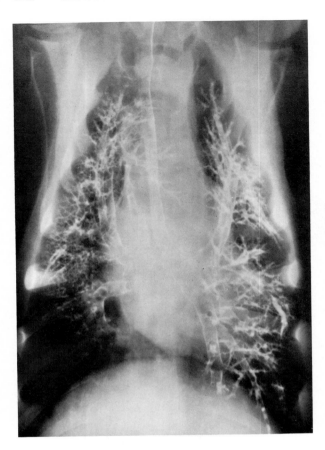

Figure 12-30. Bronchogram of both lungs seen in ventrodorsal projection. The right caudal and accessory lobes are incompletely outlined in this radiograph.

main stem bronchi can be outlined together, but a complete procedure should be confined to one lung at a time. A waiting period of 2 to 3 days is advisable before performing the procedure in the other lung.

The animal is placed first in sternal or dorsal recumbency and the catheter introduced into the appropriate main stem bronchus, ideally, under fluoroscopic control. Then the animal is placed in lateral recumbency with the lung to be studied downward. If a complete bronchogram is to be performed, the catheter is gently introduced as far as possible into the caudal lobe bronchus. The syringe is then attached and a small amount (½ cc) of contrast material is injected. The catheter is then slowly withdrawn while injecting just enough contrast material to coat the bronchial wall. The material will be seen to spread quite readily over the mucosal surfaces, moving distally with each inspiration.

The caudal lobe bronchus can be easily coated with the animal in the lateral position. However, in order to fill the middle lobe bronchus, the animal must be in sternal recumbency, since this bronchus is directed ventrally. To fill the cranial lobe bronchus, the animal should be in a lateral position, while a small amount (2 to 3 ml) of material is deposited at the opening of the bronchus. The dog is then moved into an oblique, sternally recumbent position (approximately 20 degrees) with the lobe to be studied downward. The hindquarters are then elevated and held for a few minutes to allow the contrast agent to spread ventrally and cranially by gravity.

Aftercare

The animal should be placed with the opacified lung upward and the head down-

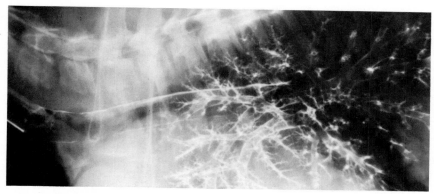

Figure 12–31. Bronchogram of both lungs in lateral projection. The superimposition of the structures creates confusion in this view, which makes simultaneous left and right sided bronchography undesirable in clinical patients.

ward to promote postural drainage, and suction should be used to remove as much of the contrast material as possible. Good postural drainage is difficult to obtain in dogs (Figs. 12–32 and 12–33). The angulating drainage methods used in human patients are not effective in the dog because of the acute angles at which the main bronchi leave the trachea.

The contrast is usually completely cleared from the lungs in three to four days by the ciliary-mucous transport system and by coughing and/or swallowing (Upham et al., 1971). In the event of alveolization into the distal nonciliated areas, clearance is by lymphatic or blood-vascular transport and by macrophages.

There may be a transient rise in temperature, which usually recedes in 24 to 48 hours without treatment. Alveolization of the contrast medium usually is not of clinical importance.

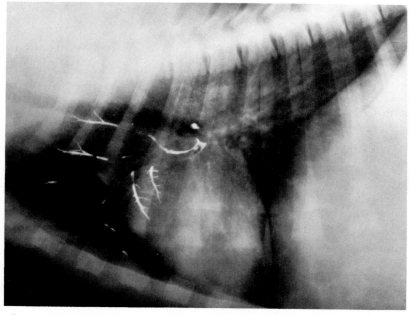

Figure 12–32. Bronchogram taken 24 hours after bronchography of left lung, lateral view. Note retention of medium in cranial lobe owing to lack of adequate postural drainage caused by acute angulation of the bronchial origin.

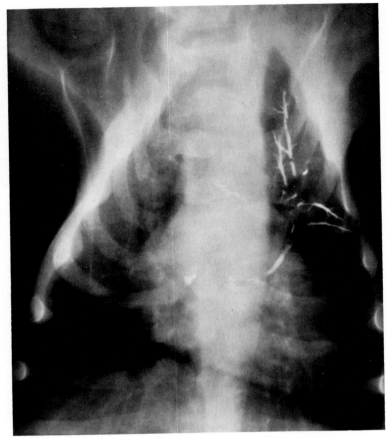

Figure 12–33. Same as Figure 12–32, ventrodorsal projection.

PRECAUTIONS WHEN PERFORMING BRONCHOGRAPHY

1. Select patient carefully.
2. Be prepared for respiratory and cardio-vascular emergencies.
3. Do not overfill lungs.
4. Monitor filling fluoroscopically.
5. Examine one lung at a time.

REFERENCES

Bishop, E. J., Medway, W., and Archibald, J.: Radiological methods of investigating the thorax of small animals, including a technic for bronchography. No. Am. Vet., 36:477, 1955.

Bjork, L., and Lodin, H.: Pulmonary changes following bronchography with dionosil oily (animal experiments). Acta Radiol., 47:177, 1957.

Christoforidis, A. J., Nelson, S. W., and Pratt, P. C.: An experimental study of the tissue reaction to the vehicles commonly used in bronchography. Am. Rev. Resp. Dis., 96:249, 1967.

Cracovaner, A. J.: Bronchography. In Naclerio, E. A. (Ed.), Bronchopulmonary Diseases. New York, Hoeber-Harper, 1957.

Douglas, S. W., and Hall, L. W.: Bronchography in the dog. Vet. Rec., 43:901, 1959.

Dyce, K. M.: Experimental bronchography of the dog. Brit. Vet. J., 111:319, 1955.

Farinas, L., and Zaldivar, R. G.: Bronchography. In Rabin, C. B. (ed.), Roentgenology of the Chest. Springfield, Ill., Charles C Thomas, Publisher, 1958.

Hellstrom, B., and Holmgren, H.: The reaction of the lung on bronchography with viscous Umbradil (Umbradil-Viskos B) (Astra), Umbradil (Astra) and Carboxymethylcellulose. Acta Radiol., 32:471, 1949.

Hersman, R., Kleine, L. J., and Gilmore, C. E.: A clinical evaluation of propyliodone bronchography. J. Amer. Vet. Radiol. Soc., 13:27, 1972.

Huston, J., Wallach, D. P., and Cunningham, C. J.: Pulmonary reaction to barium sulfate in rats. Arch. Path., 54:430, 1952.

Johnson, P. M., Benson, W. R., Sprunt, W. H., and Dunnagan, W. A.: Toxicity of bronchographic contrast media. Ann. Otolaryngol., 69:1102, 1960.

Johnson, T. H., and Howland, W. J.: Aerosol bronchography, Am. J. Roentgenol. Radium Ther. Nucl. Med., *104*:787, 1968.

Nadel, J. A., Wolfe, W. G., and Graf, P. D.: Powdered tantalum as a medium for bronchography in canine and human lungs. Invest. Radiol., *3*:229, 1968.

Nelson, S. W., Christoforidis, A. J., and Pratt, P. C.: Barium sulfate and bismuth subcarbonate suspensions as bronchographic contrast media. Radiology, *72*:829, 1959.

Nelson, S. W., Christoforidis, A. J., and Pratt, P. C.: Bronchography. *In* Felson, B. (Ed.), Roentgen Techniques in Laboratory Animals. Philadelphia, W. B. Saunders Co., 1968.

Nelson, S. W., Christoforidis, A. J., and Pratt, P. C.: Further experiences with barium sulfate as a bronchographic contrast medium. Am. J. Roentgenol. Radium Ther. Nucl. Med., *92*:595, 1964.

Nomina Anatomica Veterinaria. Vienna, Adolf Holzhausen's Successors, 1968.

Shook, C. D., and Felson, B.: Inhalation bronchography. Chest, *58*:333, 1970.

Upham, T., Graham, L. S., Steckel, R. J., and Poe, N.: Determination of in vivo persistence of tantalum dust following bronchography using reactor-activated tantalum and total body counting. Am. J. Roentgenol. Radium Ther. Nucl. Med., *111*:690, 1971.

Whitehouse, W. M.: Bronchography. *In* Potchen, E. J., Koehler, P. R., and Davis, D. O. (Eds.), Principles of Diagnostic Radiology. New York, McGraw-Hill Book Company, 1971.

Willson, J. K. V., Rubin, P. S., and McGee, T. M.: The effects of barium sulfate on the lungs. A clinical and experimental study. Am. J. Roentgenol. Radium Ther. Nucl. Med., *82*:84, 1959.

Angiocardiography

GARY L. WOOD,
STEPHEN J. ETTINGER,
EDWARD A. RHODE

INTRODUCTION

Angiocardiography refers to the production of radiographs by exposing a sequence of films during the circulation of contrast medium through the heart and blood vessels. This valuable diagnostic tool is utilized primarily by veterinarians in large practices or institutions. Because of the specialized equipment required, angiocardiography usually is not a procedure utilized by the general practitioner. Angiocardiography can provide information relevant to the diagnosis and prognosis of most congenital and some acquired cardiac diseases.

Before contrast radiography is done, it is imperative that a complete cardiovascular examination be performed. Such a work-up should include a complete physical examination, an electrocardiogram, thoracic radiographs and routine blood tests. Special procedures such as phonocardiograms, vectorcardiograms or blood gas studies may also be indicated. This section describes the indications, contraindications, procedures and results of angiocardiography.

INDICATIONS

Selective angiocardiography involves placing the catheter as close as possible to a suspected lesion in the heart or great vessels for delivering contrast medium. Its indications are threefold: (1) to obtain a specific diagnosis when routine methods have failed, (2) to better define a known lesion, or (3) to provide information complementary to hemodynamic studies. Nonselective angiocardiography, although its results may be inconsistent, may be indicated to demonstrate lesions in or near the heart and great vessels in a limited number of disease conditions.

Noninvasive diagnostic methods often do not prove a specific diagnosis in congenital heart lesions. For example, the diagnosis of ventricular septal defect, a valvular insufficiency or a combination of heart defects may be confusing, but can be positively identified by selective angiocardiography. Less often selective contrast studies are indicated for the diagnosis of an acquired disease in veterinary medicine.

Sometimes, although the diagnosis is known, the lesion may be more accurately defined through angiocardiography. For the potential surgical patient, selective contrast radiography can demonstrate the exact morphology of the defect. It may also reveal additional complicating lesions.

Selective angiocardiography used as an adjunct to other cardiovascular studies is usually confined to a research situation. As an example, it may be used to follow the pathogenesis of experimentally produced heart defects in animals.

CONTRAINDICATIONS

There are six relative contraindications to angiocardiography: (1) inadequate indication, (2) congestive heart failure, (3) serious respiratory disease, (4) life-threatening arrhythmias, (5) foci of infection (especially cardiovascular or respiratory) and (6) hypersensitivity to any agents to be used. Some are relative contraindications because they may be controlled by appropriate therapy. For example, heart failure due to a congenital defect may be temporarily controllable

324

TABLE 12–1

INSTRUMENTS USED FOR
CARDIAC CATHETERIZATION

Operating scissors
Curved Iris scissors
Straight Iris scissors
Scalpel handle and blades
Collier needleholder
2 Bulldog clamps
Iris forceps (more than 2)
Iris dressing forceps (2 or 3)
4 Backhaus clamps
4 Straight Halstead mosquito forceps
4 Curved Halstead mosquito forceps
Vessel dilator
Sponge bowl
Saline bowl
Assorted tapered and cutting edge needles
4 × 4 Gauze sponges
5–0 Silk with taper cardiovascular needle
3–0 Medium chromic gut
2–0 Nonabsorbable suture
Umbilical tape
Rubber bands
4 Surgical towels
Assorted glass and plastic syringes

with digitalis, diuretics and a low-sodium diet. Arrhythmias and infections may likewise be controlled medically. Prior to angiocardiography, all patients must be carefully evaluated with a complete medical and cardiovascular examination.

EQUIPMENT

Zimmerman (1966) describes four kinds of equipment used in angiocardiography: (1) that for preparing and catheterizing the patient, (2) that for monitoring the patient, (3) that for producing the image, and (4) that for handling emergencies. In addition, in veterinary medicine, preparation of the patient for selective catheterization usually includes general anesthesia.

Equipment for preparing and catheterizing the patient includes instruments and equipment necessary to perform aseptic vascular surgery. An ample and varied supply of catheters and guide wires is a prerequisite. Some instruments and catheters used by

TABLE 12–2

CATHETERS USED FOR CARDIAC CATHETERIZATION AND ANGIOCARDIOGRAPHY IN THE DOG

Type	Sizes	Description and Tip Styles	Use
NIH (National Institutes of Health)	5F–8F	Closed distal tip with 6 round openings within the first cm. Pediatric types preferred for small and medium-sized dogs	Angiocardiography, mainly aorta and left ventricle.
Odman-Ledin (Kifa)	Red–1 Green–2 (Yellow–3 and Grey–4 not used in dogs)	Tubing bought in coils. Length, curves, and tips are shaped according to the proposed procedure. Requires flange or fittings. Thermoplastic (polyethylene).	Tapered end for percutaneous catheterization. End-hole for measuring of pulmonary wedge pressure. End- and side-holes for pressure recordings and left and right ventricular angiocardiography. For contrast injections, tip should be tapered.
Goodale-Lubin	5F to 8F	One pair of side-holes close to the open tip. Flexible catheter.	Pressure recordings, angiocardiography, and angiography. Widely used for metabolic studies.
Cournand		End-hole only	Pressure recordings, withdrawal of blood, determination of pulmonary capillary wedge pressure.
Lehman Ventriculography	5F to 8F	Thin, flexible blind tip designed to bend at the aortic valve and then to snap into the ventricle. Closed end, 4 side-holes.	Retrograde aortic catheterization and left ventricular angiocardiography. Long tip might keep the holes in the vicinity of the aortic valve cusps.
Swan-Ganz	4, 5, 7F	Flexible catheter with an inflatable balloon tip to help carry the catheter through the right heart into the pulmonary artery. End-hole or side-hole.	Pulmonary artery blood samples and pressures, wedge pressures and angiography.

Ettinger and Suter (1970) are listed in Tables 12–1 and 12–2.

The patient parameters monitored or recorded during cardiac catheterization include the electrocardiogram, arterial blood pressure, pressure at the catheter tip and blood oxygen tension. A multichannel medical recorder adapted for electrocardiography and blood pressure measurements, special transducers and blood gas analyzers are part of the basic equipment needed.

The apparatus for producing the image is sophisticated and varies considerably among institutions. The expense of such equipment is one of the main reasons that angiocardiography is limited to large institutions. At a minimum, it requires a conventional x-ray machine and fluoroscopic equipment with image intensification. If the image is recorded on conventional x-ray film, a rapid film changer is used. Such changers are designed for either cut film or roll film. These films are exposed in either a single or biplane manner. If the image is recorded as a moving picture, a cinefluoroscopic unit or video tape recorder may be used. An automatic programmed high powered injector is needed to infuse the dye through the catheter into the heart or vessel. Usually the contrast medium selected is a sodium or methylglucamine diatrizoate (Hypaque, 50%, Hypaque-M, 75%, Renovist, 69%, or Renografin, 76%).

The equipment necessary for handling cardiovascular emergencies includes a direct current defibrillator and an adequate supply of emergency drugs (See Table 12–3).

Proper anesthetic management of patients with cardiovascular disease requires inhalation equipment, whether or not inhalation agents are the primary anesthetic. In addition, respiration assist apparatus should be available. Anesthetic programs may vary

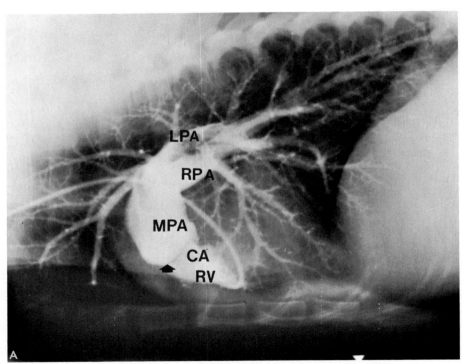

Figure 12–34. Lateral and dorsoventral angiocardiograms exposed simultaneously using a biplane roll-film changer. Selective right ventricular injection of a normal, 3 year old male dog of mixed breed.

A, Lateral angiocardiogram. The dog was placed in a prone position, and a horizontal beam was used. The angiocardiogram demonstrates that the details of the right ventricle (RV) and the main pulmonary artery (MPA) can be outlined much better with a selective than with a nonselective technique. The catheter was inserted into the right ventricle via the jugular vein. The pulmonic valve (arrow) separates the funnel-shaped conus arteriosus (CA) from the main pulmonary artery (MPA). Notice the slight curve of the normally branching peripheral pulmonary arteries. (Courtesy of Ettinger, S. J., and Suter, P. F.: *Canine Cardiology.* Philadelphia, W. B. Saunders Co., 1970.)

(*Figure 12–34 continued on the opposite page.*)

widely, but must be carefully designed to minimize the dose of cardiotopic agents.

CATHETERIZATION PROCEDURE

A team of skilled, experienced personnel is necessary to perform angiocardiography safely. Catheterization teams vary considerably; however, a basic team includes a catheterizer (ideally with an assistant), an anes-thetist, a physiologic monitor and a radiologist or radiographic technician.

The patient is prepared for general anesthesia in the usual manner. After anesthesia has been accomplished, the skin over the common carotid artery and jugular vein or femoral artery and vein is prepared for aseptic surgery. Direct cardiac puncture should be reserved only for those patients in whom selective approach through a vessel is impossible. Generally, a cut-down is performed on

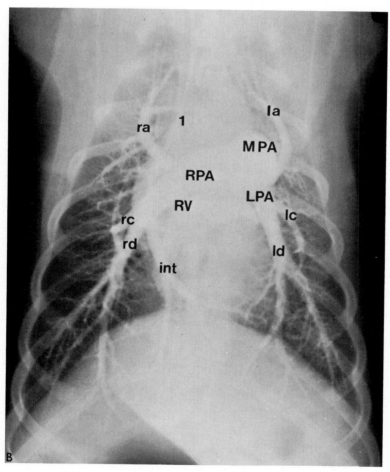

Figure 12–34 *Continued.* *B*, Catheter (1) was passed via the cranial vena cava into the right atrium and curves medially into the right ventricle (RV). The right pulmonary artery (RPA) is superimposed on the right ventricle; it branches into the right cranial lobar artery (ra), the right middle lobar artery (rc), the right caudal lobar artery (rd), and the artery to the intermediate or azygos lobe (int). Because the exposure was made at the end of systole, the main pulmonary artery (MPA) is very large. The bulge caused by the main pulmonary artery is also referred to as the pulmonary artery segment of the cardiac silhouette. The left pulmonary artery (LPA) branches into the left cranial lobar artery (la), the left middle lobar artery (lc), and the left caudal lobar artery (ld). Notice the slight curvature of the small arterial branches in the caudal lobar area. In addition, notice that the inclination of the heart can also be seen in this view. Normally, the right ventricle would be nearly completely obscured by the right pulmonary artery. (Courtesy of Ettinger, S. J., and Suter, P. F.: *Canine Cardiology*. Philadelphia, W. B. Saunders Co., 1970.)

the desired pair of vessels, which are gently isolated and occluded. Using the fluoroscopic image and pressure tracings as a guide to catheter placement, the catheter is passed along the vessel to the desired position. Anticoagulant flushes are used frequently. Some of the patients are treated with systemic anticoagulants.

If arrhythmias occur, slight catheter withdrawal will usually result in a return to normal rhythm. These are most often single atrial or ventricular premature contractions. If arrhythmias persist or advance to more serious disturbances (i.e., ventricular tachycardia), additional steps should be taken. Reducing the anesthetic level and increasing oxygen flow are imperative. Short-acting antiarrhythmic drugs such as lidocaine may be indicated. Ventricular fibrillation requires immediate corrective measures, including

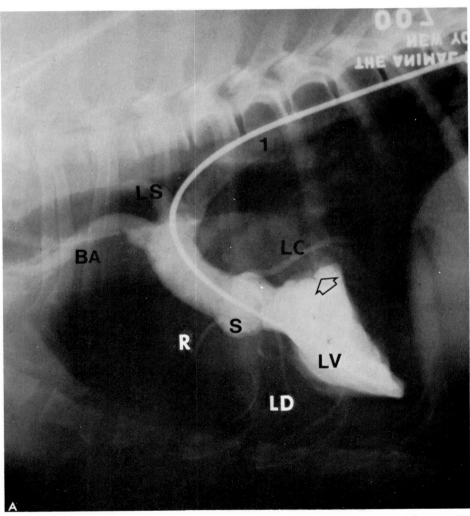

Figure 12–35. *A,* Left lateral angiocardiogram, selective left ventricular injection, normal Basset-mixed breed dog of unknown age. Notice the catheter (1), which was advanced retrograde from the femoral artery, through the descending aorta, and into the left ventricle. Both the mitral valve (open arrow) and the aortic valve are closed, and the ventricular outline (LV) is relatively small and well delineated, indicating that the exposure was made at the beginning of diastole (isometric relaxation). The sinuses of the aorta (S) are filled with contrast medium. The right coronary artery (R) leaves the cranial sinus. The left coronary artery, which is about twice the size of the right coronary artery, branches almost immediately into the left circumflex coronary artery (LC), lying in the left coronary sulcus, and the left descending branch (LD), lying in or near the left longitudinal sulcus. At the aortic arch, the origin of the larger brachiocephalic artery (BA) is just ventral to the origin of the smaller left subclavian artery (LS). (Courtesy of Ettinger, S. J., and Suter, P. F.: *Canine Cardiology.* Philadelphia, W. B. Saunders Co., 1970.)

(Figure 12–35 continued on the opposite page.)

external cardiac massage and direct current defibrillation, as detailed by Kirk and Bistner (1969).

Once the catheterization of the heart or vessel has been performed, the physiologic data are collected. Pressures and blood gases from all locations catheterized and dye dilution studies may substantiate the diagnosis without the use of contrast medium injections. Ettinger and Suter (1970) have given examples of such data and have summarized the findings of others.

When physiologic data collection is completed, the contrast medium is injected at selected locations. Its flow is followed by several radiographs or cinefluoroscopic film. Special care must be taken to choose the proper dose, pressure and duration of injection and appropriate film sequence to demonstrate the suspected lesion. The films

(*Text continued on page 334.*)

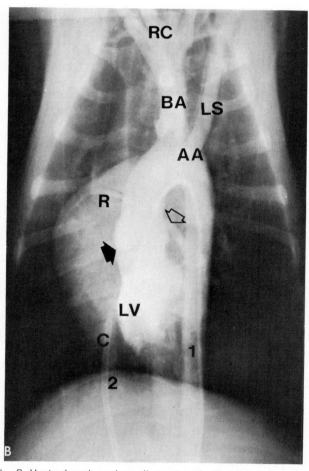

Figure 12–35 *Continued.* *B,* Ventrodorsal angiocardiogram, selective left ventricular injection, normal male Collie-mixed breed dog approximately 1 year old. Notice the catheter (1) which has been advanced retrograde from the femoral artery into the aorta and the left ventricle. A second catheter (2), introduced via the femoral vein, is seen entering the right atrium from the caudal vena cava (C). Hypaque-M 75% (1 ml/kg body weight) was injected over a period of 1.5 sec. This exposure was made 2 sec after the beginning of the injection. The left ventricle (LV) is in diastole, and the caudal portion of the ventricle has filled with blood containing no contrast medium, which entered from the left atrium. The aortic valve (black arrow) is closed. The left coronary artery (open arrow) originates from the sinuses of the aorta. The right coronary artery (R), which is smaller than the left coronary artery, is barely visible. The brachiocephalic artery (BA) and the left subclavian artery (LS) originate from the aortic arch (AA). The brachiocephalic artery then divides into the right common carotid artery (RC), the left common carotid artery (to the left of RC), and the right subclavian artery (to the right of RC). The heart has rotated to the right side despite the correct positioning of the thorax; this is due to the normal mobility of the heart. The rotation makes the aortic arch look wider than usual. (Courtesy of Ettinger, S. J., and Suter, P. F.: *Canine Cardiology.* Philadelphia, W. B. Saunders Co., 1970.)

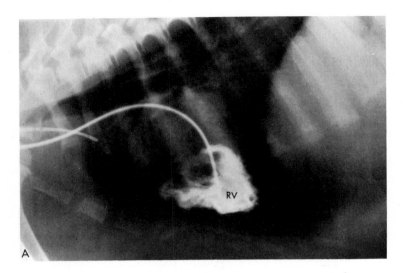

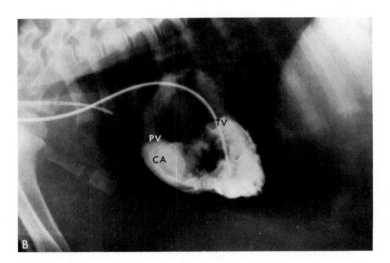

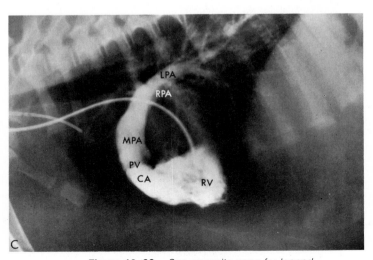

Figure 12–36. *See opposite page for legend.*

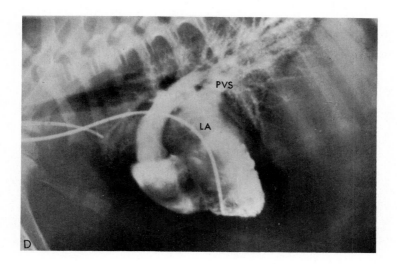

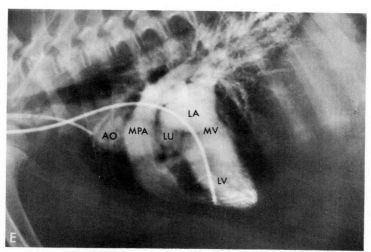

Figure 12-36. Right lateral angiocardiogram, after selective right ventricular injection, of 3 month old New-foundland female. A 5F Swan-Ganz catheter was passed down the right jugular vein, through the right atrium, and into the right ventricle. (Usually a less flexible side-hole catheter is used for ventricular injections). A 5F Lehman ventriculography catheter lies in the brachiocephalic artery. Film A was exposed 5/6 sec after beginning an injection of 9 cc Hypaque-M 75% at 150 psi. Film B was exposed 2 sec post injection, film C at 4 sec, film D at 5 sec and film E at 5.5 sec post injection. *A,* The catheter tip is in the right ventricle (RV) whose trabeculae will cause a roughened border. *B,* The right ventricular cavity is more completely filled as contrast medium enters the conus arteriosus (CA). The pulmonic valve (PV) is closed. The level of the tricuspid valve is marked by TV. The ventricle is in diastole. Lucency in the center of the ventricle is caused by unopacified blood entering from the right atrium. *C,* The ventricle is in early systole. The tricuspid valve (TV) is closed across the top of the full ventricle and the pulmonic valve (PV) is beginning to open. An earlier contraction has filled the main pulmonary artery (MPA) and has begun to outline the left and right pulmonary arteries (LPA, RPA). Superimposition of the pulmonary arteries is due to slight rotation of the thorax. Compare with Figure 12–34*A. D,* Contrast medium remains in the previously outlined structures and has entered the pulmonary venous circulation. Pulmonary arteries and veins are seen simultaneously. Contrast medium is approaching the left atrium (LA) through the pulmonary veins (PVS). *E,* The left atrium (LA) is filled, and contrast medium has moved through the mitral valve (MV) to outline the left ventricle (LV). Contrast medium remains in the conus arteriosus and among the trabeculae of the right ventricular wall which wraps around the left ventricle caudally. The left auricle (LU) is seen over the area occupied by the sinuses of the aorta. In addition, the aorta (AO) is seen over the main pulmonary artery (MPA). In nonselective angiocardiography these superimpositions are further complicated by the presence of the cranial vena cava and right auricle, thus making diagnosis of lesions in this area extremely difficult by that method. (Angiocardiogram courtesy of Dr. Richard D. Park).

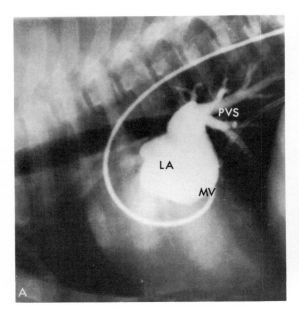

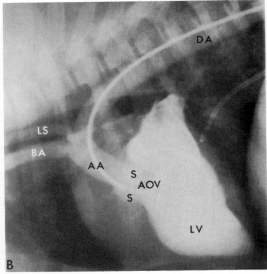

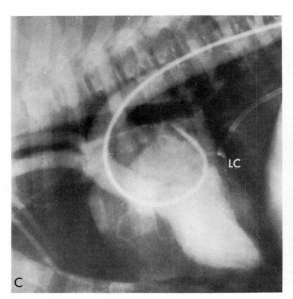

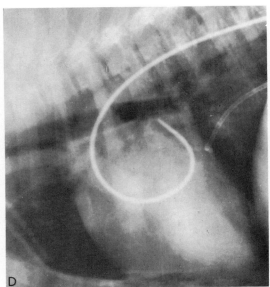

Figure 12–37. Right lateral angiocardiogram, after selective left atrial injection, of female Chesapeake Bay Retriever approximately 10 weeks old. A 5F Kifa catheter was fashioned so that it could be passed from the femoral artery through the aorta, left ventricle, and into the left atrium. Another Kifa catheter lies in the caudal vena cava. Six milliliters of Hypaque-M 75% was injected. Film A was exposed immediately after injection, film B 2 sec later, film C 3 sec, and film D 4 sec after film A. *A,* The left atrium (LA) is filled with contrast medium. It has a smooth wall. The left auricle is not well seen in this series. The pulmonary veins (PVS) are filled briefly in a retrograde manner. The mitral valve (MV) is closed because the ventricle is in systole.

B, The mitral valve has opened and the diastolic left ventricle (LV) is filled. It has a smooth, cone-shaped outline. Contrast medium has been ejected through the aortic valve (AOV), which is now closed. A previous contraction has outlined the sinuses of the aorta (S), the ascending aorta (AA), and descending aorta (DA) with contrast medium. The brachiocephalic artery (BA) and left subclavian artery (LS) branch from the aortic arch.

C, The ventricle is in systole. Its diameter is less. Contrast medium in the left atrium is diluted with fresh blood. The left circumflex coronary artery (LC) is seen; the left descending and right coronary arteries are not well outlined. (See Fig. 12–35A.)

D, The left atrium is nearly empty. Contrast medium in the left ventricle and aorta is barely visible, as it has nearly all been carried away with unopacified blood. (Angiocardiogram courtesy of Dr. Peter F. Suter.)

TABLE 12–3

DRUGS FOR CARDIAC EMERGENCIES

Cardiovascular Support and Cardiac Arrhythmia

Isoproterenal HCl (Isuprel) — Dilute 1 mg in 250 ml of dextrose and water solution. Use intravenous drip to maintain heart rate between 80 to 140 beats/minute.

Epinephrine HCl (1:10,000) — Administer 1 cc intracardiac to convert cardiac standstill to coarse ventricular fibrillation, or weak bradycardia to rapid stronger beat. Coarse ventricular fibrillation may be converted by DC shock.

Lidocaine HCl (Xylocaine) — This preparation is without epinephrine in a 20 mg/cc strength. To control ventricular arrhythmias, give 2 to 4 mg/lb by slow IV bolus and follow with quinidine sulfate, administered orally if indicated.

Fluid Retention and Pulmonary Parenchymal Fluid

Diuretics

Lasix — $\frac{1}{2}$ to 1 mg/lb IV, IM, SC, or orally.

Hydrodiuril — 1 mg/lb every 12 hours orally.

Bronchodilators

Aminophylline — 250 mg/cc; give 2 to 4 mg/lb IM.

Analgesia

Demerol — 1 to 5 mg/lb IM: if shock is present, give 1 mg/lb IM.

Morphine — 1 mg/lb IM or SC in dogs. 0.1 mg/lb IM or SC in cats.

Tranquilizers

Acepromazine — 1 mg/20 lb IM or IV. It may cause vasodilation; therefore, do not use in shock states.

Chlorpromazine (Thorazine) — $\frac{1}{4}$ to $\frac{1}{2}$ mg/lb IM. If necessary, it can be used when shock is present because it functions as an α-blocker. It can be given after 15 cc/lb of lactated Ringer solution has been given IV.

Supplemental O₂

Administer by mask, intubation, tracheostomy, or in a modified O_2 cage (Kirschner).

Intravenous Fluids

Ringer's lactate — Use 7 cc sodium bicarbonate (44.6 mEq/50 cc) per 250 ml to neutralize; use 10 to 12 cc/250 ml if treating shock. Use 20 to 40 ml/lb, monitoring central venous pressure as the fluids are administered.

Saline — Use 7 cc sodium bicarbonate to neutralize.

Dextrose and saline.

Whole fresh blood.

Antibiotics

Broad-spectrum antibiotics should be given to all injured animals.

Shock States

Crystalline sodium penicillin — 1 to 5 million units in initial IV drip. Give IM penicillin and streptomycin simultaneously.

Chloromycetin IV — 10 to 25 mg/lb initially.

Intravenous Liquamycin — 25 mg/lb.

Nonshock States

Crystalline penicillin — SC or IM, 10,000 units/lb twice daily.

Penicillin — streptomycin IM.

Liquamycin — 25 mg/lb.

Chloromycetin IV — 10 to 25 mg/lb initially; then orally, 10 mg/lb qid for follow up.

Sodium Bicarbonate (44.6 mEq/50 cc)

Give $\frac{1}{2}$ to 1 cc/10 lb of body weight for shock and acidosis. Give in IV drip unless emergency such as cardiac arrest dictates that it be given directly. Often it is given as part of the IV drip solution as outlined above.

Corticosteroids (for shock)

Dexamethasone (Azium) — 1 to 5 mg/lb IV in association with 20 to 40 cc/lb of IV fluids for the first hour depending on cardiopulmonary function and urine output.

Hydrocortisone sodium succinate (Solu-Cortef) — 10 to 20 mg/lb IV.

For Strengthening Myocardial Contraction and Increasing Myocardial Excitability

Calcium gluconate — 10 per cent solution, 3 to 10 cc intravenously or intracardially.

Calcium chloride — 1 to 2 cc intravenously or intracardially.

From Ticer, J. W., and Brown, S. G.: Thoracic trauma. *In* Ettinger, S. J.: Textbook of Veterinary Internal Medicine: Diseases of the Dog and Cat. Philadelphia, W. B. Saunders Co., 1975.

are developed (preferably in an automatic processor) and studied for completeness. Before removing the catheters and closing the surgical site, it is important to ensure that all desired information has been collected. The patient is monitored while recovering from anesthesia. All equipment is serviced properly to avoid damage to sensitive transducers or clotting within the catheters and stopcocks.

RESULTS

To diagnose cardiac lesions by angiocardiography one must first be familiar with the normal angiocardiogram. The easiest way to acquire this understanding is to follow the circulation of contrast medium through each side of the heart. Refer to Figures 12–34 thru 12–37 for an understanding of the normal circulatory pattern.

Contrast medium injected into the right ventricle outlines its irregular cavity (Figs. 12–34 and 12–36). Next the dye is seen in the conus arteriosus of the ventricle. It crosses the pulmonic valve, entering the main pulmonary artery. This vessel branches immediately into the left and right pulmonary arteries. Contrast material then outlines the respective arteries of each lung lobe. In many studies, circulation of dye through the lungs presents enough of a bolus of contrast medium to the pulmonary veins to produce reasonable opacification of the left heart circulation. However, the clarity needed for diagnostic films of the left side must usually come from selective injection there. For the same reason, nonselective studies are usually not diagnostic for lesions in the left heart or between the two circulations.

If contrast medium is injected in the left atrium (Figs. 12–35 and 12–37), some of the pulmonary veins may be briefly outlined in a retrograde manner. This is followed by rapid filling of the left ventricle as the dye crosses the mitral valve. The normal left ventriculogram is smooth and cone-shaped. Systole ejects the dye across the aortic valve, outlining the three bulging sinuses of the aorta and the ascending and descending aorta. The coronary arteries may be seen just above the aortic sinuses. The contrast medium leaves the vascular structures in the same order in which it enters them, although usually less dramatically because of blood dilution.

REFERENCES

Buchanan, J. W.: Selective angiography and angiocardiography in dogs with acquired cardiovascular disease. J. Amer. Vet. Radiol. Soc., 6:5, 1965.

Buchanan, J. W., and Patterson, D. F.: Selective angiography and angiocardiography in dogs with congenital cardiovascular disease. J. Amer. Vet. Radiol. Soc., 6:21, 1965.

Detweiler, D. K., Hubben, K., and Patterson, D. F.: Survey on cardiovascular disease in dogs: preliminary report on the first 1000 dogs screened. Amer. J. Vet. Res. 21:329, 1960.

Detweiler, D. K.: Cardiovascular disease in animals. A. Trisala (ed.), Encyclopedia of the Cardiovascular System, Vol. 5. New York, McGraw-Hill, 1961.

Ettinger, S. J., and Suter, P. F.: Canine Cardiology. Philadelphia, W. B. Saunders Co., 1970.

Fabian, L. W., and Short, C. E.,: Anesthesia for the patient with acquired and congenital heart disease. Vet. Clin. N. Amer., 3:33–44, 1973.

Felson, B. (ed.): Roentgen Techniques in Laboratory Animals. Philadelphia, W. B. Saunders, 1968.

Friedberg, C. K.: Diseases of the Heart, Philadelphia, W. B. Saunders Co., 1966.

Grossman, W. (ed.): Cardiac Catheterization and Angiography. Philadelphia, Lea and Febiger, 1974.

Hamlin, R. L.: Angiocardiography for the clinical diagnosis of congenital heart disease in small animals. J. Amer. Vet. Med. Assoc. 135:112, 1959.

Hamlin, R. L.: Radiographic anatomy of the heart and great vessels in healthy living dogs. J. Amer. Vet. Med. Assoc., 136:265, 1960.

Kirk, R. W. and Bistner, S. I.: Handbook of Veterinary Procedures and Emergency Treatment. Philadelphia, W. B. Saunders, Co., 1969.

Knight, D. H.: Principles of catheterization. In R. W. Kirk (ed.): Current Veterinary Therapy V. Philadelphia, W. B. Saunders, 1971.

Kory, R. C., Tsagans, T. J., and Bustamonte, R. A.: A Primer of Cardiac Catheterization. Springfield, Ill. Charles C Thomas, 1965.

Kraner, K. W.: Angiocardiography in acquired heart disease. J. Amer. Anim. Hosp. Assoc., 8:308, 1972.

Moscovitz, H. L., Donoso, E., Gelb, I. J., and Wilder, R. J.: An Atlas of Hemodymanics of the Cardiovascular System. New York, Grune Stratton, 1963.

Patterson, D. F.: Angiocardiography. J. Amer. Vet. Radiol. Soc., 1:26, 1961.

Pyle, R. L.: Angiocardiography in congenital cardiovascular diseases of the dog. J. Amer. Anim. Hosp. Assoc., 8:310, 1972.

Rushmer, R.: Cardiovascular dynamics. 4th ed. Philadelphia, W. B. Saunders Co., (in press).

Rhodes, W. H., Patterson, D. F., and Detweiler, D. K.: Radiographic anatomy of the canine heart. Part I. J. Amer. Vet. Assoc., 137:283, 1960.

Rhodes, W. H., Patterson, D. F., and Detweiler, D. K.: Radiographic anatomy of the canine heart. Part II. J. Amer. Vet. Med. Assoc., 143:137, 1963.

Rising, J. L., and Lewis, R. E.: A technique for arterial catheterization in the dog. Amer. J. Vet. Res., 31: 1309, 1970.

Tashjian, R. J., and Albanese, N. M.: A technique of canine angiocardiography. J. Amer. Vet. Med. Assoc., 136:359, 1960.

Wallace, C.: Cardiac catheterization to aid in diagnosis of cardiovascular disease. Small Anim. Clin., 2:324, 1962.

Zimmerman, H. A. (ed.): Intravascular Catheterization, 2nd ed. Springfield, Ill., Charles C Thomas, 1966.

13
ABDOMEN

Radiographic examination of the abdomen requires careful technique. Excellent radiographic quality is essential for providing accurate diagnostic information.

Patient Preparation

Radiographic visualization of abdominal structures is very difficult, if not impossible, in the presence of a large amount of ingesta within the gastrointestinal tract (Root, 1974a). A 12-hour fast should precede most routine abdominal radiographic examinations. In patients with a history of emesis or anorexia for 12 hours or more, this fasting period may be omitted. Generally, routine examinations do not require that an enema be given. Water may be given during the fasting period, but the patient should not be allowed excessive consumption immediately prior to radiography.

In severely debilitated patients and patients with life-threatening metabolic disorders, such as diabetes mellitus, fasting may be contraindicated. In these cases, a diet of low residue foods, such as baby foods or dietary concentrates (Pet Kalorie, Haver-Lockhart Laboratories; Nutri-cal, EVSCO Pharmaceutical Corp.), may be fed 12 to 24 hours prior to radiographic examination.

Mild cathartics or enemas may be used in the preparation of patients for abdominal radiography, especially if there is a relatively good chance that a special contrast procedure will be performed after the initial radiographs are produced. Generally, gravity flow, water or isotonic saline enemas are superior to hypertonic enema preparations (Root, 1974a). The enema fluid temperature should be less than that of the body since this seems to stimulate expulsion of much of the gas that usually remains in the colon after warm enemas (Root, 1974a).

Exposure Technique

Marked loss of radiographic detail occurs if exposures are made during normal diaphragmatic excursions. Exposures are best made during the pause that occurs at the end of expiration. At this point in the respiratory cycle, the diaphragm is cranially displaced and the body wall is relaxed (Root, 1974a). This avoids crowding of abdominal viscera and ensures adequate time to make the exposures without the blurring effect produced by diaphragmatic movements. By producing radiographs of the abdomen during the expiratory pause, there is an added benefit in that there is maximum separation of the kidneys in the lateral projection, thus enhancing visualization (Grandage, 1975).

Measurement for determining exposure technique is usually best made over the caudal rib cage, where the greatest width of the abdomen occurs. This will avoid underexposure of the relatively dense structures of the cranial abdomen. In extremely deep-chested dogs, additional radiographs produced with a decreased exposure may be necessary to examine the caudal abdomen.

Procedure

Right Lateral View. The patient is placed in right lateral recumbency, with the sternum elevated to the same height above the x-ray table as the lumbar spine, and the femurs are placed at approximately 90 degrees to the vertebral column (Fig. 13–1).

The x-ray beam is centered midabdominally and is collimated to include the region between the xyphoid and the pubis. The radiograph is produced during the expiratory pause.

Figure 13–2 illustrates the normal radiographic anatomy of the canine abdomen in right lateral recumbency.

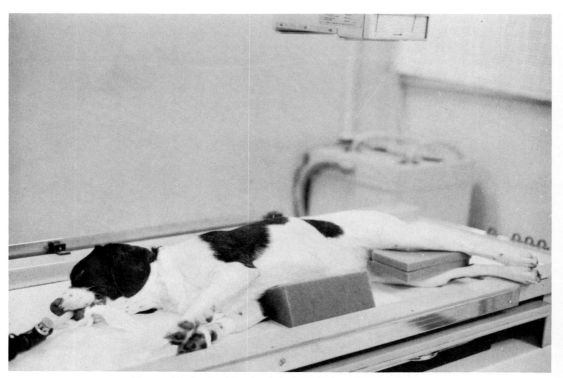

Figure 13–1. Position for right lateral view of the abdomen.

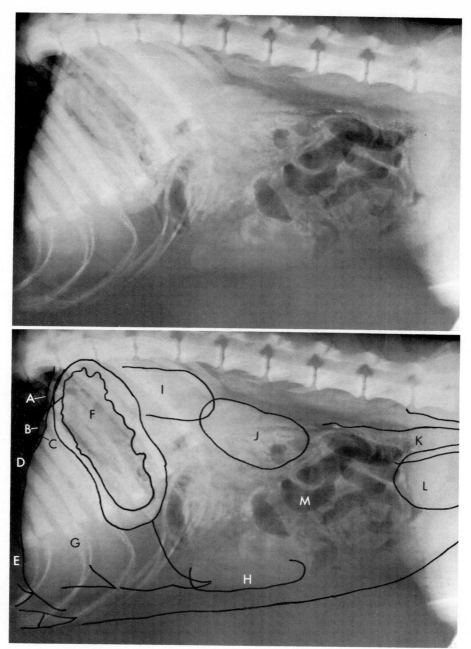

Figure 13–2. Right lateral view of the canine abdomen. Note that the right crus *(A)* is cranially displaced and the vena cava *(D)* is more dorsally located compared to the left lateral view (Fig. 13–4). The liver *(G)* also appears moderately larger in right lateral view. The left kidney is bean-shaped in right lateral view (see text). Gas pattern of the stomach outlines the fundus and body *(F)* in the right lateral view.

A. Right diaphragmatic crus
B. Intercrural cleft
C. Left diaphragmatic crus
D. Caudal vena cava
E. Heart
F. Fundus and body of the stomach
G. Liver
H. Spleen
I. Right kidney
J. Left kidney
K. Descending colon
L. Urinary bladder
M. Small bowel

337

Left Lateral View. The patient is placed in left lateral recumbency, with the sternum elevated to the same height above the x-ray table as the lumbar spine, and the femurs are placed at approximately 90 degrees to the vertebral column (Fig. 13–3). The x-ray beam is centered midabdominally and is collimated to include the region between the xyphoid and the pubis. The radiograph is produced during the expiratory pause.

Figure 13–4 illustrates the normal radiographic anatomy of the canine abdomen in left lateral recumbency.

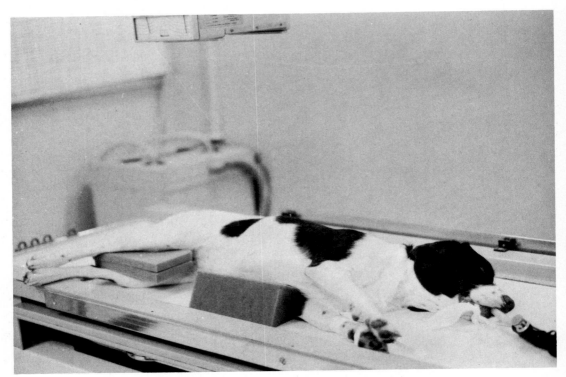

Figure 13–3. Position for left lateral view of the abdomen.

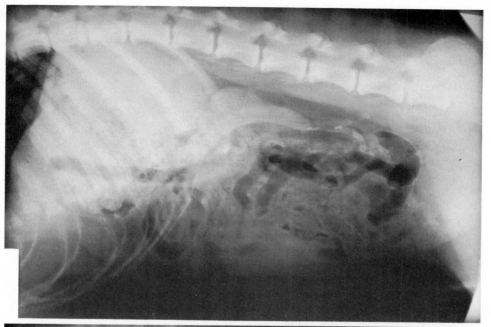

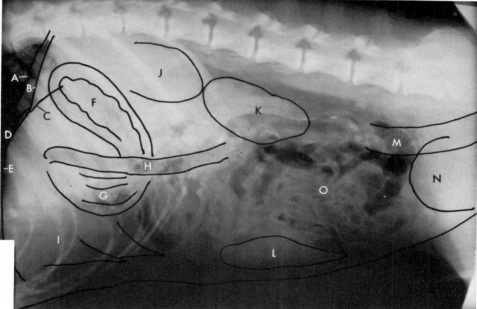

Figure 13–4. Left lateral view of the canine abdomen. Note that the left crus *(A)* is cranially displaced and the vena cava *(D)* is more ventrally located compared to the right lateral view (Fig. 13–2). The liver *(I)* appears smaller compared to the right lateral view. The gas pattern of the stomach shows a decreased volume in the fundus *(F)* and increased volume in the pyloric antrum *(G)* compared to the right lateral view (Fig. 13–2).

A. Left diaphragmatic crus
B. Right diaphragmatic crus
C. Intracrural cleft
D. Caudal vena cava
E. Diaphragmatic cupula
F. Fundus of the stomach
G. Pyloric antrum of the stomach
H. Descending duodenum
I. Liver
J. Right kidney
K. Left kidney
L. Spleen
M. Colon
N. Urinary bladder
O. Small bowel

Ventrodorsal View. The patient is placed in dorsal recumbency with the rear limbs in a "frog leg" position (Fig. 13–5). This will prevent stretching of the inguinal flank folds, thus avoiding the artifacts frequently caused by those structures (Root, 1974*a*). The x-ray beam is centered at the umbilicus and is collimated to include the region between the xyphoid and the pubis. The radiograph is produced during the expiratory pause.

Figure 13–6 illustrates the normal radiographic anatomy of the canine abdomen in VD recumbency.

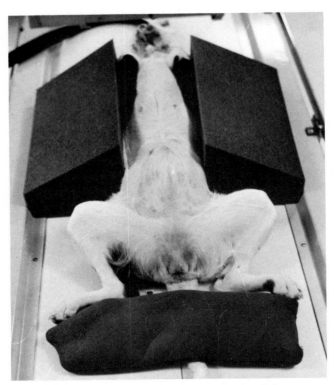

Figure 13–5. Position for the VD view of the abdomen.

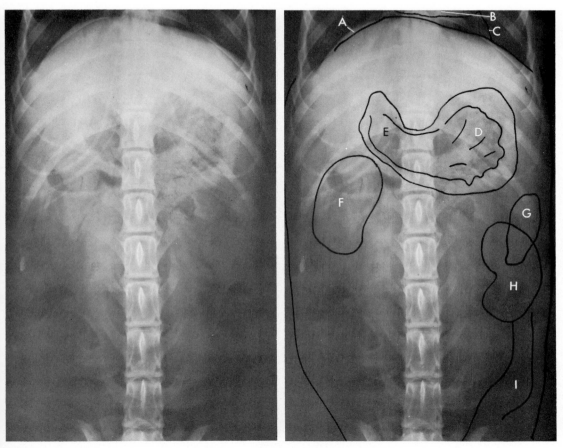

Figure 13–6. VD view of the canine abdomen. Note the increased volume of gas in the pyloric antrum *(E)* compared to the DV view (Fig. 13–8).

A. Diaphragm
B. Heart
C. Cardiophrenic ligament
D. Fundus of the stomach
E. Pyloric antrum of the stomach
F. Right kidney
G. Spleen
H. Left kidney
I. Descending colon

Dorsoventral View. The patient is placed in ventral recumbency, with the rear limbs in "frog leg" position (Fig. 13–7). The x-ray beam is centered just caudal to the thirteenth rib arch and collimated to include the xyphoid and the pubis. The radiograph is produced during the expiratory pause.

Figure 13–8 illustrates the normal radiographic anatomy of the canine abdomen in DV recumbency.

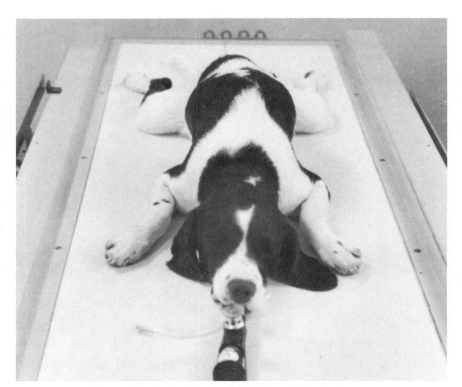

Figure 13–7. Position for the DV view of the abdomen.

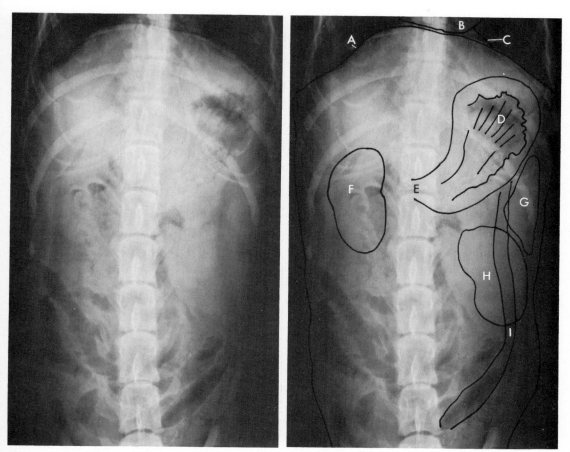

Figure 13–8. DV view of the canine abdomen. Note the decreased volume of gas and medical displacement of the pyloric antrum *(E)* compared to the VD view (Fig. 13–6).

A. Diaphragm
B. Heart
C. Cardiophrenic ligament
D. Fundus of the stomach
E. Pyloric antrum of the stomach
F. Right kidney
G. Spleen
H. Left kidney
I. Descending colon

Interpretation

The position and appearance of the normal abdominal viscera vary, depending on postural relationships, respiratory cycle, physiological state, body type, and x-ray beam geometry. Generally the most variable position is observed in the structures of the cranial abdomen: diaphragm, liver, stomach, descending duodenum, spleen and kidneys.

Stomach and Diaphragm

The body and fundus of the stomach are located on the left side of the midline and are in direct contact with the left hemidiaphragm. In lateral projection, the air- or ingesta-filled stomach may be seen in direct contact with the left diaphragmatic crus. Since the dependent crus sags cranially in lateral recumbency, the left crus and stomach will be projected cranial to the right crus in left lateral recumbency (Grandage, 1974; Root, 1974a). The crural lines tend to cross at the intracrural cleft. In right lateral recumbency, the crura appears parallel with the right crus, displaced cranially when the x-ray beam is centered at the midabdomen. A line drawn through the fundus, body and pylorus on the lateral recumbent radiograph may be perpendicular to the vertebral column, may run parallel to the ribs or may lie in between these extremes in normality (Root, 1974a).

In the VD view, a line drawn through the fundus to the pylorus should be perpendicular to the vertebral column.

Fluid gastric contents are extremely mobile and tend to move to the dependent portions of the stomach during postural changes.

In right lateral recumbency, gas is seen in the fundus and body of the stomach, and in left lateral recumbency, gas is seen in the fundus and pylorus.

Ventrodorsal views of the stomach show air in the fundus, body, and pylorus of the stomach and descending duodenum, while in the DV view, most of the air is in the fundus. The VD abdominal view tends to show the diaphragmatic outline as a single dome-like shadow with the right hemidiaphragm slightly displaced cranially (Grandage, 1974). There may be a distinct cardiac depression seen slightly to the left of the midline, particularly in small, barrel-chested dogs.

In deep-chested dogs, the DV abdominal view projects the diaphragm as a trilobed shadow with the right and left crus located lateral to a centrally located cupula.

Spleen

The splenic shadow may also vary in location and appearance with postural changes. The head of the spleen is attached to the stomach, and the body and tail are very mobile. In left lateral recumbency, the entire splenic shadow may be hidden beneath the small intestines and may not be visualized radiographically. In right lateral recumbency, a portion of the spleen is usually seen on the ventral abdomen just caudal to the liver margin. The most usual projection shows a crescent-shaped or curved triangular shadow produced as the x-ray beam is absorbed by a portion of the spleen that is tangential to the central ray. The remaining portion of the spleen is presented with its flat surface to the x-ray beam, thereby not absorbing sufficient x-rays to produce a distinct shadow.

In the VD or DV projection, the spleen appears as a small triangle just caudal to the stomach fundus.

Liver

The position and size of the liver vary with postural changes and respiration. Right lateral recumbency allows the left lateral liver lobe to slide caudally, causing the projection of a larger shadow than that seen in left lateral recumbency (Grandage, 1974). Moderate rotation of the trunk may allow the increased obliquity of the x-ray beam to produce a falsely rounded caudoventral margin (Root, 1974a). The fat-laden falciform ligament of the liver appears larger on exhalation and smaller on inhalation.

Kidneys

Kidney size may be estimated by comparing the kidney length to the length of a vertebral body (Kneller, 1974). The normal canine kidney length is roughly three times the length of the second lumbar vertebra (Finco et al., 1971). A range of from 2½ to 3⅓ times the length should be considered within normal limits (Osborn et al., 1972). The normal feline kidney is 2½ to 3 times the length of the L_2 (Barrett and Kneller, 1972). Very young kittens and large male cats have relatively large kidneys (Hall and MacGregor, 1937).

The width and shape of the kidney may vary with postural changes. In lateral recumbency, the uppermost kidney will rotate on its longitudinal axis, profiling the hilar notch and appearing bean-shaped (Grandage, 1974). This appearance is due to the relative mobility of the kidney that allows the lateral aspect to fall downward in lateral recumbency.

This rotation also allows the region of kidney that is well covered by adipose tissue to be presented tangentially to the x-ray beam, thus allowing better radiographic contrast between the perirenal fat and the kidney capsule. Therefore, when one of the kidneys is of particular interest, it should be placed up in at least one of the lateral recumbent positions.

Passive movements of the diaphragm may allow a shift in the location of the kidneys by 2 cm or more (Grandage, 1974). In right lateral recumbency, the right kidney may be displaced cranially ½ to 1 vertebral length when compared to left lateral recumbency, because of the cranial displacement of the dependent diaphragmatic crus. The normally staggered arrangement of the kidneys, with the left kidney slightly caudal to the right, is therefore usually accentuated in right lateral recumbency and reduced in left lateral recumbency (Grandage, 1975). Therefore, survey radiographs of the kidneys are best produced in right lateral recumbency in order to provide maximum kidney separation.

Small Bowel

The small bowel occupies nearly all of the abdominal space not taken up by the less mobile viscera. Displacement usually indicates the presence of a pathologic process, such as a space-occupying mass or a specific intestinal disorder.

Colon

The ascending colon and cecum are usually located on the right side of the abdomen, and the descending colon is located on the left side when viewed in VD or DV projection. The descending colon may be displaced to the right by a distended urinary bladder. When viewed in lateral projection, the ascending and descending sections of the colon are usually superimposed and located approximately halfway between the vertebral column and the ventral abdomen.

Urinary Bladder and Prostate Gland

A distended urinary bladder may displace abdominal viscera cranially and the descending colon to the right. The prostate gland should be mostly contained in the pelvic canal but may be cranially displaced by moderate benign prostatic hypertrophy that is without clinical significance.

Other Viscera

Normally the adrenal glands, mesentery, mesenteric lymph nodes, omentum, pancreas, abdominal aorta, abdominal vena cava, gallbladder, ovaries and uterus are not seen radiographically (Root, 1974a).

Recumbent VD View With Horizontal X-ray Beam

The patient is placed in left lateral recumbency and a horizontal x-ray beam is used to produce a VD view (Fig. 13–9). The x-ray beam is centered at the cranial abdomen and the exposure is made during the expiratory pause.

This examination is indicated when free air is suspected in the peritoneal space because of ruptured viscus.

Figure 13–10 illustrates the normal radiographic anatomy of the canine abdomen in the recumbent VD view with a horizontal x-ray beam.

Figure 13–11 illustrates the appearance of free air in the peritoneal space as a result of a ruptured small bowel segment.

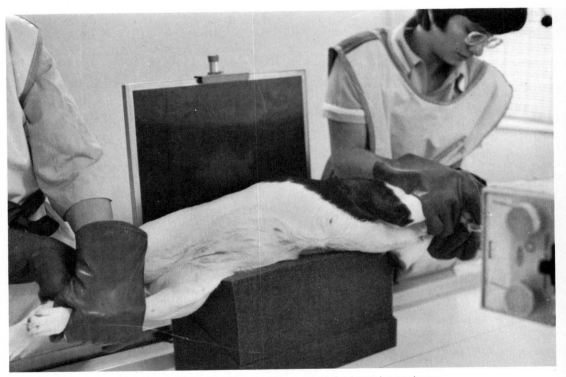

Figure 13–9. Position for VD view with horizontal x-ray beam.

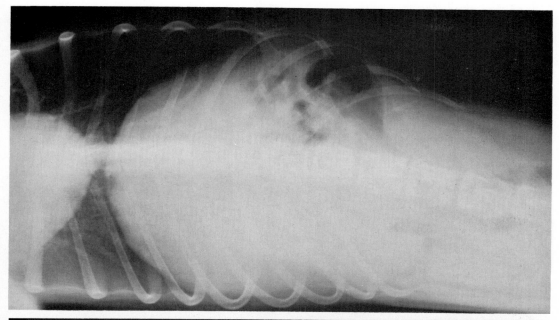

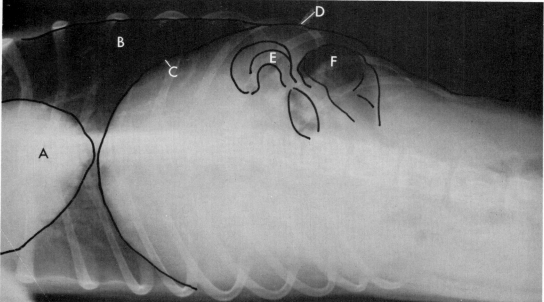

Figure 13–10. VD view with horizontal x-ray beam of the canine abdomen, right side down.

A. Heart
B. Left lung
C. Diaphragm
D. Right craniolateral abdominal wall
E. Gas in small bowel loops
F. Gas in cecum

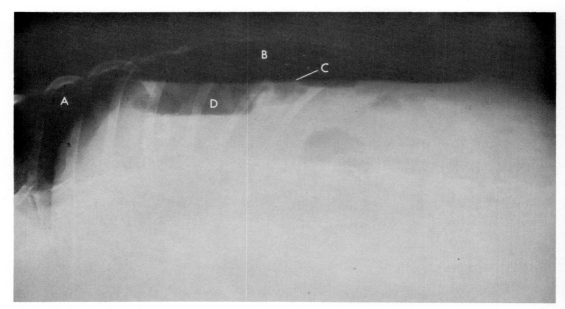

Figure 13–11. VD view with horizontal x-ray beam illustrating the appearance of free air in the peritoneal space due to a rupture of a small bowel segment, right side down.

        A. Left lung
        B. Free air in the peritoneal space
        C. Air-fluid interface
        D. Gas in the stomach

Pneumoperitonography

Pneumoperitonography is a negative contrast medium examination of the abdominal cavity after the introduction of a gas into the peritoneal space for the purpose of increasing subject contrast.

Indication

Pneumoperitonography is indicated when the demonstration of an organ or mass is not possible with routine radiography because of an inherent lack of subject (patient) contrast. These situations exist when there is insufficient abdominal adipose tissue to cause contrast and may also be caused by many physiologic or pathologic states, the most common being an accumulation of excessive peritoneal fluid.

Contraindication

Contraindications for pneumoperitonography are limited to those that preclude profound sedation or anesthesia. In some cooperative patients, this contraindication may be overcome by performing the procedure with local anesthesia.

Technique

Patient Preparation

Generally a 12-hour fast and profound sedation or anesthesia are necessary. Local anesthesia at the injection site is sometimes sufficient, but this method should be reserved for those patients for whom chemical restraint is contraindicated.

The midventral abdomen should be clipped and prepared surgically.

Materials

A large syringe, three-way valve and an 18-gauge indwelling catheter (Sovereign Indwelling Catheter, Sherwood Medical; Jelco I.V. Catheter Placement Unit, Jelco Laboratories) are used for patients without peritoneal fluid. Compressed gases (such as oxygen, CO_2, or nitrous oxide) may be used instead of room air, but these must be administered with caution to avoid overdistention of the abdomen. The advantage of CO_2 and nitrous oxide is their increased rate of absorption from the peritoneal space.

If peritoneal fluid is present, a small rubber feeding catheter (Brunswick Feeding Catheter) with several previously placed holes in the side of the tube near the end is used to facilitate drainage prior to air injection.

Dosage

Generally 200 to 1000 cc of gas provides sufficient contrast for most pneumoperitonograms; however, if gross displacement of mobile viscera is desired for horizontal x-ray beam studies, the volume of gas may be increased until moderate abdominal distention is obtained (Carlson, 1967).

Medium Injection

The patient is placed in left lateral recumbency, theoretically to permit any inadvertent vascular air introduction to be trapped in the right atrium. This is said to allow slow liberation of the air into the pulmonary circulation, preventing air embolism (Root, 1974b). If no peritoneal fluid is present, the indwelling catheter is introduced into the abdomen approximately 1 cm lateral to the umbilicus. To assure that no organ is penetrated, the needle and catheter assembly are directed at a 70 to 90 degree angle to the sagittal plane (vertebral-sternal axis) of the abdomen (Barrett, 1975).

The catheter and needle assembly should just penetrate the parietal peritoneum. The needle is then withdrawn approximately 1 cm from the catheter before the assembly is advanced into the peritoneal space to the full length of the catheter. The needle is then withdrawn fully and a 3-way valve and syringe are attached. The use of the indwelling catheter instead of a needle for medium injection has the advantage of being less traumatic during subsequent manipulations. This technique will also decrease the incidence of medium injection into the falciform ligament, small bowel, spleen or vasculature. Splenic or vascular injection will result in air embolism. Gas is then injected, while respiration is monitored. Simultaneous pneumothorax may be produced in patients with a ruptured diaphragm. Demonstration of a ruptured diaphragm may be accomplished by performing pneumoperitonography with 10 to 20 cc of air and radiographing in an erect VD view, using a horizontal x-ray beam (Roenigk, 1971; Ticer and Brown [in press]). In the presence of an intact diaphragm, the injected air will accumulate under the diaphragm and allow the liver to fall away in a caudal direction. If diaphragmatic rupture is present, the air will be found at the pleural space cranial to the cranial lung lobes.

Excessive peritoneal fluid accumulation necessitates drainage prior to pneumoperitonography. This is accomplished by the insertion of a catheter into the peritoneum through a small incision made immediately lateral to the umbilicus. This procedure is best accomplished by making a stab incision with a No. 11 blade and introducing the catheter tip through the hole while holding the catheter between the jaws of a small forceps. The forceps is then retracted and the catheter is inserted approximately 3 to 4 cm and fixed in place with a single suture. Drainage of peritoneal fluids will then occur without aspiration. Upon completion of drainage, a sufficient amount of air will have been aspirated into the peritoneal space to impart adequate radiographic contrast to the serosal surfaces (Fig. 13–12). A small addi-

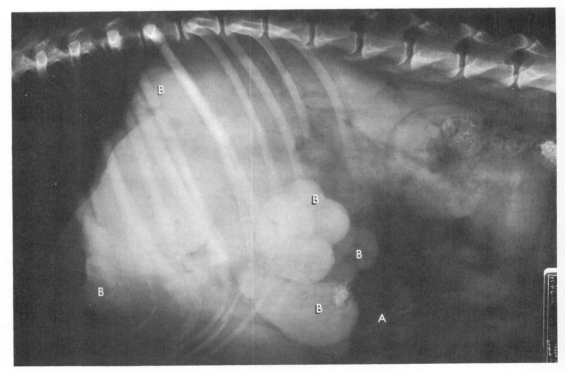

Figure 13–12. Lateral view of a nine year old female airedale abdomen with pneumoperitonogram produced after drainage of 9 liters of serosanguinous fluid and injection of 1 liter of air via an indwelling catheter (A). Radiographs produced prior to drainage and air injection were undiagnostic because the serosal surfaces were rendered indistinct by the peritoneal fluid. The pneumoperitonogram shows multiple globular masses on the liver and spleen (B). Histological diagnosis was hemangiosarcoma.

tional amount of air (200 to 500 cc) may be injected if desired.

Radiography

Routine VD and lateral views are produced upon completion of medium injection. A DV view may be needed if the structures in the dorsal abdomen are of interest.

Erect, inverted and standing radiographs may be produced using a horizontal x-ray beam if a specific demonstration of a given abdominal region is desired.

Interpretation

Interpretation of pneumoperitonograms is essentially the same as for routine abdominal radiography. Care should be taken not to mistake normal structures not usually seen on routine radiographs (such as the normal ovarian bursa) for abnormalities.

Figures 13–13 through 13–19 show the normal radiographic anatomy of the canine abdomen seen with pneumoperitonography.

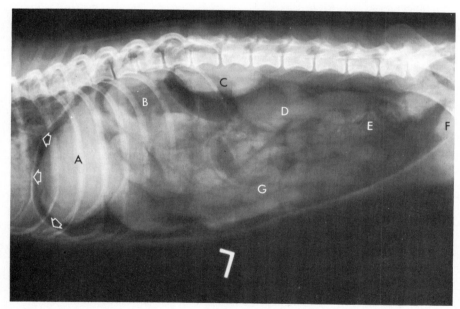

Figure 13–13. Left lateral view of a canine pneumoperitonogram. Arrows indicate diaphragm.
A. Liver
B. Fundus of the stomach
C. Right kidney
D. Left kidney
E. Colon
F. Urinary bladder
G. Small bowel

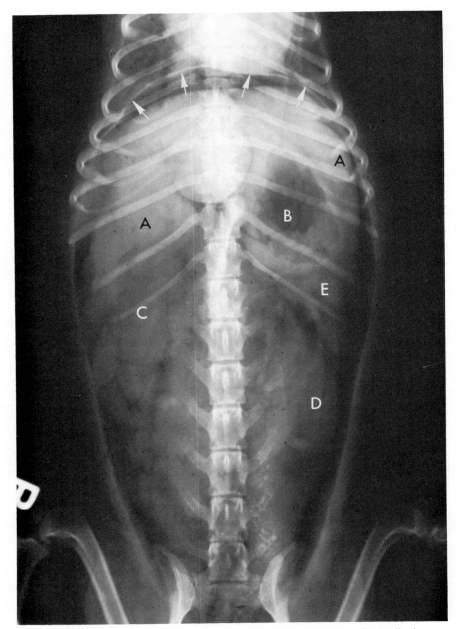

Figure 13–14. VD view of a canine pneumoperitonogram. Arrows indicate diaphragm.
A. Liver
B. Fundus of the stomach
C. Right kidney
D. Left kidney
E. Spleen

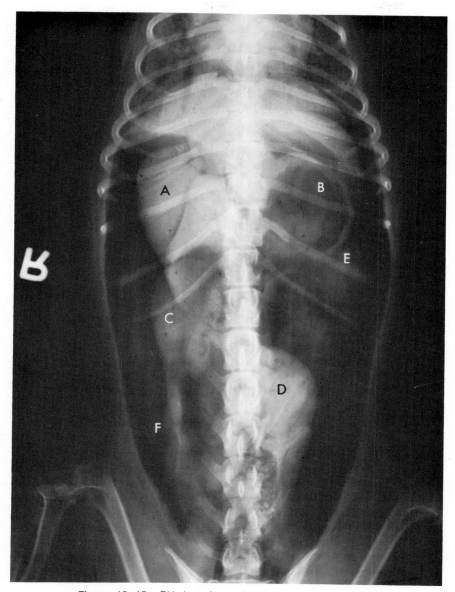

Figure 13–15. DV view of a canine pneumoperitonogram.
   A. Liver
   B. Fundus of the stomach
   C. Right kidney
   D. Left kidney
   E. Spleen
   F. Small bowel

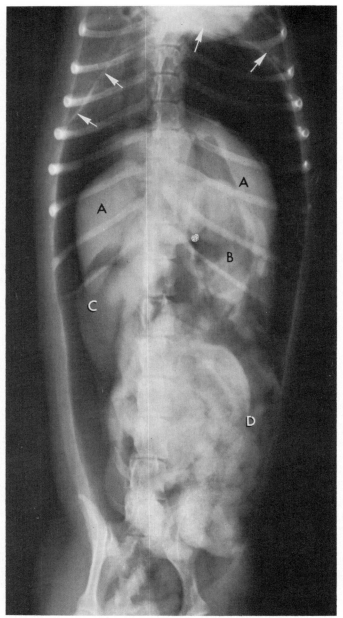

Figure 13–16. VD view of a canine pneumoperitonogram using an erect posture (patient suspended by forelimbs) and a horizontal x-ray beam. Arrows indicate diaphragm.

A. Liver
B. Fundus of the stomach
C. Right kidney
D. Small bowel

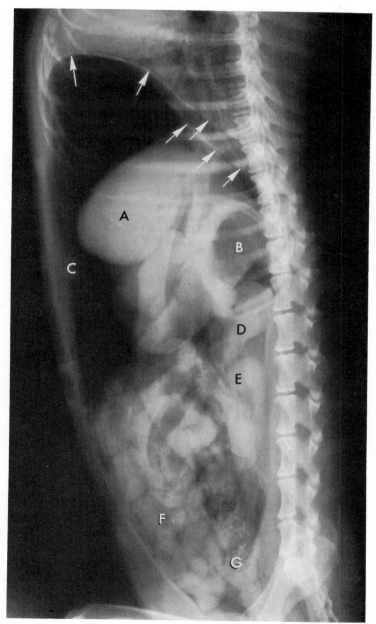

Figure 13–17. Lateral view of a canine pneumoperitonogram using an erect posture (patient suspended by forelimbs) and a horizontal x-ray beam. Arrows indicate diaphragm.

A. Liver
B. Fundus of the stomach
C. Falciform ligament of the liver
D. Right kidney
E. Left kidney
F. Small bowel
G. Colon

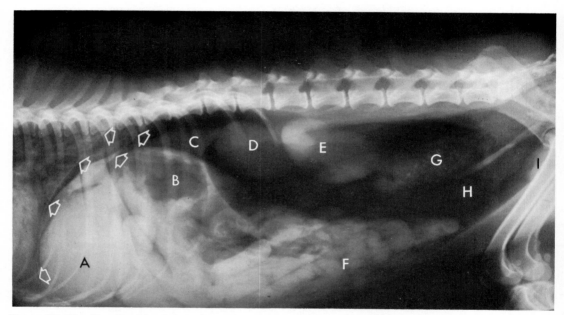

Figure 13–18. Standing lateral view of a canine pneumoperitonogram using a horizontal x-ray beam. Arrows indicate diaphragm.

A. Liver
B. Fundus of the stomach
C. Caudate lobe of the liver
D. Right kidney
E. Left kidney
F. Small bowel
G. Colon
H. Uterus
I. Urinary bladder

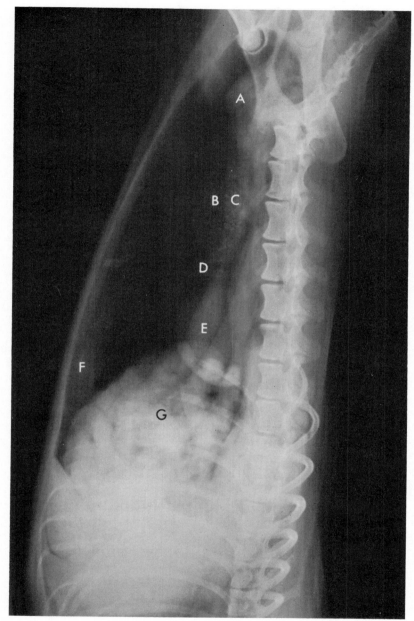

Figure 13–19. Lateral view of a canine pneumoperitonogram using an inverted posture (patient suspended by rear limbs) and a horizontal x-ray beam.

A. Urinary bladder
B. Uterus
C. Colon
D. Ovary
E. Left kidney
F. Falciform ligament of the liver
G. Small bowel

Cholecystography

Cholecystography is the radiographic examination of the main bile ducts and gallbladder after uptake of a radiodense medium.

Indications

Cholecystography may be indicated to visualize the bile ducts and gallbladder when there is evidence of biliary tract or gallbladder disease, such as cholangiectasis, cholecystitis, cholelithiasis, or gallbladder or bile duct neoplasia.

Contraindications

The use of meglumine iodipamide is contraindicated in patients with hypersensitivity to organic iodides. This condition is rare in dogs and cats. Administration of the salts of iodipamide are also contraindicated in patients with severe impairment of renal or liver function or in cases of hyperthyroidism.

Technique

Materials

The preferred medium for cholecystography in the dog and cat is Meglumine Iodipamide U.S.P. (Cholografin Meglumine, Squibb & Sons), injected intravenously.

Dosage

An intravenous dose of 0.2 cc/kg body weight is usually adequate.

Procedure

Survey radiographs of the cranial abdomen are produced in at least the lateral and VD projections. The medium is injected into the cephalic vein over a period of approximately 3 minutes. Rapid injection may produce discomfort and retching. Radiographs of the cranial abdomen are then produced at approximately 30 minutes, 60 minutes, and, if necessary, 90 minutes after injection.

If post-emptying study of the gallbladder is desired, a small fatty meal may be fed and radiographs produced in approximately 15 minutes.

Interpretation

The main bile ducts and gallbladder should be well opacified by the contrast medium (Fig. 13–20). Alterations in margination or content should be considered signs of disease. The radiographic appearance of bile duct and gallbladder disease has not been adequately described in dogs and cats; however, this should not discourage the use of the technique.

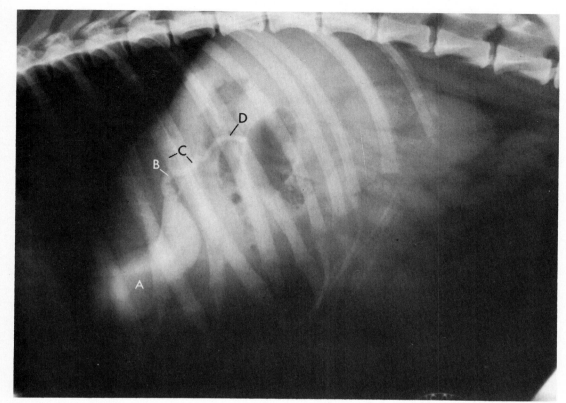

Figure 13–20. Lateral view of a canine cranial abdomen with a cholecystogram. This radiograph was produced 60 minutes after an intravenous injection of 0.2 cc/kg body weight of meglumine iodipamide.

  A. Gallbladder
  B. Cystic duct
  C. Hepatic ducts
  D. Common bile duct

REFERENCES

Amberg, J. R., and Roenigk, W. J.: In Felson, B. (Ed.): Roentgen Techniques in Laboratory Animals: Radiography of the Dog and Other Experimental Animals. Philadelphia, W. B. Saunders Co., 1968.

Barrett, R. B., and Kneller, S. K.: Feline kidney measuration. Acta Radiol. Suppl., *319*:279, 1972.

Barrett, R. B.: A new method of abdominal and thoracic pericentesis in the dog and cat. Vet. Med./Sm. Anim. Clin., *70*:76, 1975.

Carlson, W. D.: Veterinary Radiology. Philadelphia, Lea & Febiger, 1967.

Douglas, S. W., and Williamson, H. D.: Principles of Veterinary Radiography. 2nd Ed. Baltimore, Williams & Wilkins Co., 1972.

Finco, D. R., Stiles, N. S., and Kneller, S. K.: Radiologic estimation of kidney size of the dog. J. Amer. Vet. Med. Ass., *159*:995, 1971.

Grandage, J.: The radiology of the dog's diaphragm. J. Small Anim. Pract., *15*:1, 1974.

Grandage, J.: Some effects of posture on the radiographic appearance of the kidney of the dog. J. Amer. Vet. Med. Ass., *166*:165, 1975.

Hall, V. E., and MacGregor, W. W.: Relation of kidney weight to body weight in the cat. Anat. Rec., *69*:319, 1937.

Kneller, S. K.: Role of the excretory urogram in diagnosis of renal and ureteral disease. Vet. Clin. N. Amer., *4*:843, 1974.

Miller, M. E., Christensen, G. C., and Evans, H. E.: Anatomy of the Dog. Philadelphia, W. B. Saunders Co., 1964.

Osborne, C. A., Low, D. G., and Finco, D. R.: Canine and Feline Urology. Philadelphia, W. B. Saunders Co., 1972.

Roenigk, W. J.: Injuries to the Thorax. J. Amer. Anim. Hosp. Assoc., *7*:266, 1971.

Root, C. R.: Interpretation of Abdominal Survey Radiographs. Vet. Clin. N. Amer., *4*:763, 1974a.

Root, C. R.: Abdominal masses: The radiographic differential diagnosis. J. Amer. Vet. Radiol. Soc., *15*:26, 1974b.

Schebitz, H., and Wilkins, H.: Atlas of Radiographic Anatomy of Dog and Horse. Berlin, Paul Parey, 1968.

Ticer, J. W., and Brown, S. G.: Thoracic trauma. In Ettinger, S. J. (Ed.): Textbook of Veterinary Internal Medicine; Diseases of Dog and Cat. Philadelphia, W. B. Saunders Co., (in press).

Contrast Radiography of the Alimentary Tract

Charles R. Root

Few practicing veterinarians have access to equipment that will permit clinical evaluation of the dynamics of the alimentary tract. Fluoroscopy or its modern counterpart, image intensified fluoroscopy, enables one to thoroughly evaluate the upper gastrointestinal tract (esophagus, stomach and small bowel) with respect to peristalsis, transit time, mucosal integrity, and luminal size, shape and content. Of these factors, only peristalsis cannot be satisfactorily evaluated by routine radiography. The type of equipment necessary for appreciation of the dynamics of the gastrointestinal tract is expensive and usually is found only in teaching institutions, large private practices or specialty practices. Therefore, the following discussion of contrast radiography of the alimentary tract will not include the use of fluoroscopy or image intensification. The emphasis will be upon screening studies or those procedures most likely to yield a large amount of information. Special studies using barium-impregnated food or different concentrations of barium will not be discussed.

ESOPHOGRAM (BARIUM SWALLOW)

Indications

In general the esophagus should be evaluated every time barium sulfate suspension is administered. In most instances this is not done, making examination of the upper alimentary tract technically incomplete.

Specific indications for esophageal contrast studies include regurgitation of undigested food, persistent gagging or vomiting, and suspected esophageal foreign bodies (Douglas and Williamson, 1970, 1972; Morgan, 1964). Breed and age predisposition for megaesophagus should be borne in mind, especially if the clinical history specifically includes regurgitation rather than vomiting. Gagging, as an independent sign, often accompanies pharyngeal or tracheal disease. However, when gagging is accompanied by swallowing motions or excessive salivation or both, esophageal lesions are more likely. Positive history of the ingestion of any type of foreign body, accompanied by compatible signs, such as mild to severe dysphagia, salivation, gagging, hematemesis or anxiety, provides ample justification for contrast radiography of the esophagus. Delay in clinical detection of an esophageal lesion or detection of such a lesion at necropsy cannot be excused for economic reasons, either those of the client or those of the veterinarian.

True vomiting which is not responsive to symptomatic treatment is often indicative of lesions in the stomach or in the orad portion of the small bowel. However, even when the stomach and intestinal tract are the organs of primary interest, an esophageal study may demonstrate contributory secondary or simultaneous lesions.

Contraindications

Barium sulfate contrast radiography of the esophagus has not been recommended if there is reason to suspect rupture or perforation. However, it has been shown that neither barium sulfate nor organic iodides adversely affect existing periesophageal mediastinitis (Vessal, 1973). The presence of bronchoesophageal or similar fistulae is also a contraindication for esophageal contrast study. A small amount of pure barium sulfate suspension is well tolerated by normal lungs and bronchi (Dunbar, 1959; Nelson et al., 1964; Nice, 1964; Shook and Felson, 1970), but if introduced into diseased lung tissue, it may not be cleared normally. Another major contraindication for contrast radiography of the esophagus is the inability to swallow, since the danger of aspiration is increased when a large amount of barium is present in the caudal pharynx.

Preparation of Patient

The animal should be fasted for at least 12 hours before the administration of contrast material. Fasting permits the esophagus to empty, should it contain ingesta, which is often seen on survey films of the thorax in patients with one of the various forms of congenital or acquired megaesophagus. Fasting is advised even when esophageal dilation is not suspected, to reduce the possibility of artifacts caused by adherence of a small amount of ingesta to luminal masses or mucosal defects.

Scout films should be made in VD and lateral projections immediately before the contrast material is administered. Films made one to two days before giving the opaque agent will not suffice, since lesions may change appreciably in the interim.

Materials

No specific special equipment is required for esophageal contrast studies, but a large syringe facilitates administration of the contrast material. Esophageal contrast materials are supplied commercially in many forms, including $BaSO_4$ U.S.P., and micropulverized $BaSO_4$ powder (Micropaque, Barium Sulfate Powder, Damancy & Co., Ltd.), suspension (redi-FLOW Gastric and Colonic Barium Sulfate Suspensions, Flow Pharmaceuticals, Inc.; Novopaque, Barium Sulfate Suspension, Picker X-ray Corp.) and paste (Esophotrast, Barium Sulfate Esophageal Cream, Barnes-Hind Diagnostics). If the esophageal study is part of a complete upper gastrointestinal series, one of the liquid suspensions is preferred. Thick paste alone is not satisfactory for upper G.I. series and mixes poorly with the additional thin suspension necessary for the study of the stomach and small bowel. If, however, the study is specifically for opacification of the esophagus, one of the thicker suspensions or one of the esophageal pastes is recommended. Such preparations tend to coat the esophageal mucosa better than the thin or watery media (Douglas and Williamson, 1970). It is the author's opinion that $BaSO_4$ U.S.P. (Carlson, 1967; Crags, 1960; Seward, 1951) is worthless for any meaningful contrast study and should not be used, despite the fact that it is cheap. Barium-impregnated food should be given only if a routine esophogram is negative and clinical signs are strongly suggestive of an esophageal lesion.

Dosage of Contrast Material. If the study is being done at the beginning of an upper G.I. series, the dose is not important. The dose necessary for opacification of the stomach and small bowel will coat the mucosal surface of the esophagus sufficiently for radiographic evaluation. In instances in which a specific study of the esophagus is desired, enough esophageal paste or thick barium sulfate suspension should be administered to distend or completely coat the esophagus. Since megaesophagus requires more contrast material than a normal esophagus, and since it is impossible to overdistend the normal esophagus, it is best to give enough barium suspension to distend the esophagus if it will distend. A rough guide appears to be 1.0 to 3.0 ml of contrast medium per pound of body weight. Passage of this amount of contrast material will surely coat the mucosal surface if distention does not occur. If the radiographs show incomplete distention of the esophagus, give more contrast medium and repeat the study. Much more contrast material may be required for adequate demonstration of the degree of dilation and for evaluation of the terminal portion of the esophagus in animals with long-standing achalasia.

Procedure (Table 13–1)

The contrast material is administered slowly orally, via the buccal pouch, with a large syringe. Even the thickest of pastes may be successfully given in this way.

TABLE 13-1

SUMMARY OF PROCEDURE FOR
ESOPHAGEAL CONTRAST STUDIES

1. Fast the animal for at least 12 hours.
2. Obtain current survey radiographs of the thorax.
3. If the purpose of the study is to delineate only the esophagus:
   a. Slowly administer enough barium sulfate paste or similar thick barium suspension orally via the buccal pouch to distend or coat the esophagus. The dosage is extremely variable; unless extreme esophageal dilation is present, 1 to 3 ml per pound of body weight is usually satisfactory.
   b. Make lateral, VD and right VD oblique radiographs of the thorax.
4. If the study is made as part of an upper G.I. series:
   a. Administer 3 to 5 ml of the liquid barium suspension orally per pound of body weight.
   b. Immediately make lateral and VD or right VD oblique radiographs of the thorax.

Rapid delivery of the contrast material should be avoided, since aspiration of the agent may lead to coughing, anxiety and delayed administration time. Thick barium paste may be given with a tongue depressor or similar object, but delivery time is slow.

As the last of the contrast medium is being swallowed, radiographs of the thorax are made in both projections. If the study is to be specifically of the esophagus, a right VD oblique radiograph of the thorax is also made. This view projects the esophagus away from the spine, upon which it is normally superimposed in the VD view. This oblique view also may be performed in conjunction with the upper G.I. series, but it is usually not considered necessary unless the esophagus is of primary interest. If lesions are demonstrated in such survey films, an esophogram should be done with the esophageal paste for better visualization.

Complications

Aspiration of contrast material is most often due to hasty administration. This is usually not disastrous if only a small amount of the medium is inhaled, but a large amount can result in fatal pneumonia if alveolar flooding occurs.

Extraluminal deposition of barium sulfate may result if the esophagus is ruptured or perforated. However, animals with such ruptures or perforation die from infection rather than from the ectopic barium (Vessal, 1973). In the presence of broncho-esophageal fistulae (which are admittedly rare) barium sulfate may be cleared slowly and further aggravate a seriously diseased lung lobe.

Normal Findings

Barium sulfate suspension or paste coats the esophagus and appears radiographically as a series of regular, parallel lines of nearly uniform width (Carlson, 1967; Douglas and Williamson, 1970, 1972), which correspond to longitudinal crypts between folds of the esophageal mucosa (Fig. 13-21). This appearance is better appreciated if one recalls that the surface area of the mucosa of the esophagus greatly exceeds that of the serosa. Further, the muscular wall of the esophagus can stretch to accommodate a bolus of food, while the epithelial lining, relatively much less capable of stretching, allows passage of boluses by passive flattening of its multiple redundant longitudinal folds. At the thoracic inlet, the esophagus may be transiently roughened and irregular, probably because of slight delay in bolus passage of that site. In cats, the caudal third of the esophagus usually is transversely striated (Kneller and Lewis, 1973), in addition to having longitudinal folds. This produces a striking "herringbone" or "burlap" pattern (Fig. 13-22), which often has been mistaken for a cloth foreign body or a fish skeleton within the caudal esophagus.

GASTROGRAPHY (NEGATIVE CONTRAST GASTROGRAPHY, DOUBLE CONTRAST GASTROGRAPHY)

Indications

Specific radiographic study of the stomach is indicated when there is strong suspi-

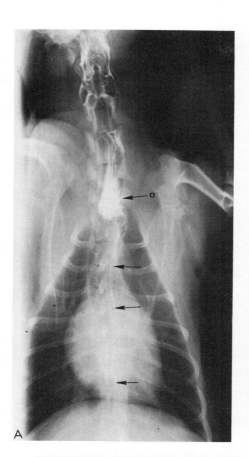

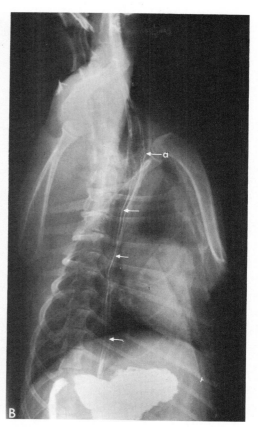

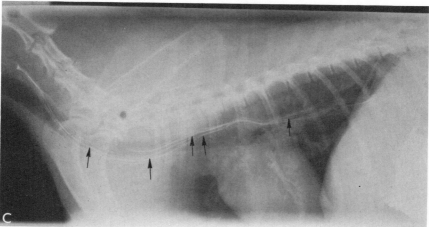

Figure 13–21. Normal esophogram (dog). *A,* VD; *B,* right VD oblique; and *C,* lateral views of a normal canine thorax after administration of barium sulfate paste. Notice the parallel opaque lines (arrows) formed by barium collected between multiple longitudinal mucosal folds. At the thoracic inlet, the esophageal mucosa may be transiently roughened and irregular *(A).* The oblique view allows visualization of the esophagus without interference by the spine.

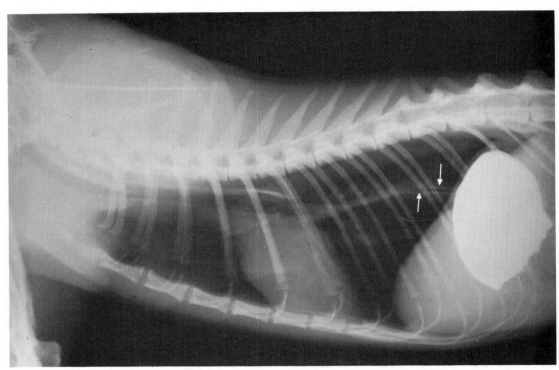

Figure 13–22. Normal esophogram (cat). Lateral view of a normal feline thorax after administration of barium sulfate paste. Parallel opaque lines are present in the cranial portion of the thoracic esophagus. The caudal esophagus is only faintly opacified, and the longitudinal parallel lines are interrupted by transverse striations creating a "herringbone" or "burlap" pattern (arrows).

cion of gastric masses or radiolucent foreign bodies. This study is most often done for further evaluation of the stomach after suspicious or equivocal findings are noted during a complete gastrointestinal series, but it can be performed as an independent study if desired (Morgan, 1964; Schnelle, 1950).

Contraindications

Gastrography is contraindicated in the presence of massive gastric fluid accumulation. If the animal has diarrhea, a greater amount of information will be gained by performing a complete upper G.I. series. Selective study of the stomach can be performed if necessary, after evaluation of the stomach and small bowel with positive contrast material.

Preparation of Patient

A 12-hour fast and routine radiographs of the abdomen should precede gastrography.

Materials

The necessary materials for gastrography depend upon the method selected for introduction of gas into the stomach. The preferred method requires only a highly carbonated beverage. Use of room air requires a stomach tube, a large syringe with a catheter adapter and a three-way valve. Another method (Ferrucci and Benedict, 1971; Geltand and Hachiya, 1969) utilizes effervescent tablets or granules (E-Z-Zoru Tablets or Granules, E-Z-Em Corp.).

Dosage of Contrast Material. If a carbonated beverage is used as the source of gas for distention of the stomach, the recommended dose is 30 to 90 ml. If room air is introduced into the stomach via a stomach tube, 3 to 5 cc per pound of body weight is used. The effervescent tablets may dissolve too slowly in the stomach to liberate a significant quantity of gas. However, the granules can be dissolved in water and administered via the buccal pouch or by stomach tube. In the author's experience, effervescent substances are markedly infe-

rior to carbonated beverages or room air for gastrography.

Procedure (Table 13–2)

Negative Contrast Gastrography. If a carbonated beverage is used, it is administered with a large syringe into the buccal pouch, rather than by a stomach tube. The swallowing action of the patient permits most of the gas to be liberated by the time the carbonated beverage reaches the stomach. Four standard projections are made of the cranial abdomen (ventrodorsal, dorsoventral, right lateral and left lateral).

If air is the chosen medium, a gastric tube is introduced and the calculated volume of air is introduced (3 to 5 cc/lb). After the air is introduced, the catheter is removed and the gastric region is radiographed in the four standard projections.

Effervescent granules (mixed with water) should be administered into the buccal pouch from an open container rather than from a large syringe, because the effervescence may become uncontrolled in the relatively enclosed syringe barrel, resulting in loss of much of the foaming solution before it can be administered.

TABLE 13–2

SUMMARY OF PROCEDURE FOR GASTROGRAPHY

1. Fast the animal for 12 to 24 hours.
2. Obtain current radiographs of the abdomen.
3. *Negative contrast gastrography:* Administer 3 to 5 cc. of air per pound of body weight with a stomach tube, or administer 30 to 90 ml. of a highly carbonated beverage via the buccal pouch.
4. *Double contrast gastrography:* Mix a small amount of barium sulfate suspension with the effervescent material, give barium sulfate prior to administration of air or gas-liberating substances, or distend the stomach with gas after an upper G.I. series has been commenced.
5. Immediately make VD, DV, right lateral and left lateral radiographs of the cranial abdomen.

Double Contrast Gastrography. If a double contrast study is desired, a small amount of BaSO$_4$ can be given prior to the gas or gas-producing agents, gas may be introduced after commencement of an upper G.I. series, or effervescent substances may be mixed with barium suspension before administration (Geltand and Hachiya, 1969).

Complications

No adverse effects have been noted with this procedure to date.

Normal Findings

The stomach should be uniformly and evenly distended with gas, and the width of the crypts between rugae should be at least as wide as the rugae themselves (Figs. 13–23 and 13–24). The wall and rugal folds should not be distorted, either intrinsically or extrinsically. The lumen should be free of filling defects, and the gastric wall should be of uniform thickness. Better visualization of the wall of the distended stomach occurs with double contrast gastrography (Fig. 13–24) than with negative contrast gastrography.

(*Text continued on page 371.*)

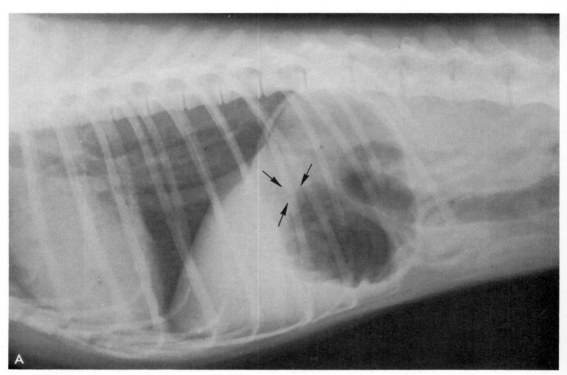

Figure 13–23. Normal pneumogastrogram. *A*, Lateral, and *B*, VD *(opposite page)* views of the abdomen of a small dog given 30 ml of a highly carbonated beverage. The rugal folds are regular, even, smooth, and nearly parallel. The crypts between adjacent rugal folds in the distended stomach are normally at least as wide as the rugal folds. The gastric wall is uniform in thickness. The pylorus (arrows) is entirely to the right of the midline in the VD view and is superimposed upon the midportion of the fundus in the lateral projection.

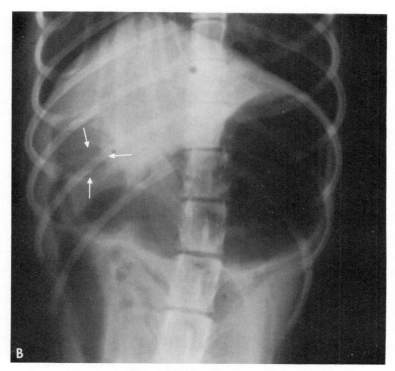

Figure 13–23. *Continued.*

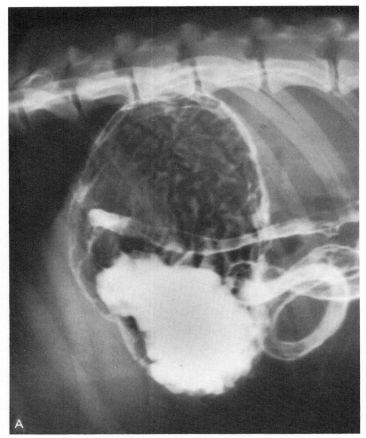

Figure 13–24. Normal double contrast gastrogram. *A*, Right lateral; *B*, left lateral; *C*, VD; and *D*, DV views of the abdomen of a dog given 3 ml/lb of room air via gastric intubation 10 to 15 minutes after being given 3 ml/lb micro-pulverized barium sulfate suspension. Superior visualization of the gastric mucosal surface results from this technique, as the stomach is not only coated with barium but also is distended with gas. Under the influence of gravity, the barium remaining in the lumen of the stomach changes location in each view.

(Illustration continued on opposite page.)

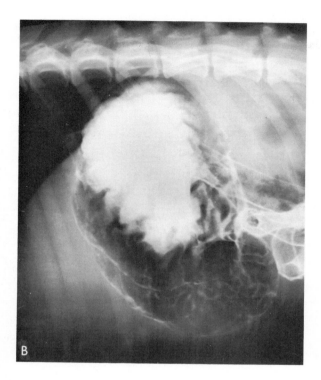

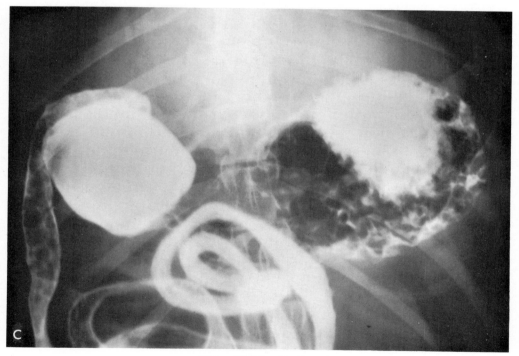

Figure 13–24. *Continued.*

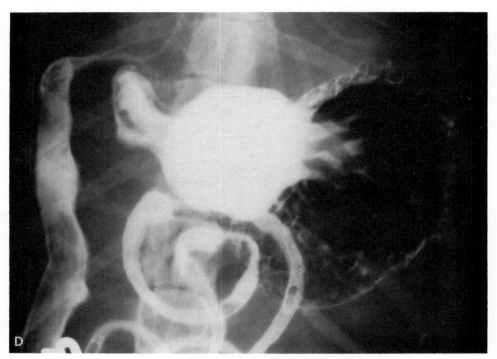

Figure 13–24. *Continued.*

UPPER GASTROINTESTINAL SERIES (BARIUM SERIES, SMALL BOWEL SERIES)

Indications

The major indications for performing contrast radiography of the upper G.I. tract are recurrent or nonresponsive vomiting, refractory or recurrent diarrhea, hematemesis, suspected gastric or enteric foreign bodies or neoplasms, suspected intestinal obstruction, the need for assistance in localization and identification of certain abdominal masses, or confirmation of various types of herniae (Barrett, 1968; Douglas and Williamson, 1970; Morgan, 1964; Schnelle, 1950).

In the instances in which the dog or cat is vomiting or has diarrhea, and has not responded to rigorous symptomatic treatment, contrast radiography of the stomach and small bowel is indicated.

Hematemesis is rare in dogs and cats. When it does occur, contrast radiography of the upper G.I. tract is definitely indicated. Ulcerated gastric or duodenal neoplasms are sometimes found, and radiographic assessment of such lesions is a rapid and direct approach.

Suspected radiolucent foreign bodies, partial obstructions or early complete obstructions of the gastrointestinal tract justify performing an upper G.I. series. In these situations, the rapid appraisal of the gastrointestinal tract provided by enteric contrast studies can mean the difference between life and death.

Abdominal masses which cannot readily be separated from the gut on the basis of survey radiographs may be better appreciated after the intestinal tract is opacified (Morgan, 1964). This use of the upper G.I. series should be limited to cases with special medical problems, such as severe pneumonia or lesions leading to respiratory distress which preclude the use of pneumoperitonography (a study which is more likely to yield information about several organ systems).

Various forms of herniae can be confirmed by contrast radiography of the gut if portions of the gut have passed through the hernial ring but have not strangulated. Examples are diaphragmatic, ventral, umbilical, inguinal and perineal herniae in which the gut is involved.

Contraindications

Barium contrast radiography of the upper G.I. tract should be avoided in patients suspected of having perforation or rupture of the stomach or gut, since barium sulfate in the peritoneal cavity may lead to the formation of granulomata. Without concomitant sepsis, however, extravasated barium sulfate is rarely fatal. Water soluble contrast media, such as the oral diatrizoates, may be used without fear of producing granulomata when there is suspicion of ruptures or perforations of the stomach or small bowel.

A barium sulfate suspension should not be administered when there is a strong indication of obstruction of the lower bowel. Resorption of water from the colonic contents may lead to inspissation of the barium and may result in severe obstipation if a blockage is already present in the lower bowel (Nelson et al., 1965). Severe debility is a contraindication for use of one of the oral diatrizoates because of their hyperosmolality and consequent dehydrating effect (Nelson et al., 1965). These agents also become progressively diluted as they pass through the intestinal tract, and are of little value in demonstrating lesions of the lower jejunum and ileum.

Preparation of Patient

The animal should be fasted for 24 hours prior to the administration of contrast material. A thorough flushing enema with tepid water or saline should be given until clear fluid returns. The various hypertonic commercial enema preparations are inadequate because they tend to cause evacuation of only the terminal portion of the colon. As in all other contrast procedures of the abdominal viscera, current survey radiographs should be made in VD and lateral projections. Unless absolutely necessary, no tranquilizers should be given prior to upper G.I. radiography, as these drugs modify gastrointestinal motility (Zontine, 1973) and therefore alter small bowel transit time. Anticholinergic drugs should not have been administered within 24 hours of the radiographic examination.

Materials

Types of contrast material for the G.I. tract are numerous. Of the barium sulfate suspensions, one of the micropulverized preparations is preferred. These are supplied in several dry powder forms (Baroperse, Barium Sulfate U.S.P. Formulation, Mallinckrodt Pharmaceuticals) or in various concentrations of premixed liquid suspension (Micropaque, Barium Sulfate Powder, Damancy & Co.; redi-FLOW, Gastric or Colonic Barium Sulfate Suspensions, Flow Pharmaceuticals, Inc., redi-PAQUE Gastric Barium Sulfate Suspension, Burns-Biotec Laboratories). Barium sulfate U.S.P. is markedly inferior to the micropulverized products. It does not coat the mucosal surfaces, it fails to maintain a continuous column of opaque medium in the gut lumen and its passage through the small bowel is slightly slower than that of the micropulverized media (Carlson, 1967; Root and Morgan, 1969).

If there is reasonable suspicion that the lower bowel is obstructed or that the upper G.I. tract is ruptured or perforated, barium products should be avoided. Instead, the organic iodides (Gastrografin, Meglumine Diatrizoate Oral Solution, Squibb & Sons; Oral Hypaque, Sodium Diatrizoate Liquid, Winthrop Laboratories) are recommended. They are also recommended if it seems imperative to reach a radiographic conclusion quickly, because these agents pass through the small bowel very rapidly.

In addition to the contrast material, the only other item needed is a large syringe with a rubber adapter. A stomach tube, a catheter adapter and a mouth gag may be required in some cases.

Dosage of Contrast Material. In general, the volume of barium sulfate suspension administered is as important as its concentration. The object in opacification of any hollow visceral structure should be reasonable physiologic distention of its lumen without masking its contents. Contrary to the recommendations of other authors (Carlson, 1967; Douglas and Williamson, 1970, 1972; Morgan, 1964), a small volume of a very concentrated contrast material is considered

by the author to be ineffective in evaluation of the stomach and gut. A larger volume of relatively dilute material is much more satisfactory because the lumen of the G.I. tract is adequately distended, and radiolucent luminal filling defects are not obscured. The recommended concentration of barium sulfate preparations is 20 to 25 per cent for G.I. opacification. The dosage should be 3 to 5 ml $BaSO_4$ suspension per pound of body weight (Barrett, 1968; Root and Morgan, 1969).

The water-soluble organic iodine solutions (Gastrografin, Meglumine Diatrizoate Oral Solution, Squibb & Sons; Oral Hypaque, Sodium Diatrozoate Liquid, Winthrop Laboratories) should be administered at the rate of 1 ml per pound of body weight. Their concentrations are usually fixed. Further dilution is ill-advised because these solutions lose density as they pass through the G.I. tract (Nelson et al., 1965). This type of contrast material is also available in powdered form (Oral Hypaque, Sodium Diatrizoate Powder, Winthrop Laboratories). The irritant and hyperosmolal properties of the organic iodides make it inadvisable to exceed the recommended concentrations.

Procedure (Table 13–3)

Administer the contrast material per os by the buccal pouch or through a stomach tube. When using the buccal pouch, allow the patient to swallow slowly in order to avoid aspiration of contrast material into the trachea and lungs. The organic iodide preparations should be administered by stomach tube only, because they are extremely bitter. Cats seem to find the taste of these latter agents especially unpleasant.

With barium products, lateral and ventrodorsal radiographs of the abdomen are made immediately, at 15 minutes, at 30 minutes, at 60 minutes and at hourly intervals until the contrast material reaches the colon. (If desired, DV rather than VD radiographs may be made immediately and at 15 minutes, theoretically permitting better visualization of the wall of the body of the stomach). Additional radiographs may be made at 24 hours if desired. If an organic iodide is administered, lateral and VD radiographs of the abdomen should be made immediately, at 5 minutes, at 15 minutes, at 30 minutes

TABLE 13-3

SUMMARY OF PROCEDURE FOR UPPER
G.I. SERIES

1. Fast the animal for 24 hours and give a cleansing tepid water or saline enema.
2. Obtain current survey radiographs of the abdomen.
3. If barium sulfate suspension is used:
   a. Slowly administer 3 to 5 ml of 20 to 25% (W/V) micropulverized barium sulfate suspension per pound of body weight orally via the buccal pouch.
   b. If screening radiographs of the esophagus are to be omitted, the contrast medium may be administered with a stomach tube.
   c. Make lateral and VD radiographs of the abdomen immediately, at 15 minutes, 30 minutes, 1 hour, 2 hours, 3 hours, etc., until the colon contains contrast material. The immediate and 15 minute radiographs may be DV rather than VD, if desired.
4. If an organic iodide solution is used:
   a. Administer 1 ml of the medium per pound of body weight, by stomach tube.
   b. Radiograph the abdomen at 0, 5, 15, 30 and 60 minutes and every half hour thereafter until the colon is opacified.

and every half-hour thereafter until the colon is visualized.

Complications

Aspiration of a small amount of pure barium sulfate suspension into the lungs during oral administration is of little serious consequence, as proved by the fact that certain commercial barium sulfate preparations have been used successfully as bronchographic agents (Dunbar, 1959; Nelson et al., 1964; Nice, 1964; Shook and Felson, 1970). However, aspiration of a large amount of any barium sulfate preparation may be fatal, since the alveoli may be flooded. Aspiration of vomited barium, even in small quantities, is potentially a very serious situation, probably due to the action of acid gastric content upon airway epithelium.

Peritoneal granulomata may be the sequela to leakage of barium through perforated or ruptured G.I. lumen. If leakage of ingesta with concomitant infection is suspected, barium preparations should be avoided. Usually this may be determined by critical examination of the survey radiographs or analysis of the clinical and hematologic findings, or both.

The presence of barium sulfate preparations in the lumen of the G.I. tract might be considered by some to be a contraindication to gastric or intestinal surgery. Peritoneal contamination with barium obscures natural color and interferes with normal texture of the mucosal surface. However, the value of the information obtained from upper G.I. series usually far outweighs the inconvenience, and careful surgical technique minimizes the possibility of peritoneal contamination with barium.

Administration of organic iodides has proved to be deleterious to the patient which is already dehydrated and debilitated (Nelson et al., 1965). Further dehydration can be brought about by the hyperosmolality of these products. Additional loss of body fluids is caused by enteric hypermotility, which results from the irritation caused by this type of contrast medium. As the contrast medium progresses through the G.I. tract, it becomes more dilute because of its hyperosmolality, and its radiopacity is often unsatisfactory by the time it reaches the terminal small bowel. In some animals, especially cats, the irritant property of organic iodides causes severe pylorospasm, which results in gastric retention of the medium until it is vomited.

Normal Findings

The normal small bowel transit time for micropulverized barium sulfate suspensions (Fig. 13-25) is two to three hours (Barrett, 1968; Root and Morgan, 1969). Barium sulfate U.S.P. requires, on the average, one hour longer to reach the colon (Root and Morgan, 1969). The organic iodides (McAlister and Margulis, 1964; Nelson et al., 1964) pass through the small bowel in 45 minutes to one hour (Fig. 13-26).

With both the micropulverized agents and the organic iodides (Figs. 13-25 and 13-26), a smooth halo is seen surrounding the

(*Text continued on page 386.*)

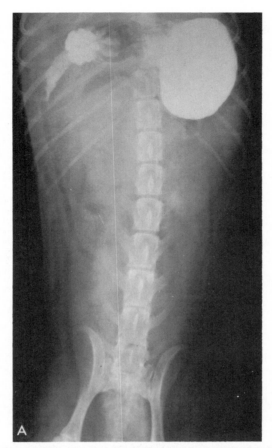

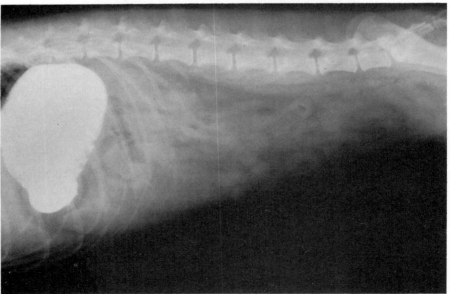

Figure 13–25. Normal upper G.I. series—micropulverized barium sulfate. Lateral and VD radiographs of the abdomen of a normal dog, made immediately *(A)*, 15 minutes *(B)*, 30 minutes *(C)*, 60 minutes *(D)*, 2 hours *(E)* and 3 hours *(F)* after oral administration of 3 ml 20% (weight per volume) micropulverized barium sulfate suspension per pound of body weight.

Immediately after administration of contrast material the stomach is distended. Its wall is of uniform thickness

(*Illustration and legend continued on the opposite page.*)

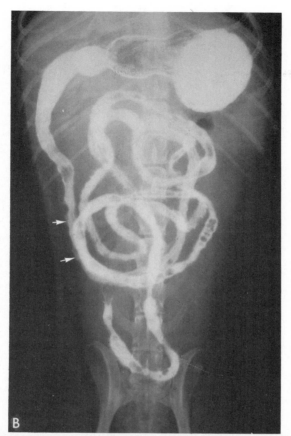

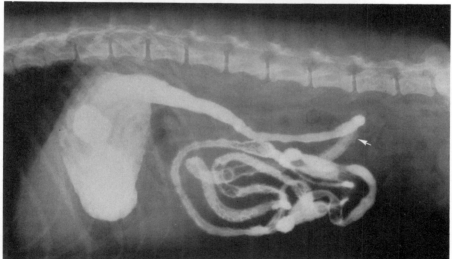

Figure 13–25. *Continued.*

and rugal folds are regular, even, smooth and nearly parallel. The crypts between adjacent rugal folds in the distended stomach normally are at least the same width as the rugae. The mucosal surface of the small bowel should be smooth and is usually outlined by a faint halo or a slightly roughened edge. There may be ulcer-shaped defects ventrally and laterally in the mucosa of the duodenum (arrows). These are called pseudoulcers and are of no clinical significance.

Between 15 minutes and 2 hours after administration, contrast material should progressively opacify and distend the duodenum, jejunum and ileum. Segmental constrictions in the gut represent peristalsis. There is no definite line of demarcation between jejunum and ileum, but the mucosal surface of the ileum lacks the mucosal halo common to the jejunum. The ileum terminates at the ileocolic valve *(a)* near the cecum *(b)* (page 379). In many animals, approximately 1 hour before the contrast material enters the colon, it collects and becomes more concentrated in the caudal jejunum and ileum. Normal small bowel transit time is 2 to 3 hours with this type of contrast medium.

(Illustration continued on the following page.)

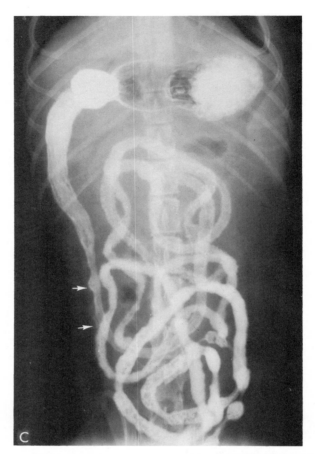

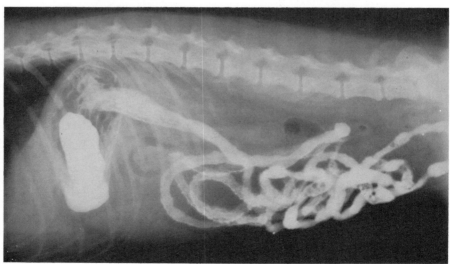

Figure 13–25. *Continued.*

(Illustration continued on the opposite page.)

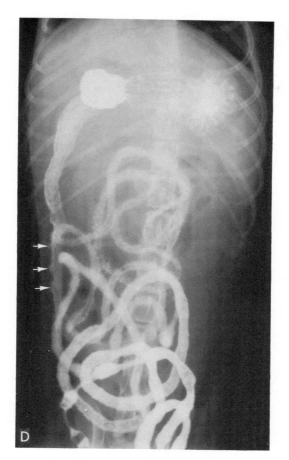

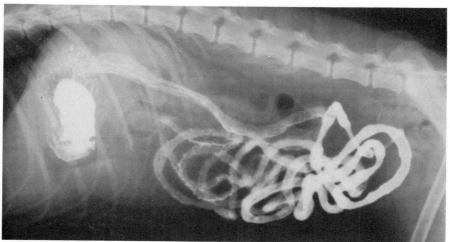

Figure 13–25. *Continued.*

(Illustration continued on the following page.)

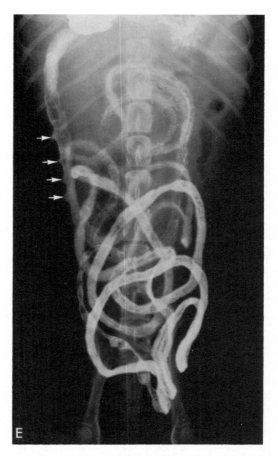

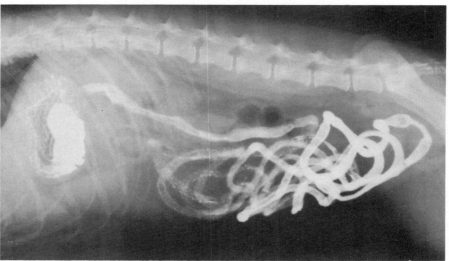

Figure 13–25. *Continued.*

(*Illustration continued on the opposite page.*)

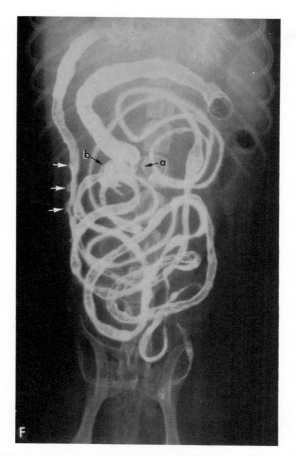

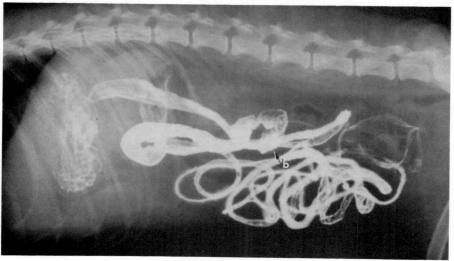

Figure 13–25. *Continued.*

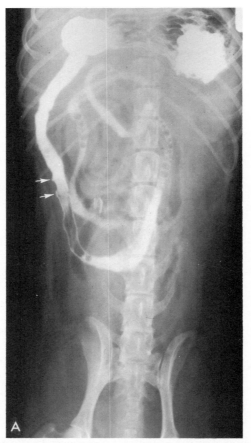

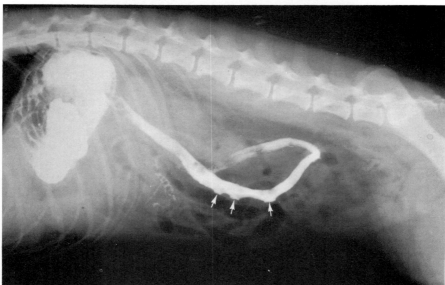

Figure 13–26. Normal upper G.I. series—water-soluble contrast media. Lateral and VD radiographs of the abdomen of a normal dog, made immediately *(A)*, 5 minutes *(B)*, 15 minutes *(C)*, 30 minutes *(D)*, 45 minutes *(E)* and 1 hour *(F)*, after gastric administration of 1 ml/lb of a water-soluble gastrointestinal contrast medium. As in Figure 13–25, all the normal anatomic structures and relationships can be appreciated. The periluminal halo and peristaltic segmentation may be much more pronounced when using one of the water-soluble products than when using a

(*Legend and illustration continued on the opposite page.*)

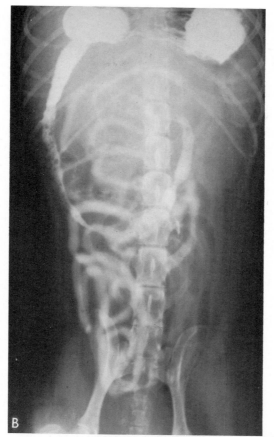

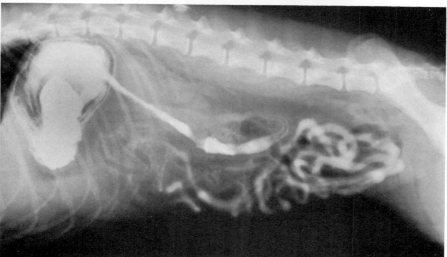

Figure 13–26. *Continued.*
barium sulfate suspension. The contrast material is usually well into the small bowel by 15 minutes. By 30 minutes, it has proceeded into the terminal portion of the small intestine. In the normal animal, this type of medium has usually entered the colon by 45 minutes to 1 hour. By this time, however, its density may have been markedly diminished by dilution due to its hyperosmolality. Pseudoulcers (arrows), the ileocolic valve *(a)* and the cecum *(b)* may be seen (page 385). Renal pelvic opacification may be seen in radiographs made near the end of the study.

(*Illustration continued on the following page.*)

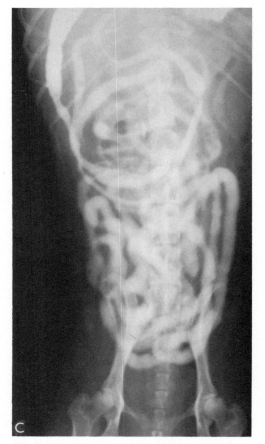

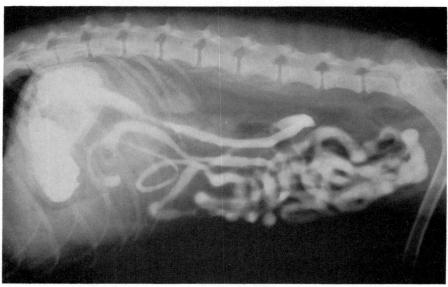

Figure 13–26. *Continued.*
(Illustration continued on the opposite page.)

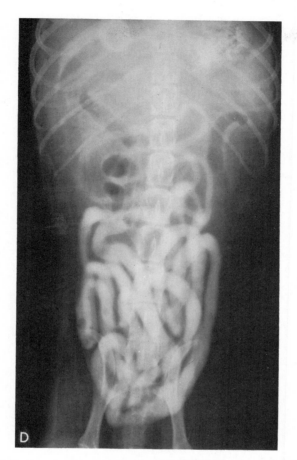

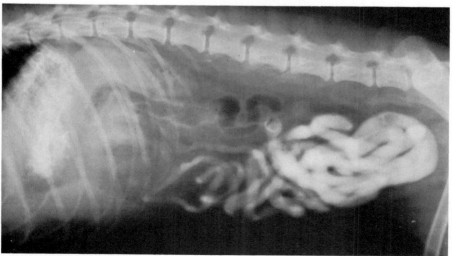

Figure 13–26. *Continued.*

(Illustration continued on the following page.)

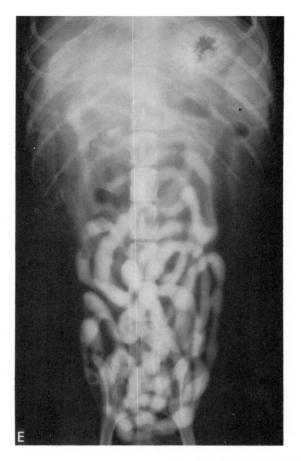

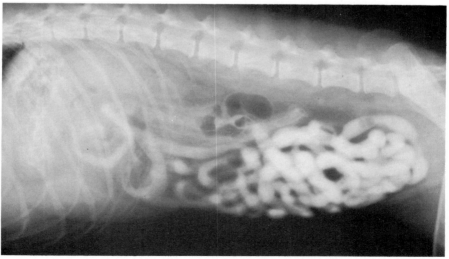

Figure 13–26. *Continued.*
(Illustration continued on the opposite page.)

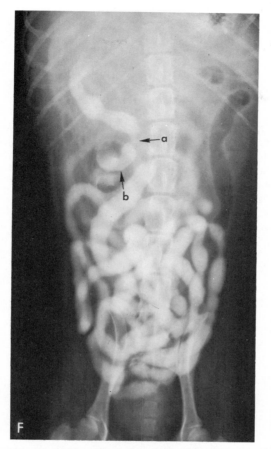

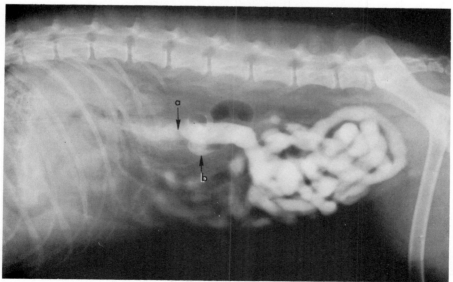

Figure 13-26. *Continued.*

luminal column of contrast material, except in the ileum, where the wall is very smooth. The halo is presumed to be caused by the presence of these contrast agents in the crypts between the intestinal villi (Barrett, 1968; Root and Morgan, 1969). This halo effect is much more pronounced with organic iodide (Fig. 13–26) than with one of the micropulverized barium agents. Barium sulfate U.S.P. is too coarse to produce this effect, and often flocculates rather than causing uniform opacification of the gut lumen (Fig. 13–27).

Regardless of the agent employed in contrast radiography of the G.I. tract, the small bowel should always appear to be evenly dispersed throughout the peritoneal cavity. No extrinsic masses should displace the small bowel. The mucosal borders should be uniform, except in the duodenum, where crater-shaped pseudoulcers (Fig. 13–25) are often seen (O'Brien et al., 1969). There should be no filling defects, either in the lumen or originating from the gastric or gut wall. The wall of the small bowel should be no thicker than one fourth to one third the width of the distended lumen. The rugal folds of the distended stomach should be roughly parallel, and their individual widths should not exceed the distance between adjacent rugae. Occasional segmental constrictions should be seen, but excessive segmentation, as evidenced by numerous constrictions in the lumen, may indicate unorganized hypermotility. The lumen of the small bowel should generally be uniform in width. There should be no extensive areas of luminal narrowing. In many animals, the sphincters of the ileocolonic (Kelly, 1967) and cecocolonic junctional zones may be seen as these regions become opacified (Fig. 13–25F).

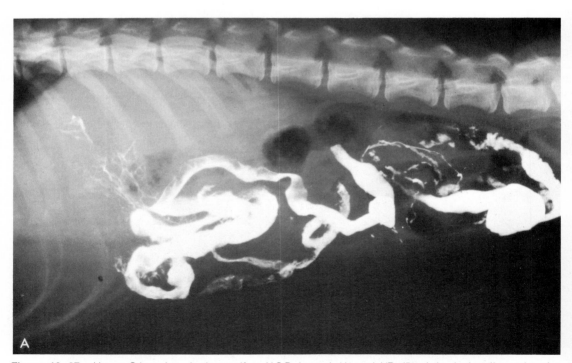

Figure 13–27. Upper G.I. series—barium sulfate U.S.P. Lateral *(A)* and VD *(B)* abdominal radiographs of a young dog 1 hour after oral administration of 3 ml/lb of 30% (weight per volume) barium sulfate U.S.P. This material is an unsatisfactory gastrointestinal contrast medium due to its tendency to flocculate and its inability to outline the normal enteric mucosal pattern.

(Illustration continued on the opposite page.)

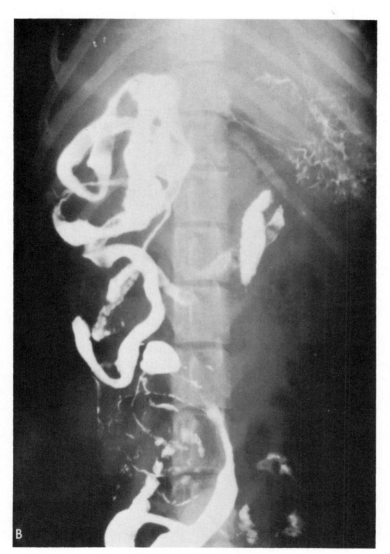

Figure 13-27. *Continued.*

CONTRAST RADIOGRAPHY OF THE COLON (BARIUM ENEMA, LOWER BOWEL SERIES, DOUBLE CONTRAST RADIOGRAPHY OF THE COLON)

Indications

Refractory or recurrent bloody diarrhea probably is the most common indication for performing contrast radiography of the colon. Rectal tenesmus, if severe or chronic, is another common justification for lower bowel studies. Ileocolonic intussusception is thought by some to be best demonstrated by opacification of the large bowel (Carlson, 1967; Douglas and Williamson, 1970). However, this lesion commonly can be seen well during contrast radiography of the upper G.I. tract, provided that obstruction of the ileum is incomplete. It is sometimes possible to reduce ileocolonic intussusceptions during inflation of the colon with contrast material. If reduction occurs, demonstration of the lesion from below may be impossible; in such a case, an upper G.I. series is indicated.

Contraindications

Barium sulfate suspension should never be given if obstruction of the colon is suspected (Nelson et al., 1965) and immediate surgery is not contemplated. Inspissation of the barium suspension may lead to severe constipation, and in some animals has resulted in the same type of obstipation caused by ingestion of a large amount of bony material. In these instances, positive contrast radiography of the colon can be done with one of the water-soluble iodine preparations, but the advantages of double contrast are lost.

Rupture or perforation of the colon or recent biopsy of the colonic wall also contraindicates the use of barium sulfate suspension. Rupture or perforation of the lower bowel is more likely to result in sepsis than is rupture or perforation of the stomach or small bowel. If such a lower bowel lesion is suspected, the contrast radiographic study should be avoided.

Contrast radiographic evaluation of lesions which are clinically limited to the rectum or terminal colon should not be attempted, since lesions in this region will be obscured by the inflated cuff of the catheter.

Preparation of Patient

The animal must be fasted for at least 24 hours prior to the contrast study (Watters, 1970). A mild cathartic should be administered at least 12 hours before the colon is opacified. A flushing enema must be given, using either water or saline, until the returning fluid is absolutely clear. Tepid, rather than warm enema solutions are recommended, since they seem to result in less gas retention in the colon. Commercial hypertonic enema kits are rarely thorough enough for satisfactory preparation of the patient. Current survey radiographs in both VD and lateral projection are necessary before the colon is opacified.

General anesthesia is required for this study, since inflation of the bulb of the cuffed catheter induces discomfort and stimulates violent tenesmus in the conscious animal.

Materials

The most important item required for contrast radiography of the colon is the catheter through which the contrast material is introduced. Cuffed rectal catheters (Bardex Cuffed Rectal Catheters, 24 to 38 French and Bardex Cuffed Pediatric Rectal Catheter, 18 French, Bard Hospital Division, C. R. Bard, Inc.) have been used successfully in medium-sized and large dogs. Cats and small dogs require smaller catheters. However, any other type of cuffed rectal catheter may be used, provided that the cuff can be distended adequately to occlude the lumen of the terminal colon. Disposable enema nozzles with removable inflatable cuffs (Dispoa-A-Tube Enema Tips and Disposable Cath-Cuffs, Picker X-Ray) may be used, but due to their size, they are not suitable for cats and smaller dogs. An adapter and a three-way valve are also required, regardless of the type of catheter used.

The concentration of the contrast medium is as important in opacifying the colon as it is in visualizing the stomach and small intestine. However, because larger volumes of contrast medium are used in studies of the colon, the concentration should be less to prevent obliteration of luminal masses. Dilute barium sulfate suspension may be prepared from powder (Micropaque, Barium Sulfate Powder, Damancy & Co., Ltd.) or may be made from commercially available liquid suspensions (redi-FLOW, Gastric or Colonic Barium Sulfate Suspensions, Flow Pharmaceuticals; redi-PAQUE, Gastric Barium Sulfate Suspension, Burns-Biotec Laboratories) or powdered products (Baroperse, Barium Sulfate U.S.P. Formulation, Mallinckrodt Pharmaceuticals). The final concentration of barium sulfate suspension should be 15 to 20 per cent (W/V). Some type of reservoir should be provided for the contrast material. This may be a used intravenous fluid bottle with its attached tubing or merely a standard enema can. If an emptied parenteral fluid bottle is used, a large disposable syringe is necessary for alternate aspiration of the contrast medium from the hanging bottle and injection of the material into the rectal catheter through the three-way valve. If the enema can is used, a clamp should be used to control the speed of gravity flow of the contrast material from the can into the colon. The disadvantage of the latter method is the relatively poor control or estimation of the volume of contrast material instilled into the colon at any time.

Dosage of Contrast Material. The object is to distend the colon to its normal physiologic capacity, but it should not be overfilled. A rough guide for dosage is 10 to 15 ml barium sulfate suspension per pound of body weight. Because the volume needed to fill the colon is extremely variable, the contrast material should be administered in several smaller increments until the desired effect is seen radiographically.

Procedure (Table 13-4)

After the patient is anesthetized, the cuffed catheter or disposable enema nozzle is inserted into the rectum so that the cuff is cranial to the pubis. The cuff should be inflated only enough to occlude the lumen firmly, and the catheter or nozzle should be pulled caudally to seat the inflated cuff against the cranial portion of the anal sphincter.

The colon is slowly filled with contrast

TABLE 13-4

SUMMARY OF PROCEDURE FOR CONTRAST RADIOGRAPHY OF THE COLON

1. Fast the animal for at least 24 hours.
2. Mild catharsis is recommended beginning at least 12 hours before the procedure is performed.
3. Give a flushing enema with tepid fluid (water or saline) until the returning fluid is clear.
4. Obtain current survey radiographs of the abdomen.
5. Anesthetize the patient.
6. Using an appropriate cuffed rectal catheter or cuffed enema nozzle with the inflated bulb or cuff seated slightly cranial to the anal sphincter:
   a. Slowly instill 5 ml (15 to 20% W/V) dilute micropulverized barium sulfate suspension per pound body weight into the colon, with the animal in right lateral recumbency.
   b. Make a VD radiograph of the abdomen to determine if the colon is adequately distended. If it is not, instill more contrast material and repeat the radiograph.
   c. When the colon is adequately distended, note the total volume of contrast material used and radiograph the abdomen in VD and lateral projections.
   d. Leaving the bulb or cuff of the rectal catheter inflated, remove as much of the contrast material as possible and radiograph the abdomen in both projections.
   e. Replace the recovered contrast material with an equal volume of air and repeat the radiographs of the abdomen.
   f. Deflate the bulb or cuff and remove the catheter or enema nozzle from the rectum.

material at body temperature with the patient in right lateral recumbency. At this point, a fluoroscope or an image intensifier is very useful but is rarely available. Without the benefit of such equipment, 5 ml of contrast material per pound of body weight should be instilled slowly and the abdomen radiographed in the VD projection. If the radiograph shows that the colon is not adequately distended, another 5 ml per pound of body weight is instilled, and the abdomen is radiographed again. This procedure must be repeated until the colon and cecum become uniformly distended. The abdomen is then radiographed in both the VD and lateral projections. The total volume of contrast material used should be noted.

Next the contrast material is removed from the colon via the catheter. An attempt should be made to recover as much of the contrast material as possible. At this point, the importance of proper cleansing of the colon will be appreciated (Zezulin, 1971). If preparation was inadequate, the catheter will become occluded with fecal material and it will be impossible to remove a significant portion of the contrast material. If the colon was properly cleansed, most of the contrast agent may be retrieved by massage and manipulation of the abdomen during gentle aspiration or by the effect of gravity. Placing the animal in left lateral recumbency is also helpful because it permits most of the contents to gravitate into the descending colon. When the lower bowel is satisfactorily emptied, the abdomen is radiographed in the VD and lateral projections. This is known as the post-evacuation study.

The final step in this procedure is the filling of the colon with a volume of air equal to the amount of contrast material recovered. Ventrodorsal and lateral radiographs of the abdomen are then made. This study provides double contrast opacification of the colon and probably produces the most valuable radiographs in the entire series, because they provide superior visualization of the mucosal surface.

At the conclusion of the study, the cuff is deflated and catheter or nozzle is removed.

Complications

The most common "complication" in contrast radiography of the colon, although it is of no significance to the patient, is flooding of the tabletop with contrast material if the cuff is not properly inflated or if the patient expels the cuff because of improper anesthesia.

Another complication is retrograde filling of the ileum and jejunum (Fig. 13–29),

which is also of no serious consequence to the patient. In as many as one third of patients, this filling occurs without overdistention. If this reflux is massive, however, it can obscure visualization of portions of the colon.

It is possible to rupture the colon in several ways if proper care is not taken. The catheter cuff can be overinflated, causing a rent or rupture to occur in the terminal colon. Rupture can occur anywhere in the colon wall if it is subjected to severe overdistention. This can be avoided by making monitoring radiographs during the filling procedure. Also, the colon can rupture without overdistention if it has been recently biopsied proctoscopically, or if its wall is otherwise weakened by disease or surgery.

Normal Findings

During the positive contrast study (Fig. 13–28A), the colon is uniformly distended and smooth in outline (Barrett, 1968; Morgan, 1964; Watters, 1970). It forms the outline of a question mark or a shepherd's crook in the VD view. In normal animals, the colon usually lies in a plane nearly parallel to the spine in the lateral projection and is located roughly halfway between the spine and the ventral body wall, the cecum, the ascending colon and the cranial descending colon being superimposed. The colon may be redundant; that is, it may appear to be too long and may have a convoluted appearance (Fig. 13–29). This is a normal variant.

In the post-evacuation radiographs (Fig. 13–28B), the only variations in the appearance of the colon are the lumen size and the appearance of the wall. The lumen narrows and the wall becomes collapsed and irregular.

After the addition of air (Fig. 13–28C), the colon is once again completely distended, but the mucosal surface of the colon is doubly contrasted with air and barium. This study is of little value when using one of the water-soluble agents, because no appreciable coating of the mucosa occurs.

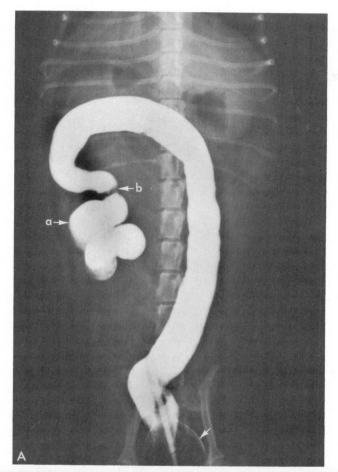

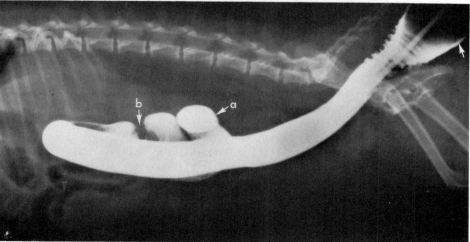

Figure 13–28. Opacification of the colon. *A*, Positive contrast study. The wall is smooth in outline and the lumen is uniform in width. The colon assumes a "shepherd's crook" or "question mark" configuration in the VD view. In this study, the cecum *(a)* and cecocolic valve *(b)* are seen. Cecal opacification during radiography of the colon is not always satisfactory. Note the air-filled cuff of the Bardex catheter (arrows). *B*, Post-evacuation study. After as much of the contrast medium as possible is removed from the colon, the lower bowel is found to be collapsed. It should not have changed in general location however. *C*, Double contrast study. A volume of air equal to the amount of contrast medium recovered prior to the post-evacuation study adequately distends the barium coated large bowel. The wall is well visualized and is normally smooth and of uniform thickness. The cecum *(a)* and cecocolic valve *(b)* are seen.

(*Illustration continued on the following page.*)

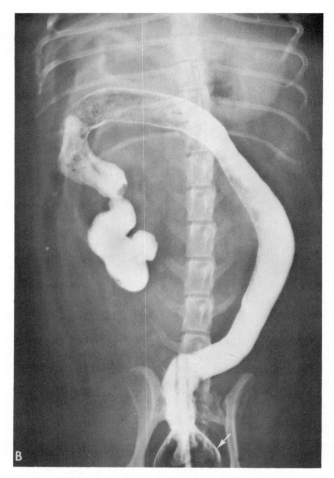

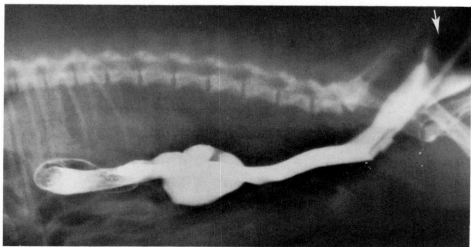

Figure 13–28. *Continued.*

(*Illustration continued on the opposite page.*)

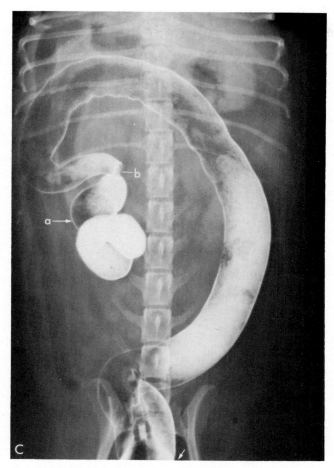

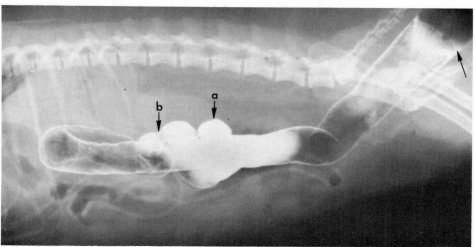

Figure 13–28. *Continued.*

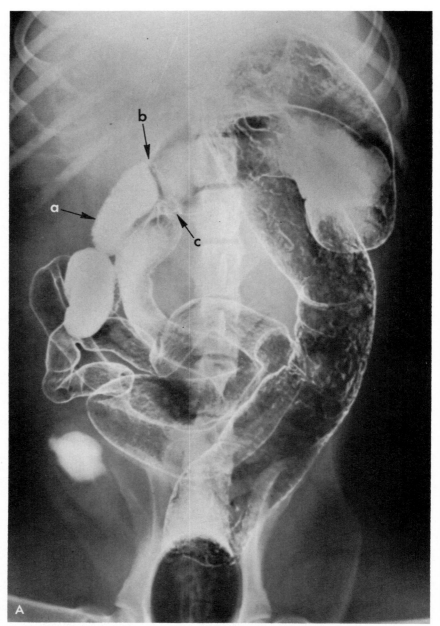

Figure 13–29. Normal variant canine colon. VD projection of double contrast study of a redundant canine colon. Retrograde filling of the ileum and terminal jejunum has occurred. This is not unusual and may be due merely to overfilling of the colon. It is otherwise unremarkable, and is considered a variation of normal. The smooth "shepherd's crook" configuration seen in Figure 13–28 is not present. The cecum *(a)*, cecocolic valve *(b)* and ileocolic valve *(c)* are seen. Because of the presence of the multiple convolutions, it is sometimes difficult to remove enough contrast material to perform satisfactory post-evacuation and double contrast studies in patients with this type of colon.

REFERENCES

Barrett, R. B.: Radiography of the small bowel and colon. Scientific Program, American Veterinary Radiology Society, Boston, 1968.

Carlson, W. D.: Veterinary Radiology. 2nd ed. Philadelphia, Lea & Febiger, 1967.

Crago, W. R.: Use of contrast media in radiological diagnosis. J. Amer. Vet. Rad. Soc., 1:6, 1960.

Douglas, S. W., and Williamson, H. D.: Principles of Veterinary Radiography. 2nd ed. Baltimore, Williams & Wilkins Co., 1972.

Douglas, S. W., and Williamson, H. D.: Veterinary Radiological Interpretation. Philadelphia, Lea & Febiger, 1970.

Dunbar, J. S.: An investigation of effects of opaque media on the lungs with comparison of barium sulfate, lipiodol and dionosil. Amer. J. Roentgen., 82:902, 1959.

Ferrucci, J. T., and Benedict, K. T.: Anticholinergic-aided study of the gastrointestinal tract using effervescent substances. Radiol. Clin. N. Amer., 9:25, 1971.

Geltand, D. W., and Hachiya, J.: The double contrast examination of the stomach using gas-producing granules and tablets. Radiology, 93:1381, 1969.

Kelly, M. L.: Silicone-foam molding of the canine ileocolonic junctional zone. Amer. J. Dig. Dis., 12:813, 1967.

Kneller, S. K., and Lewis, R. E.: Contrast radiography of the normal cat esophagus. J. Amer. Anim. Hosp. Assoc., 9:50, 1973.

McAlister, W. H., and Margulis, A. R.: Small bowel transit time of barium sulfate preparations and iodine contrast media in dogs. Am. J. Roentgen., 91:814, 1964.

Morgan, J. P.: Normal radiographic anatomy of the gastrointestinal tract of the dog. Scientific Proceedings, American Veterinary Medical Association, 101st Annual Meeting. Vol. 155, 1964.

Nelson, S. W., Christoforidis, A. J., and Pratt, P.: Further experience with barium sulfate as a bronchographic contrast medium. Amer. J. Roentgen., 92:595, 1964.

Nelson, S. W., Christoforidis, A. J., and Roenigk, W. J.: Dangers and fallibilities of iodinated radiopaque media in obstruction of the small bowel. Am. J. Surg., 109:546, 1965.

Nice, C. M.: Bronchography in infants and children: Barium sulfate as a contrast agent. Amer. J. Roentgen., 91:564, 1964.

O'Brien, T. R., Morgan, J. P., and Lebel, J. L.: Pseudoulcers in the duodenum of the dog. J. Amer. Vet. Med. Assoc., 155:713, 1969.

Root, C. R., and Morgan, J. P.: Contrast radiology of the upper gastrointestinal tract in the dog—a comparison of micropulverized barium sulfate and U.S.P. barium sulfate suspensions in clinically normal dogs. J. Small Anim. Pract., 10:279, 1969.

Schnelle, G. B.: Radiology in Small Animal Practice. 2nd ed. Evanston, Ill., The North American Veterinarian, Inc., 1950.

Seward, C. O.: The use of barium in studying the digestive tract of the dog. J. Amer. Vet. Med. Assoc., 119:125, 1951.

Shook, C. D., and Felson, B.: Inhalation bronchography. Chest, 58:333, 1970.

Vessal, K.: Evaluation of barium and gastrografin as contrast media for suspected esophageal perforation and rupture. 59th Scientific Assembly and Annual Meeting of the Radiological Society of North America, Scientific Program. Vol. 70, 1973.

Watters, J. W.: Radiography of the canine colon using different contrast agents. J. Amer. Vet. Med. Assoc., 156:423, 1970.

Zezulin, W.: Effective 24-hour preparation for the radiologic examination of the colon. Surg. Clin. N. Amer., 51:799, 1971.

Zontine, W. J.: Effect of chemical restraint drugs on the passage of barium sulfate through the stomach and duodenum in dogs. J. Amer. Vet. Med. Assoc., 162:878, 1973.

Contrast Radiography of the Urinary System

CHARLES R. ROOT

In small animal practice, the urinary system is easier to evaluate radiographically than the gastrointestinal tract. None of the techniques requires general anesthesia, and most of them are less time-consuming than those used for the G.I. tract. Special or expensive equipment is not needed. Contrast radiography can be used to outline the urinary system and can yield valuable information about form, location and function (in the case of excretory urography). All of the contrast radiographic examinations described below may be used by the practitioner and are limited only by the capability to produce good radiographs of the abdomen.

EXCRETORY UROGRAPHY (INTRAVENOUS PYELOGRAPHY, I.V.P., INTRAVENOUS UROGRAPHY)

Indications

Abnormal renal size or shape (determined by palpation or radiography) is a common indication for contrast radiography of the kidneys (Carlson and Gillette, 1967; Douglas and Williamson, 1970; Goldman and Freedman, 1971; Lord et al., 1974; McEwan, 1971; Osborne et al., 1969). Contrast radiography of the kidneys, ureters and urinary bladder is also justified when there are suspected renal masses, sublumbar masses, prostatic masses or intrapelvic masses, or when there is persistent hema-

turia. This study can be used to verify the presence of renal or ureteral calculi (Finco et al., 1970; Walker and Douglas, 1970). Other conditions, such as hydronephrosis (either congenital or acquired), ureteral ectopia (Pearson and Gibbs, 1971; Walker and Douglas, 1970) and ureterocele (Pearson and Gibbs, 1971; Scott et al., 1974) can also be demonstrated by excretory urography. Traumatic rupture of ureters may be visualized and characterized (Burt and Root, 1971; Lord et al., 1974). When catheterization is impossible or difficult (as in female cats), excretory urography can be used to evaluate the urinary bladder (Borthwick and Robbie, 1971).

Contraindications

In man, excretory urography is contraindicated in severely debilitated patients, especially in the presence of marked dehydration (Talner, 1972). Presumably, the same is true in animals. High arterial concentrations of certain older types of intravascular contrast materials have been shown to be contraindicated because of renal damage (Andrew et al., 1964; Dean et al., 1964; Killen et al., 1962; Luttwak et al., 1961; Stokes and Bernard, 1961), but there is little, if any, danger of renal toxicity with today's contrast media even if given in high doses (Lord et al., 1974; Stokes and Bernard, 1961) or to an uremic patient, unless that patient is severely dehydrated (Talner,

1972). In fact, diagnostic excretory urography in man is possible and safe even in the presence of markedly elevated creatinine or blood urea nitrogen (B.U.N.) levels using dosages in excess of 400 mg/lb of body weight (Bosniak and Schweizer, 1972).

Preparation of Patient

Standard clinical pathologic tests should be completed if they have not been done as part of the animal's medical work-up. Recent survey radiographs of the abdomen are necessary. The animal should be fasted for 24 hours and should have a thorough enema. Water should be withheld for 12 hours if the patient is not severely dehydrated, since mild dehydration facilitates opacification of the renal system (McClennan and Becker, 1971; McClennan et al., 1971; Talner, 1972).

Materials

Many different types of intravenous infusion devices are satisfactory for delivery of the contrast material. One of the longer indwelling devices (Angiocath Intravenous Placement Unit, Deseret Pharmaceutical Co.; Intrafusor, McGaw Laboratories) should be used, since the contrast materials must not be injected perivascularly.

The type of contrast material used is a matter of personal preference. Mixtures of sodium and meglumine diatrizoates are recommended (Renovist II, Sodium and Meglumine Diatrizoate Injection, Squibb & Sons; Hypaque-M, 75%, Sodium and Meglumine Diatrizoates, Sterile Aqueous Injection, Winthrop Laboratories), since they seem to provide an acceptable combination of radiopacity and patient tolerance. Although certain types of intravascular contrast materials have been found to be nephrotoxic if injected into the aorta or renal arteries (Andrew et al., 1964; Dean et al., 1964; Luttwak et al., 1961; Stokes and Bernard, 1961), the diatrizoate salts are safe even in uremia, provided the patient is not severely dehydrated (Talner, 1972). It has been found that satisfactory opacification of the urinary system of an uremic patient often can be accomplished by increasing the

dose of contrast material (Voltz et al., 1971), since renal opacification is directly related to the amount of contrast material in the blood (Dure-Smith et al., 1972; McEwan, 1971). Sodium diatrizoate alone may cause the patient to vomit, but (possibly because of its lower molecular weight) it produces a higher renal concentration of iodine than the meglumine salt alone (Dacie and Fry, 1971). The method used will determine whether or not a 5 per cent glucose solution will be needed. If a procedure requiring abdominal compression is used, a compression device must be available. A simple compression device can be made by grooving a sponge or foam pad on one side (to accommodate the penis in male dogs). The grooved pad is placed securely on the ventral abdomen just cranial to the brim of the pelvis and is held in that position by a tight encircling elastic bandage or similar wrapping material placed around the wings of the ilia. Alternatively, conventional compression bands, which are provided as accessories to some x-ray tables, may be used. This requires that the patient be held in dorsal recumbency during the compression phase of the procedure, with the compression band passing across the ventral abdomen, immediately cranial to the pubis (Douglas and Williamson, 1972; Suter, 1973).

Dosage of Contrast Material. The dosage of contrast material depends upon several factors—the concentration of iodine in the contrast medium (Table 13–5), the type of excretory urography to be done (Table 13–6), and the renal function of the patient (as evaluated by determination of B.U.N. and/or creatinine levels). If the contrast material is delivered rapidly or as a bolus, the dose should be 425 to 850 mg I/kg of body

TABLE 13–5

IODINE CONCENTRATIONS OF VARIOUS EXCRETORY UROGRAPHIC MEDIA

Product	mg I/ml
Hypaque, 50% (Winthrop Laboratories)	300
Hypaque-M, 75% (Winthrop Laboratories)	385
Renovist II (Squibb & Sons)	310
Renographin-60 (Squibb & Sons)	288
Renographin-76 (Squibb & Sons)	370

TABLE 13–6

SUMMARY OF EXCRETORY
UROGRAPHY PROCEDURES

1. Fast the animal for 24 hours and give a thorough enema.
2. Obtain current survey radiographs of the abdomen.
3. *Low volume, rapid infusion technique with abdominal compression:*
   a. Place an indwelling catheter in a convenient peripheral vein.
   b. Apply a compression band just cranial to the pubis.
   c. Rapidly administer 425 mgI/kg of one of the mixtures of sodium and meglumine diatrizoates intravenously.
   d. Make lateral and VD radiographs of the abdomen immediately and at 1, 3 and 5 minutes.
   e. Remove the compression band immediately prior to the 10 minute radiographs and make lateral and VD abdominal radiographs at 10 and 15 minutes.
   f. VD oblique radiographs of the pelvis made immediately after removal of the compression band are necessary for visualization of the terminal ureters.
4. *Low volume, rapid infusion technique without abdominal compression:*
   a. Place an indwelling catheter in a convenient peripheral vein.
   b. Position the animal over the cassette in dorsal recumbency.
   c. Inject 850 mgI/kg of one of the mixtures of sodium and meglumine diatrizoate intravenously as rapidly as possible.
   d. The first radiograph (VD only) is made 10 seconds after injection is commenced.
   e. Make VD and lateral abdominal radiographs as soon as possible and at 1 minute, at 3 to 5 minutes and at 15 minutes following injection.
   f. VD oblique views of the pelvis may be made if terminal ureters are of special interest.
5. *Low volume, slow infusion technique without abdominal compression:*

   a. Place an indwelling catheter in a convenient peripheral vein.
   b. Over a 2 to 3 minute period of time, infuse 425 mgI/kg of one of the mixtures of sodium and meglumine diatrizoates intravenously.
   c. When the contrast material has been injected, make lateral and VD radiographs of the abdomen immediately and at 3, 5, 10 and 15 minutes after completion of injection of the contrast material.
   d. VD oblique views of the pelvis may be made if terminal ureters are of special interest.
6. *High volume, drip infusion technique with abdominal compression:*
   a. Place an indwelling catheter in a convenient peripheral vein.
   b. Mix 1200 mgI/kg body weight of one of the mixtures of sodium and meglumine diatrizoates (maximum dose, 35 g) with an equal volume of 5% dextrose and water.
   c. By drip infusion, administer the mixture over a 10 minute period of time, accelerating the rate of infusion near the end of this period if necessary to insure injection of all the contrast material within the specified time.
   d. At the end of the infusion, make radiographs of the abdomen in both projections.
   e. Immediately apply a compression band to the caudal abdomen.
   f. If renal function was determined to be normal, repeat radiographs in both projections 10 minutes later.
   g. If renal function was abnormal, make radiographs of the abdomen 20 minutes later.
   h. Remove the compression band.
   i. Additional radiographs after removal of the compression band are optional. Oblique films of the trigone should be made at this time if the terminal ureters are of special interest.

weight. If the high volume, drip infusion technique is used, 1200 mg I/kg of body weight should be administered. Maximum dose probably should not exceed 35 g.

In uremic animals, the recommended dose may be safely doubled. Arbitrarily, this should be done if the B.U.N. is in excess of 40 mg/100 ml.

Procedure (Table 13–6)

Low Volume, Rapid Infusion Technique With Abdominal Compression. The intravenous catheter is placed in a convenient peripheral vein, and the compression device is applied. The total dose of contrast material (425 mgI/kg) is administered rapidly. Ventrodorsal and lateral films of the abdomen are made immediately and at 1, 3, 5, 10 and 15 minutes. Abdominal compression should be released just prior to the 10 minute film. The purpose of the compression device is to press the urinary bladder against the spine and occlude the terminal ureters, causing stasis and accumulation of opacified urine in the renal pelves and proximal ureters. Some feel that this method is not physiologic and introduces artifacts (Lord et al., 1974), such as tortuosity, dilation and distention of the obstructed ureters. However, in films made after the compression band is released, the normal ureteral course and diameter should be visualized. Left and right VD oblique radiographs are necessary to visualize the terminal ureters.

Low Volume, Rapid Infusion Technique, Without Abdominal Compression. Using this method (Lord et al., 1974), the contrast material (850 mgI/kg) is delivered as rapidly as possible through a large intravenous catheter after the patient has been positioned in VD recumbency over the cassette. Ten seconds after injection commences, the first exposure (VD only) is made. After the first radiograph, VD and lateral radiographs are made as soon as possible, and at 1 minute, at 3 to 5 minutes and at 15 minutes after the contrast medium was injected. Left and right VD oblique radiographs are necessary to visualize the terminal ureters. Often an arteriographic phase is seen on the radiograph made 10 seconds after beginning injection of contrast material; at the same time, the nephrogram phase is appreciated. Abdominal compression is not done, therefore avoiding ureteral distention and tortu-osity. Ureteral opacification is usually much less pronounced with this technique than with one of the techniques employing ureteral compression.

Low Volume, Slow Infusion Technique, Without Abdominal Compression. Using this technique, the contrast material (425 mgI/kg) is infused over a 2 to 3 minute period. Lateral and VD radiographs are made immediately and at 3, 5, 10 and 15 minutes after the injection is complete. Left and right VD oblique radiographs are necessary to visualize the terminal ureters. No ureteral artifacts are seen, but visualization of the collecting systems may be poor if renal clearance and ureteral function are normal.

High Volume, Drip Infusion Technique, With Abdominal Compression. This method is felt to produce the best visualization of the urinary system (Borthwick and Robbie, 1969; Suter, 1973; Walker and Douglas, 1970). It has the advantage of requiring fewer radiographs than the other procedures, allowing simultaneous visualization of the kidneys, ureters and urinary bladder. The calculated dose of contrast material (1200 mgI/kg, not to exceed 35 g) is mixed with equal volume of 5 per cent glucose solution, and is administered over a 10 minute period through a suitable intravenous catheter. The duration of infusion should be at least 10 minutes in order to allow the entire renal system to be opacified. Contrast material remaining approximately 8 minutes after the beginning of infusion should be rapidly infused within the last 2 minutes. Lateral and VD radiographs are made of the abdomen at the completion of infusion of the contrast material, and a compression device is applied. If renal function has been determined to be normal, radiographs of the abdomen are repeated 10 minutes later, and the compression band is removed. If renal clearance is abnormal, the compression band remains in place and radiographs are made 20 minutes later. If the terminal ureters are to be visualized, VD oblique radiographs of the pelvic region must be made immediately after removal of the compression device.

Complications

If the contrast material is injected too rapidly, vomiting may be induced, especially when a contrast medium containing only the sodium salt of the diatrizoate molecule is used. Vomiting is less common when a combination of the sodium and meglumine diatrizoates is used, but it can occur. Emesis will not effect the outcome of the study, but it may cause a slight delay in the filming sequence.

Because perivascular deposition or significant extravasation of the contrast material will cause a severe slough (McAlister and Palmer, 1971), an indwelling type of venous catheter is strongly recommended. If perivascular deposition of media occurs, immediate local infiltration of the perivascular swelling with sterile saline, lidocaine HCl and a corticosteroid is helpful in reducing the severity of the reaction.

Anaphylactoid reactions to the contrast agent are rare in animals and man. In human studies, most radiologists no longer administer a preliminary "test dose" of the contrast material because reactions are so uncommon and are often delayed. Reactions to the "test dose" are often no less severe than reactions to the entire dose. In man, the incidence of severe reactions may be lessened by giving atropine sulfate prior to injection of contrast material (Svendsen and Wilson, 1971).

Pancytopenia is reported to have resulted from the administration of diatrizoates in man (Stemerman et al., 1971). This has not been reported in dogs or cats.

Normal Findings (Figs. 13–30 and 13–31)

Both kidneys should be visualized. The left kidney in the dog is normally located caudomedially to the spleen adjacent to the

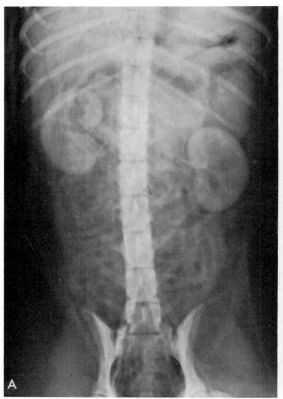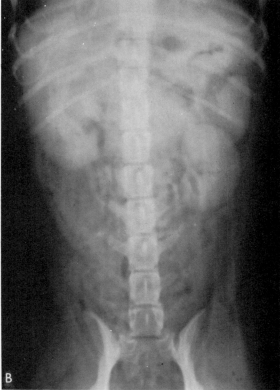

Figure 13–30. Normal excretory urogram, low volume, rapid injection without compression. Radiographs of the abdomen of a normal dog made 8 seconds *(A)*, 15 seconds *(B)*, 3 minutes *(C)*, 10 minutes *(D)*, and 15 minutes *(E)* after rapid intravenous injection of organic iodide solution containing 450 mg of organic iodine per kg of body weight (using a mixture of sodium and meglumine diatrizoates). At 8 seconds (A) and at 15 seconds (B), the renal outlines (nephrogram phase) are well visualized. At 3 minutes, faint opacification of the renal collecting systems and ureters (pyelogram-ureterogram phase) is seen. At 10 (D) and 15 minutes (E), there is progressive opacification of the urinary bladder.

(Illustration continued on the opposite page.)

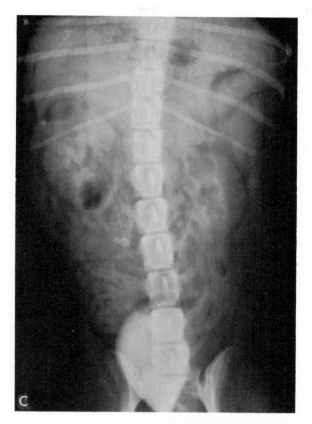

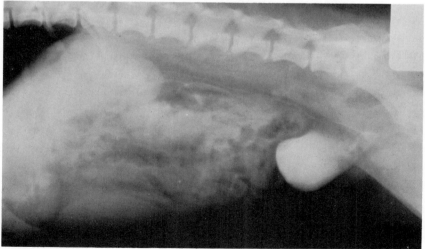

Figure 13-30. *Continued.*

(Illustration continued on the following page.)

second, third, fourth and fifth lumbar vertebrae (Osborne et al., 1969), while the right kidney normally is located approximately half its length further craniad, at the level of T_{13} to L_3. Renal position is more variable in the cat. Normal kidney length is approximately 2½ adjacent vertebral bodies in the dog (Douglas and Williamson, 1970; Root and Scott, 1971) and approximately 2 adjacent vertebral bodies in the cat (Lord et al., 1974). In both species, this measurement includes the widths of the interposed intervertebral disc spaces. The ratio of kidney length to the length of L_2 has been deter-

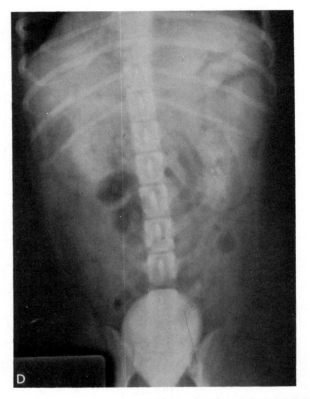

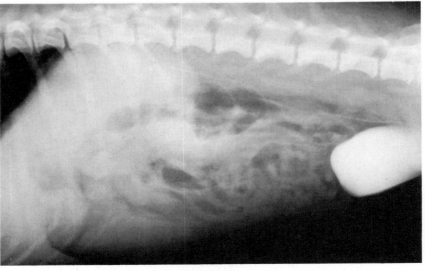

Figure 13–30. *Continued.*

(Illustration continued on the opposite page.)

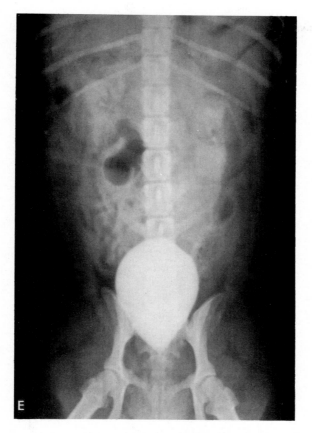

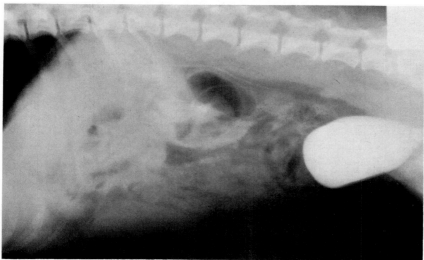

Figure 13–30. *Continued.*

mined in the dog (Finco et al., 1971), but the accuracy of this method was not compared with previous methods of evaluating kidney size. The kidneys should be smooth in outline. Feline kidneys normally are more rounded than those of the dog. The renal shadows should be uniformly opaque, indicating normal function of all areas.

Both pelves and both ureters should be visualized. If compression is not used, these structures may be difficult to see; because of long peristaltic waves, only portions of each

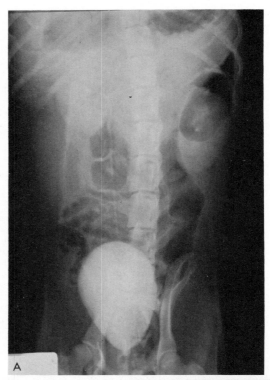

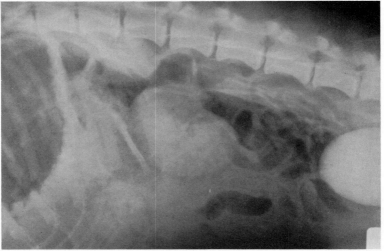

Figure 13–31. Normal excretory urogram—high volume drip infusion with compression. *A,* Lateral and VD abdominal radiographs of a normal dog at the completion of slow intravenous injection of organic iodide containing 850 mg of iodine per kg of body weight (using a mixture of sodium and meglumine diatrizoates). The kidneys, ureters and urinary bladder are faintly opacified. *B,* Lateral and VD abdominal radiographs of the same dog 20 minutes after commencement of injection (10 minutes after cessation of infusion and application of a tight compression bandage around the caudal abdomen). The renal collecting systems, ureters, and urinary bladder are distended and well visualized.

(*Illustration continued on the opposite page.*)

ureter will be visualized. The ureters should be straight in the absence of obstruction or abdominal compression. The pelves and collecting systems will be faint densities, often incomplete in outline. However, if a compression device is applied, the collecting systems, renal pelves and proximal ureters are well delineated and slightly dilated. The

ureters may be slightly tortuous, owing to their increased length from overdistention.

Whether or not abdominal compression is used, visualization of the terminal ureters is usually poor, unless supplemental oblique projections of the pelvic region are made. The urinary bladder should become progressively opaque and should contain no filling

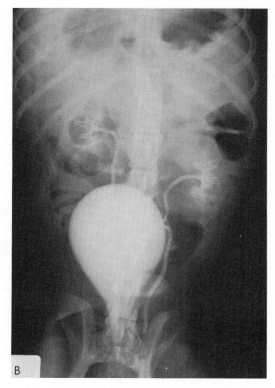

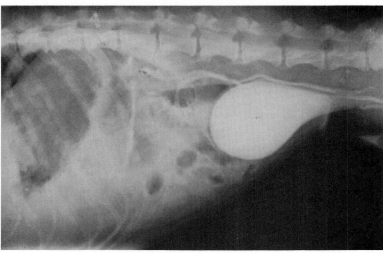

Figure 13–31. *Continued.*

defects. The bladder wall should be smooth in outline and uniform in thickness. Urinary bladder outline may reflect extrinsic pressures of adjacent structures unless fully distended.

CONTRAST RADIOGRAPHY OF THE URINARY BLADDER (CYSTOGRAPHY, PNEUMOCYSTOGRAPHY, DOUBLE CONTRAST CYSTOGRAPHY)

Indications

The most common indication for contrast radiography of the urinary bladder is hematuria, especially if it is accompanied by vesical tenesmus. However, straining to urinate without hematuria is also a valid indication for this study. In susceptible breeds of dogs, pneumocystography (Rhodes and Biery, 1967) or cystography may be the only methods by which radiolucent urinary calculi can be demonstrated. Contrast radiography is important for definitive localization of the urinary bladder in cases of perineal or other herniae (Carlson and Gillette, 1967), caudal abdominal or pelvic masses (Douglas and Williamson, 1972), prostatic enlargement (Douglas and Williamson, 1972; Leav and Ling, 1968; Pearson and Gibbs, 1971) or suspected rupture of the bladder (Carlson and Gillette, 1967). Suspected patent urachus also may be evaluated by opacification of the urinary bladder (Greene and Bohning, 1971; Pearson and Gibbs, 1971).

Contraindications

Contrast radiography of the urinary bladder is unrewarding and possibly contraindicated in the presence of massive bladder enlargement resulting from atony, since true atony is most often due to neurologic deficit rather than obstructive disease. Although contrast radiography is not contraindicated in the presence of radiopaque cystic calculi, it is usually not necessary, since the wall of the urinary bladder can be viewed directly during cystotomy.

Double contrast cystography (Osborne and Jessen, 1971) with barium sulfate as the positive contrast agent probably should not be done if fistulae, blind tracts, diverticula or similar lesions are suspected, because of the possibility that entrapment of barium in such structures may lead to granulomas.

Preparation of Patient

The patient should be fasted for 12 to 24 hours (Carlson and Gillette, 1967) and a cleansing enema should be given (Carlson and Gillette, 1967; Rhodes and Biery, 1967). As in most other contrast procedures involving abdominal viscera, commercial hypertonic enema solutions usually are not thorough enough. A current urinalysis is recommended before opacification of the urinary bladder, since it will provide information useful in differential diagnosis. Survey radiographs of the abdomen are required (Carlson and Gillette, 1967).

Materials

A three-way stopcock, a catheter adapter (Rubber Catheter Adapter, Rusch, Inc.) a male catheter (Ureteral Catheters, 3-10 French, Rusch, Inc.) and a large syringe are necessary for performing contrast radiography of the urinary bladder. Rigid female catheters are not needed because females may be easily and safely catheterized with large male catheters, with reduced risk of puncturing the urinary bladder or lacerating the urethra. Flexible male catheters also appear to be more comfortable and therefore may be allowed to remain in place during the study.

Any of the diatrizoate media (Hypaque-M, 75%, Winthrop Laboratories; Renovist II, Squibb & Son) may be used for cystography, but must be diluted to 5 to 10 per cent iodine (W/V). Room air is used for pneumocystography.

Dosage of Contrast Material. The urinary bladder must be moderately distended with contrast medium. This usually requires 3 to 5 ml of medium per pound of body weight. The desired concentration of iodine in the urinary bladder may be accomplished in several ways. The easiest and most accurate method is to empty the bladder completely before instilling a known concentration (5 to 10% iodine, W/V) of contrast material.

In double contrast cystography with barium sulfate suspension and air, the amount of barium sulfate used is not critical. The object is to thoroughly coat the mucosal surface of the bladder with barium sulfate suspension. After removal of as much of the barium sulfate as possible, the bladder is distended with 3 to 5 cc of air per pound of body weight.

Procedure (Table 13–7)

In veterinary medicine, either positive contrast cystography or pneumocystography usually is performed. Unfortunately, this often results in obtaining less than maximal information about the character of the wall of the urinary bladder. It is recommended, therefore, that pneumocystography routinely follow positive contrast cystography, since the mucosal surface of the urinary bladder is best appreciated when the bladder is opacified and the thickness of its wall is best seen when contrasted with air. Pneumocystography alone is indicated only if rupture of the urinary bladder is suspected.

A catheter is introduced and as much of the urine as possible is removed. The urinary bladder is then filled with 3 to 5 ml/lb of body weight of a 5 to 10 per cent solution (W/V) of one of the mixtures of sodium and meglumine diatrizoate. Filling of the urinary bladder should be monitored by abdominal palpation. Radiographs of the caudal abdomen are then made in the lateral and VD projections. The contrast material is then replaced with an equal volume of air, and the radiographs of the caudal abdomen are repeated.

Double contrast cystography (Osborne and Jessen, 1971), with barium sulfate suspension and air, is done as follows: The urinary bladder is catheterized and the urine is removed. A small volume of barium sulfate suspension (1 to 2 ml per pound of body weight) is then instilled into the urinary bladder. The barium sulfate suspension should be fairly dilute (15 to 20 per cent, W/V) or it will be difficult to inject and retrieve through the catheter. The patient should be rotated along its longitudinal axis several times or the bladder should be massaged by gentle abdominal palpation to allow the barium to contact the entire mucosal surface of the urinary bladder, and as much of the contrast material as possible is removed. The urinary bladder is then filled with 3 to 5 cc of air per pound of body weight and radiographs of the caudal abdo-

men are made in both VD and lateral projections.

Complications

Overdistention of the urinary bladder will lead to rupture. This is not a common sequela to contrast radiography of the urinary bladder if normal precautions are used and recommended volumes of contrast media are not exceeded. However, if there are large masses within the urinary bladder, 3 to 5 cc/lb may cause overdistention and may lead to rupture. Palpation of the urinary bladder during filling is therefore advised. Careless catheterization can lead to urethral trauma or cystitis, but these problems are easily avoided by using caution and antiseptic technique.

TABLE 13–7

SUMMARY OF CYSTOGRAPHY PROCEDURES

1. Fast the patient for 12 to 24 hours.
2. Give a cleansing enema.
3. Obtain current survey radiographs of the abdomen.
4. *Cystography–Pneumocystography:*
   a. Catheterize and empty urinary bladder.
   b. Instill 3 to 5 ml/lb of body weight of 5 to 10% organic iodide solution.
   c. Make lateral and VD radiographs of the caudal abdomen, leaving the catheter in place.
   d. Remove the iodide solution and replace it with an equal volume of air.
   e. Make lateral and VD radiographs of the caudal abdomen.
5. *Double Contrast Cystography:*
   a. Catheterize the urinary bladder with as large a catheter as possible and remove the urine.
   b. Instill a small volume (1 to 2 ml/lb of body weight) of dilute (15 to 20% W/V) barium sulfate suspension into the urinary bladder.
   c. Roll the patient over several times or massage the bladder to coat the mucosa of the urinary bladder with contrast material.
   d. Remove as much of the barium sulfate suspension as possible.
   e. Distend the urinary bladder with 3 to 5 cc of air/lb of body weight.
   f. Make lateral and VD radiographs of the caudal abdomen.

Normal Findings (Figs. 13–32 and 13–33)

The urinary bladder should be uniformly distended. Its wall should be intact and should be thin and regular in width. There should be no mural or luminal filling defects. Contrast material should be present only in the lumen of the urinary system and should not fill the prostatic ducts in the male. In the

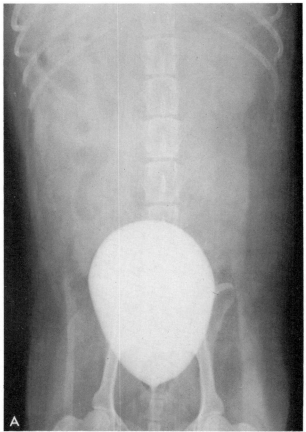

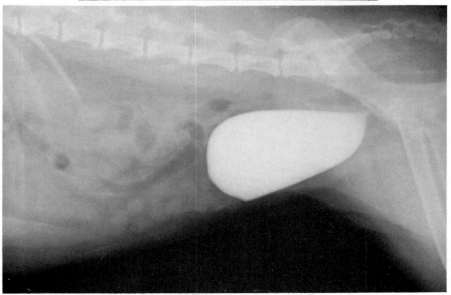

Figure 13–32. *See opposite page for legend.*

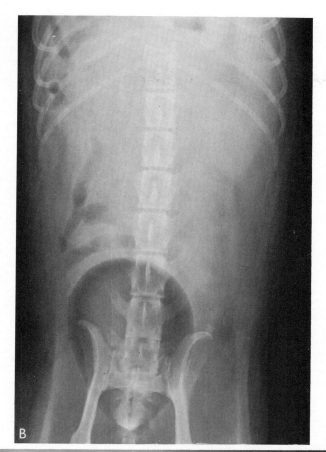

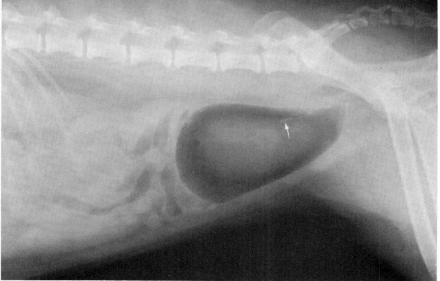

Figure 13–32. *Continued.* Normal cystogram—pneumocystogram. *A,* Lateral and VD radiographs of the abdomen of a normal female dog after distention of the urinary bladder with 4 ml of 7.5% organic iodide solution per pound of body weight. *B,* Lateral and VD radiographs of the same dog after replacement of the iodine solution with an equal volume of room air. The wall of the urinary bladder is smooth and uniform in width. No mural or luminal filling defects are seen. The tip of the catheter (arrow) is seen in the apex of the urinary bladder during the pneumocystogram.

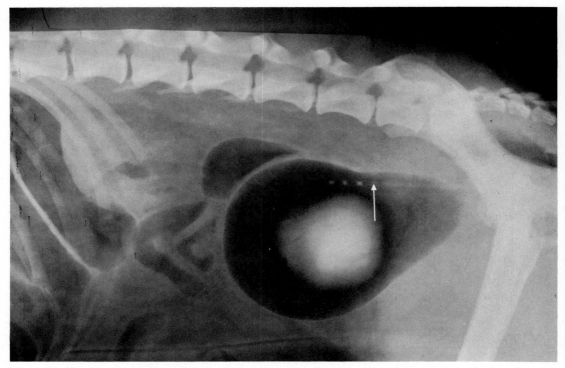

Figure 13–33. Normal double contrast cystogram. Lateral radiograph of the abdomen of a male dog after coating the urinary bladder mucosa with a small amount of barium sulfate suspension and distention of the urinary bladder with 5 cc room air per pound of body weight. A pool of barium is present in the dependent portion of the urinary bladder. The catheter tip is visible (arrow). The mucosal surface of the bladder is faintly coated with positive contrast medium. The wall is smooth and of uniform thickness. Note the air bubbles at the edge of the barium pool.

female, the apex of the urinary bladder is more pointed than in the male. The distended urinary bladder displaces the small bowel cranially and dorsally. Ventrally, the urinary bladder is usually in contact with the ventral body wall. The colon is usually displaced to the left, but in some animals it may be displaced to the right if the bladder is markedly distended. Retrograde opacification of one or both ureters may be a normal finding (Christie, 1971, 1973*a, b;* Newman et al., 1973). This finding is most common in young dogs (Christie, 1971, 1973*a, b*) and in patients positioned in lateral recumbency during distention of the urinary bladder with contrast material (Newman et al., 1973).

URETHROGRAPHY

Indications

Opacification of the urethra is usually in-

dicated when there is severe dysuria or tenesmus, which may occur with iatrogenic trauma or urethral calculi. Severe pelvic trauma, in which one or both of the pubes are fractured and displaced, is another strong indication for urethrography (Kleine and Thornton, 1971), especially in the male dog. Prostatic lesions also justify urethral opacification. In rare fractures of the os penis, opacification of the penile urethra can determine whether or not the damage includes disruption of the urethral mucosal lining.

Contraindications

There are few contraindications for urethrography. Retrograde urethral filling requiring high pressure should be avoided. In such cases, surgical exploration of the obstructed portion of the urethra is indicated. In the presence of severe urethral hemorrhage, hemostasis should be accomplished before contrast radiography of the urethra is performed. Urethrography is not contraindicated in female dogs but is very difficult to perform because the urethra is relatively short in length and wide in diameter.

Preparation of Patient

Cleansing of only the terminal colon and rectum usually is satisfactory, and the commercial hypertonic enema solutions are adequate for this purpose. Fasting is not necessary unless studies of the kidneys and urinary bladder are also needed. Survey radiography of the pelvis and perineum in the lateral and VD projections is required.

Materials

An organic iodide solution is recommended, and the diatrizoates (Renovist II, Squibb & Sons; Hypaque-M 75%, Winthrop Laboratories) are the agents of choice. Depending upon the part of the urethra to be studied, either an 8 to 12 French gauge pediatric Foley catheter (Pediatric Gilbert Foley Catheters, 8 to 12 French, Bard Hospital Divison, C.R. Bard, Inc.) or a male urethral catheter (Ureteral Catheters, 3 to 10 French, Rusch, Inc.) is needed. If the Foley catheter is chosen, 2 per cent lidocaine HCl solution and gel (Xylocaine HCl Injection or Gel, 2%, Ayerst Laboratories) are also required. With either catheter, an appropriate catheter adapter (Rubber Catheter Adapters, Rusch, Inc.) and a three-way stopcock are necessary.

Dosage of Contrast Material. The amount of contrast material is not critical, but the urethra must be distended at the time the films are made. This usually requires 5 to 10 ml of contrast material.

Procedure (Table 13-8)

Retrograde Urethrography

The Foley catheter is used to administer the medium to the extrapelvic or penile portion of the urethra. Its introduction may be facilitated through the use of a stylet to produce rigidity. Using a small amount of the lidocaine gel, for lubrication, the catheter is inserted so that its cuff is within that

TABLE 13-8

SUMMARY OF URETHROGRAPHY PROCEDURES

1. Fasting is not necessary, but cleansing the colon is advised.
2. *Retrograde Urethrography:*
   a. Introduce an appropriate Foley catheter into the penile urethra, using lidocaine HCl gel and a stylet if necessary.
   b. Instill several milliliters of lidocaine HCl solution or gel into the penile urethra through the Foley catheter. Inflate the cuff.
   c. Slowly inject 2 to 5 ml of lidocaine HCl solution into the urethra.
   d. Slowly inject 5 to 10 ml of the contrast material with the animal positioned for lateral radiography.
   e. As the injection is terminated, make an exposure, centering on the perineum.
   f. Repeat the injection with the patient in a slightly oblique VD position if desired.
3. *Prostatic Urethrography:*
   a. During positive contrast cystography, deliver 5 to 10 ml of 5 to 10% organic iodide solution or opacified urine into the prostatic urethra (the location of which is 1 to 3 cm distal to the point at which aspiration is not possible during slow withdrawal of the catheter from the urinary bladder).
   b. Radiograph the prostatic urethra in the lateral projection at the end of the injection.

portion of the urethra contained by the os penis. The stylet is removed, and 2 to 3 ml of 2 per cent lidocaine HCl solution or gel are slowly injected, and the cuff is inflated. Several more milliliters of lidocaine HCl are injected slowly. With the patient positoned in lateral recumbency, 5 to 10 ml of the contrast material are slowly injected and the film is exposed as the last of the contrast medium is infused. Additional injections may be made with the animal in right and left VD oblique positions if desired; however, the lateral projection is the most valuable.

Prostatic Urethrography

If the prostatic urethra is to be studied, a standard male catheter is used. This study should be a part of the standard positive contrast cystogram in the male dog. After the required volume of 5 to 10 per cent iodide solution has been instilled into the urinary bladder, the catheter is slowly withdrawn into the prostatic urethra while aspirating some of the opaque medium from the urinary bladder until backflow into the syringe ceases. The catheter is then withdrawn 1 to 3 cm further to ensure that the delivery holes in the catheter tip are in the prostatic urethra. Then the contrast material is slowly re-injected. At the conclusion of the injection, a lateral radiograph of the caudal abdomen and perineum is made. A slightly oblique VD projection also may be worthwhile. If the contrast medium or opacified urine is re-injected too rapidly or too far distally, micturition may be stimulated.

Complications

Overdistention of the bulb or cuff of the Foley catheter can traumatize the urethra.

Air bubbles may be difficult to differentiate from calculi; they may be prevented by injecting enough contrast medium to flush them retrograde into the urinary bladder. If, during prostatic urethrography, the tip of the standard male catheter is too distally located, the animal may be stimulated to urinate. If this occurs, and one is not quick enough to obtain a voiding urethrogram, the study may have to be repeated. If topical anesthesia is inadequate or omitted, during the Foley catheter technique a long spasm of the pelvic urethra (particularly at the ischial arch) may be seen.

Normal Findings (Figs. 13–34 and 13–35)

The urethra should be smooth in outline throughout its entire course, but in the presence of spasm of its pelvic portion it may not be uniform in width. The prostatic urethra usually is slightly wider than the ex-

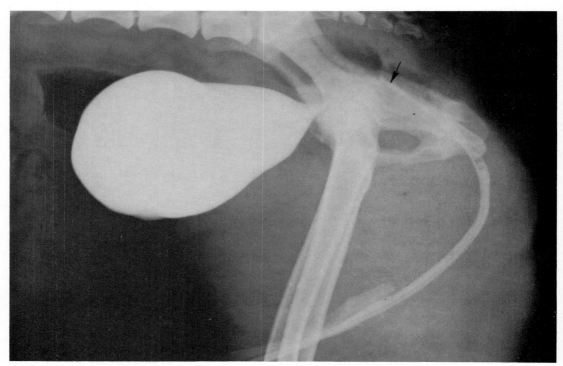

Figure 13–34. Normal prostatic urethrogram. Lateral radiograph of the caudal pelvis of a male dog, made during routine cystography after injection of 10 ml of 75% organic iodide solution into the prostatic portion of the urethra. Not only is the prostate gland totally within the pelvic canal, but no contrast material has entered the prostatic ducts. Some of the contrast material also opacifies the penile portion of the urethra. The catheter tip (arrow) is seen in the caudal prostatic urethra.

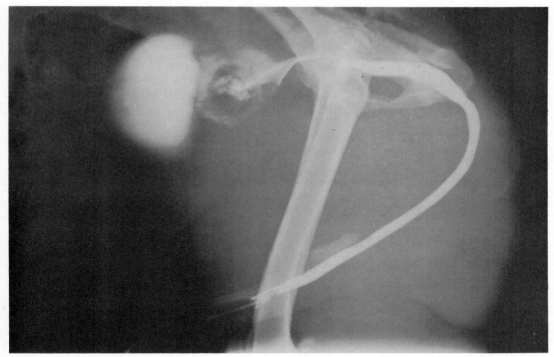

Figure 13–35. Normal retrograde urethrogram. Lateral radiograph of the caudal abdomen and perineum of a male dog at the conclusion of retrograde opacification of the urethra with 15 ml of 75% organic iodide solution injected through a Foley catheter. The urethral mucosa had been topically anesthetized by retrograde flushing of lidocaine HCl solution before instillation of contrast agent. The prostatic urethra in this animal is narrowed by spasm but may be dilated in other normal patients. The entire penile urethra is smooth in outline and uniform in width. No filling defects are present.

trapelvic urethra. No filling defects are seen in the urethral lumen, and no contrast material normally enters the prostatic ducts or glandular tissue.

REFERENCES

Andrew, J. H., et al.: Renal damage from angiographic media. Arch. Surg., *88*:812, 1964.

Borthwick, R., and Robbie, B.: Large volume urography in the cat. J. Small Anim. Pract., *12*:579, 1971.

Borthwick, R., and Robbie, B.: Urography in the dog by an intravenous infusion technique. J. Small Anim. Pract., *10*:465, 1969.

Bosniak, M. A., and Schweizer, R. D.: Urographic findings in patients with renal failure. Radiol. Clin. N. Amer., *10*:433, 1972.

Burt, J. K., and Root, C. R.: Radiographic manifestations of abdominal trauma. J. Amer. Anim. Hosp. Assoc., *7*:328, 1971.

Carlson, W. D., and Gillette, E. L.: Veterinary Radiology. 2nd ed. Philadelphia, Lea & Febiger, 1967.

Christie, B. A.: Incidence and etiology of vesicoureteral reflux in apparently normal dogs. Invest. Urol., *9*:184, 1971.

Christie, B. A.: The occurrence of vesicoureteral reflux and pyelonephritis in apparently normal dogs. Invest. Urol., *10*:359, 1973*a*.

Christie, B. A.: Vesicoureteral reflux in dogs. J. Amer. Vet. Med. Assoc., *169*:772, 1973*b*.

Dacie, J. E., and Fry, I. K.: A comparison of sodium and methylglucamine diatrizoate in clinical urography. Brit. J. Radiol., *44*:51, 1971.

Dean, R. E., Andrew, J. H., and Read, R. C.: Renal damage from angiographic media. J.A.M.A., *187*:27, 1964.

Douglas, S. W., and Williamson, H. D.: Principles of Veterinary Radiography. 2nd ed. Baltimore, Williams & Wilkins, 1972.

Douglas, S. W., and Williamson, H. D.: Veterinary Radiological Interpretation. Philadelphia, Lea & Febiger, 1970.

Dure-Smith, P., Simenhoff, M., Brodsky, S., and Zimskind, P. D.: Opacification of the urinary tract during excretory urography: Concentration vs. amount of contrast medium. Invest. Radiol., *7*:407, 1972.

Finco, D. R., Kurtz, H. J., and Porter, T. E.: Renal and ureteral urolithiasis in a dog. J. Amer. Vet. Med. Assoc., *157*:837, 1970.

Finco, D. R., Stiles, N. S., Kneller, S. K., Lewis, R. E., and Barrett, R. B.: Radiologic estimation of kidney size of the dog. J. Amer. Vet. Med. Assoc., *159*:995, 1971.

Goldman, H. S., and Freeman, L. M.: Radiographic and radioisotopic methods of evaluation of the kidneys and urinary tract. Ped. Clin. N. Amer., *18*:409, 1971.

Greene, R. W., and Bohning, R. H.: Patent persistent urachus associated with urolithiasis in a cat. J. Amer. Vet. Med. Assoc., *158*:489, 1971.

Killen, D. A., Foster, J. H., and Scott, H. W.: Toxic reactions incident to urokon aortography. Ann. Surg., *155*:472, 1962.

Kleine, L. J., and Thornton, G. W.: Radiographic diagnosis of urinary tract trauma. J. Amer. Anim. Hosp. Assoc., *7*:318, 1971.

Leav, I., and Ling, G. V.: Adenocarcinoma of the canine prostate. Cancer, *22*:1329, 1968.

Lord, P. F., Scott, R. C., and Chan, K. F.: Intravenous urography for evaluation of renal diseases in small animals. J. Amer. Anim. Hosp. Assoc., *10*:139, 1974.

Luttwak, E. M., Reed, G. E., and Breed, E. S.: Effect of aortography on renal function. Ann. Surg., *154*:190, 1961.

McAlister, W. H., and Palmer, K.: The histologic effects of four commonly used media for excretory urography and an attempt to modify the responses. Radiology, *99*:511, 1971.

McClennan, B. L., and Becker, J. A.: Excretory urography: Choice of contrast material — clinical. Radiology, *100*:591, 1971.

McClennan, B. L., Becker, J. A., and Berdon, W. E.: Excretory urography: Choice of contrast material — experimental. Radiology, *100*:585, 1971.

McEwan, A. D.: The clinical diagnosis of renal disease in the dog. J. Small Anim. Pract., *12*:543, 1971.

Newman, L., Bucy, J. G., and McAlister, W. H.: Incidence of naturally occurring vesicoureteral reflux in mongrel dogs. Invest. Radiol., *8*:354, 1973.

Osborne, C. A., and Jessen, C. R.: Double-contrast cystography in the dog. J. Amer. Vet. Med. Assoc., *159*:1400, 1971.

Osborne, C. A., Yoho, B. C., Low, D. G., and Wall, B. E.: Radiographic evaluation of the canine urinary system. J. Amer. Anim. Hosp. Assoc., *5*:136, 1969.

Pearson, H., and Gibbs, C.: Urinary tract abnormalities in the dog. J. Small Anim. Pract., *12*:67, 1971.

Rhodes, W. H., and Biery, D. N.: Pneumocystography in the dog. J. Amer. Vet. Radiol. Soc., *8*:45, 1967.

Root, C. R., and Scott, R. C.: Emphysematous cystitis and other radiographic manifestations of diabetes mellitus in dogs and cats. J. Amer. Vet. Med. Assoc., *158*:279, 1971.

Scott, R. C., Greene, R. W., and Patnaik, A. K.: Unilateral ureterocele associated with hydronephrosis in a dog. J. Amer. Anim. Hosp. Assoc., *10*:126, 1974.

Stemerman, M., Goldstein, M. L., and Schulman, P. L.: Pancytopenia associated with diatrizoate. N. Y. State J. Med., *71*:1220, 1971.

Stokes, J. M., and Bernard, H. R.: Nephrotoxicity of iodinated contrast media. Ann. Surg., *153*:299, 1961.

Suter, P. F.: Personal communication. January, 1973.

Svendsen, P., and Wilson, J.: Adverse reactions during urography and modification by atropine. Acta Radiol., *11*:427, 1971.

Talner, L. B.: Urographic contrast media in uremia; physiology and pharmacology. Radiol. Clin. N. Amer., *10*:421, 1972.

Voltz, P. W., Logan, B., and Wolff, H. L.: Adequate dose excretory urography: experience with 25,000 cases. South. Med. J., *64*:903, 1971.

Walker, R. G., and Douglas, S. W.: The use of contrast media in the diagnosis of urinary tract abnormalities in the dog, with particular reference to infusion urography: A report of two cases. Vet. Rec., *87*:287, 1970.

14
TOMOGRAPHY

Jack C. Geary

Tomography is the technique of producing radiographs of selected thin planes, or layers, of the living patient. Other names given this technique are laminagraphy (or laminography), body-section radiography, planigraphy and stratigraphy. This procedure permits radiographic visualization of anatomic features, or lesions, which normally would be obscured by other structures that lie in planes above or below the region of interest. It has been used successfully in studies of the thoracic vertebral column, the thorax, various regions of the skull, certain joints and the urinary system (Geary, 1967).

THEORY

Basically tomography is accomplished by coordinated reciprocal motion of the x-ray tube and the film/cassette combination about a center or pivot point (Kiefer, 1943) (Fig. 14–1). This pivotal point can be adjusted to various levels in reference to the x-ray table top; thus different planes within the patient can be selected for display (Figs. 14–2 and 14–3).

The x-ray exposure and tube/film motion occur at the same time, producing blurred images of the structures which lie above or below the plane selected (Figs. 14–4, 14–5 and 14–6). The equipment motion and associated long exposures make general anesthesia for the patient mandatory. It is the usual practice to make a series of exposures at different levels to ensure that the tomographs fully display the information sought.

Motion of the patient during the exposure usually destroys the diagnostic value of the film, and changes of the patient's position between exposures adversely affect any reference value of one "section" film to another.

The thickness of the plane, or layer displayed on the tomograph, can be changed by varying the amplitude of tube/film travel. Greater amplitude produces a thinner section, while a lesser range of motion produces a thicker one (General Electric X-Ray Corp., 1951).

Tomographic devices vary in the complexity of their motion patterns. Some of them provide only linear motion while others are capable of circular, elliptical and hypocycloidal as well as linear motion. Equipment commonly available at nominal cost is relatively simple in operation. These devices attach to the x-ray table with linkage between it, the x-ray tube and the Bucky tray. This performs what has been called rectilinear tomography. The more complex and expensive units are, of course, capable of producing more diagnostic tomographs in certain cases.

TECHNIQUE

The decision to perform a tomographic examination should be made only after the

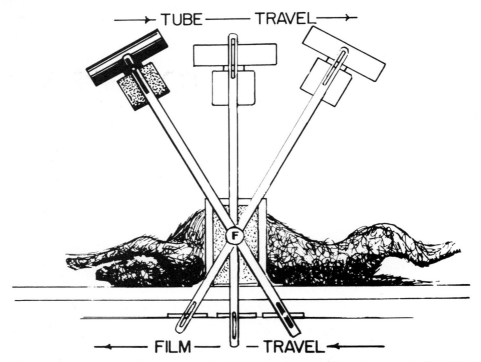

Figure 14–1. Drawing illustrating the simple mechanical principles of rectilinear tomography. The tube and Bucky tray are linked together and move in opposite directions around the pivot point "F," which can be adjusted upward or downward to selectively focus on different levels within the patient. The device is usually driven by an electric motor which moves the tubestand or ceiling mount.

preliminary survey films have been made and interpreted.

For the examination, the anesthetized patient should be positioned on the x-ray table with the site of interest centered on the table opposite the pivotal point of the device. The tube and linkage should be placed in the vertical position, which is the midpoint of its range of motion. A cassette should be placed in the tray, the exposure factors calculated and a plain film exposed. The electromechanical drive of the unit should be disconnected for this exposure. After processing, inspect the film for correctness of exposure factors and positioning. Make any necessary corrections. This first film has important reference value when interpreting the subsequent tomograms. If positioning and exposure techniques are satisfactory, determine the approximate level location of the suspected lesion from the preliminary survey views, and set this level on the adjustable pivot attachment.

Determine the desired thickness of "section" and adjust the tube/film amplitude control accordingly. Engage the electromechanical drive and make a "dry run" to ensure smooth mechanical operation. Make any necessary adjustments and begin examination.

It is usually appropriate to make a series of exposures at different levels so that the tomographic "sections" begin slightly above or below the lesion site and pass through it. This procedure usually ensures that one or two of the sections will best show the lesion. It is sometimes necessary to position the patient so that his long axis is across the table rather than parallel to it. Best displays of long, dense structures, such as the vertebral column, are produced when the plane of tube/film motion is perpendicular to them.

Multiple screen cassettes produce multiple simultaneous tomograms of levels within the patient appropriate to the spacing between the pairs of intensifying screens in the special cassette. This provides a series of tomographs with one exposure (McInnes, 1955).

Packets of nonscreen film, separated by radiolucent sheets of cardboard, can be employed in a similar manner with an appropriate increase in the exposure factors because there are no intensifying screens (McInnes, 1955). These films are especially valuable when examining complex structures in fairly small patients—for example, the stifle joint in toy breeds of dogs or in cats.

INTERPRETATION

Misinterpretation of the partially "blurred" image of a normal structure lying just outside the selected level is one of the great dangers in the reading of tomographs. These false images, when superimposed upon other structures, may appear to represent either diffuse osteolytic lesions of bone, or, perhaps, mineralization in or on the structure under investigation. Examination of a series of tomographs, rather than relying on single films, usually prevents such misinterpretation and helps the observer to gain experience and judgment regarding the significance of the false lesions.

When the basic tissue contrast of structures is low, tomography, especially "thin" sections, is disappointing. It may be necessary to employ a simultaneous contrast procedure to overcome this deficiency. Examples of this would be an excretory urogram with tomography to show small renal tumors or early changes of hydronephrosis and gaseous distension of the stomach and a tomographic study to demonstrate gastric neoplasms (Evans et al., 1955; Pagano and Laudenzi, 1966).

(*Text continued on page 421.*)

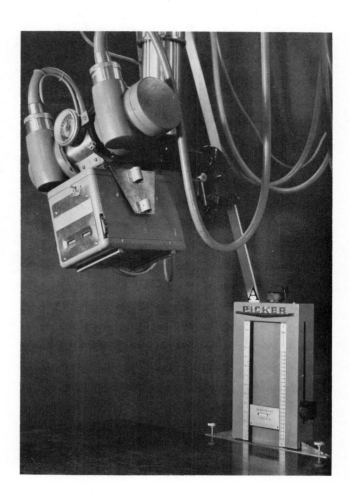

Figure 14–2. Ceiling mounted x-ray tube with collimator and the tomographic attachment clamped to x-ray table top. The flat bar, *A,* links the tube to the Bucky tray.

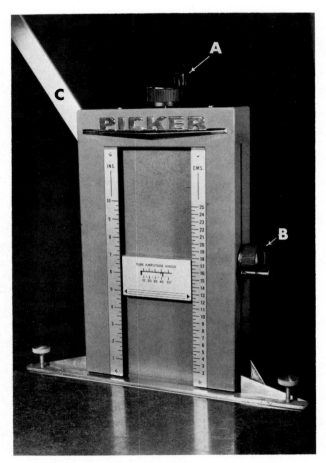

Figure 14–3. The table portion of the tomographic device, showing the adjustment controls. Control *A* varies the level of the fulcrum or pivot point. Control *B* varies the amount of tube travel and measures this as tube amplitude angle. *C* is the linking bar between tube, pivot and Bucky tray.

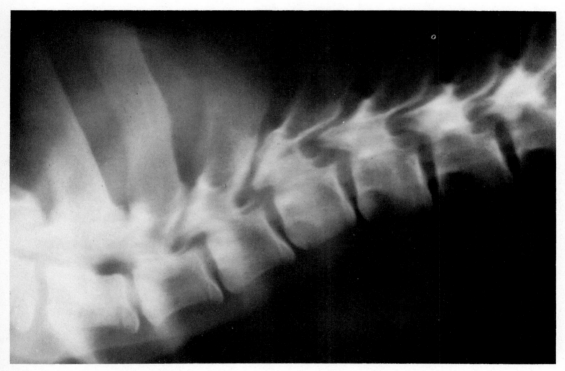

Figure 14–4. Tomogram of the cranial thoracic vertebral column, T1–6, of a year old Great Dane. Note that the scapulas and ribs have been essentially eliminated by the technique. Tube and film motion were parallel to the vertebral column.

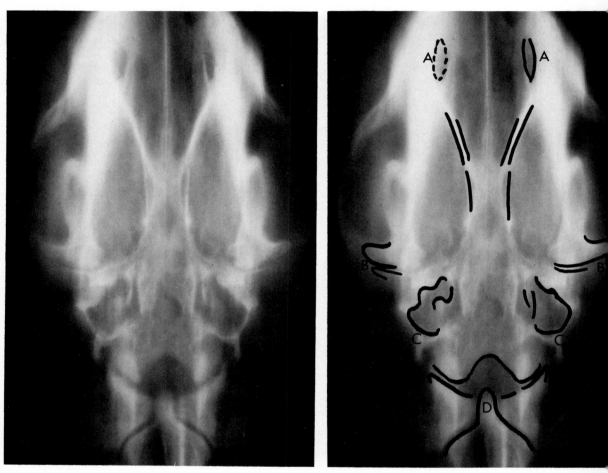

Figure 14–5. *Left*, A tomogram of a ventrodorsal projection of the skull of a dog. *Right*, The level displayed is through a part of the maxillary sinuses *(A)*, the temporomandibular articulations *(B)*, the tympanic bullae *(C)*, and the dens *(D)*.

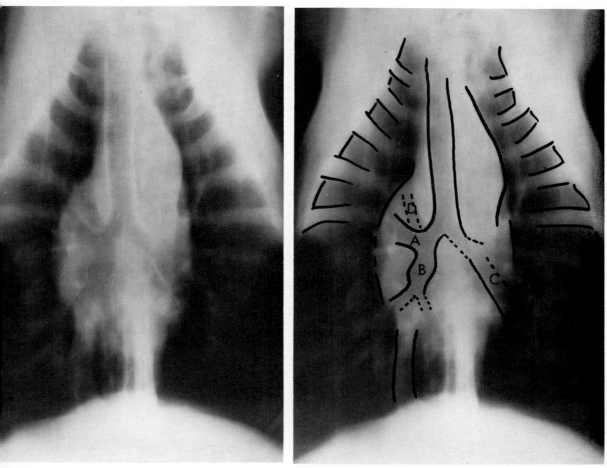

Figure 14–6. *Left,* A tomogram of a dorsoventral projection of the thorax of a three year old St. Bernard. *Right,* This level displays the terminal portion of the trachea, the beginning of the right middle lobe bronchus (*A*), and the beginning of the right caudal lobe bronchus (*B*). The left caudal lobe bronchus (*C*) is at a slightly different level and thus is less evident. The right cranial lobe bronchus (*D*) is evident but poorly defined for the same reason.

REFERENCES

Body-section radiography, its principles and application. Technical Services Bulletin, Milwaukee, General Electric X-Ray Corporation, 1951.

Evans, J. A., Monteith, J. C., and Dublier, W.: Nephrotomography. Radiology, *64*:655–663, 1955.

Geary, C.: Tomography—its place in veterinary radiology. Proceedings of the 15th Gaines Veterinary Symposium, Columbia, Missouri, pp. 4–7, 1965.

Geary, C.: Veterinary tomography. J. Amer. Vet. Radiol. Soc., *8*:32–38, 1967.

Kiefer, J.: The general principles of body section radiography. Radiog. Clin. Photog., *19*:2–10, 1943.

Littleton, J. T., and Winter, F. S.: Linear laminography. A simple geometric interpretation of its clinical limitations. Amer. J. Roentgenol. Radium Ther. Nucl. Med., *95*:981–991, 1965.

McInnes, J.: Trisection radiography. X-Ray Focus, *1*:14–15, 1955.

Pagano, C., and Laudenzi, C.: Tomography and gas distention methods in demonstrating gastric neoplasias. Radiographia, *13*:309–316, 1966.

15

SUBTRACTION RADIOGRAPHY

Roger M. Clemmons

In 1934, a photoradiographic technique was described which would produce subtraction films from two radiographs (Crittenden and Stern, 1966). "When there is a difference between two radiographs of the same part of the body, this difference can be evinced by covering one radiograph with a diapositive of the other" (Vezina and McRae, 1966). Subtraction leaves any elements not common to two superimposed radiographs enhanced in contrast and clarity by subduing or subtracting background details that are common. This technique is particularly useful when performing contrast studies of the skull, in which the removal or subtraction of the bony densities common to radiographs taken before and after contrast media injection leaves only the opacified structures visible. It is a method that can increase the scope of the human eye and "can add significantly to our armamentarium of diagnosis" (Wise, 1965).

Subtraction minimizes confusing shadows of diagnostic radiographs and is used to remove bony detail, enhance the contrast of noncommon elements and increase the recognition of small lesions. The subtraction print will have the background "greyed" out so that only differences between two radiographs will be evident (see Fig. 15–5).

Subtraction has been widely used in medical radiology for cerebral angiography, pneumoencephalography, aortography, myelography, angiocardiography, localization of ocular foreign body, examination of the heart without the use of contrast media, gas myelography and saccrography, examination of carotid-cavernous sinus lesions, examinations of cerebral tumor stains, examinations of lesions in the base of the brain, pyelography, and for many other purposes. The physiology and aberrations in the dynamics of the heart can be studied by this means. Even differences in blood flow through paired organs or between various areas of the same organ can be distinguished.

Movement of an object or part of an object, such as the borders of the heart or calcified areas of the cardiac valves, can be visualized by subtraction (Ziedes des Palantes, 1970). A lighter area in the subtraction print will show from what site a dense part moved and a darker area in the subtraction print will show the new location of the dense object. By taking two radiographs of the eye while the patient looks in different directions, ocular foreign bodies and calcifications can be localized.

Subtraction can be used to discriminate between high and low kilovoltage radiographs of the same object. A special cassette containing two sets of screens which are separated by a copper filter can be used. One pair of screens should be low speed and the other pair should be high speed. The low-speed screens should be on the tube side of the cassette and are used for the production of the low kilovoltage radiograph. The copper filter will increase the mean quantum of energy of the X rays reaching the high-speed screens, thus producing a relatively high kilovoltage radiograph. The mean densities of the soft tissues will be about the same in each radiograph, but the contrast between mineralized areas and normal soft tissues will be much higher in the low kilovoltage radiograph.

The production of a subtraction film from these two radiographs can be used to prove or disprove the presence of various types of dystrophic mineralization. The osseous system can be shown with higher contrast and clarity without the confusing soft tissue shadows. This method is very useful in delineating subtle abnormalities of the musculoskeletal system.

Subtraction will not yield information that is not already present in the radiographs, but will only distinguish between structures that have similar densities and those containing contrast media (Holman, 1966). Therefore, the densities of the radiographs must be great enough to provide sufficient contrast in the lightest areas of the radiographic image to allow for enhancement by subtraction.

INDICATIONS

Subtraction is not advocated for routine cases, but rather for the obscure case in which the information yield is lacking. Such often occurs when producing contrast studies of the skull or vertebral column, where bone densities tend to decrease contrast between the opaque or lucent media and surrounding structures. Small animal radiographic examinations that may be enhanced by subtraction technique are: ventriculography, encephalography, cerebral angiography, sialography, retrobulbar air contrast studies, infraorbital angiography, dacryocystorhinography, cranial sinus and vertebral venography.

TECHNIQUE

Equipment

Some form of a contact printer is necessary. A radiographic cassette, which has the front screen replaced with clear glass, makes a practical contact printer. A black felt surface should be placed on the metal cassette lid to ensure even pressure on the film. The overhead light in the darkroom will work effectively in making the exposures. A more elaborate printer is a 45 × 55 cm box that is 95 cm high, covered with a clear glass plate (ten Cate et al., 1966). Opal glass should be placed between the light source and the clear glass in order to diffuse the light and ensure an even exposure. A radiographic view box is necessary to view and position films. Par speed x-ray film is used for producing the scout and contrast films. A darkroom and tanks or trays are needed for developing film and making exposures. Kodak 4127 Commercial Film with estar thick base for manual processing or Kodak RP/SU X-Omat Subtraction Film for automatic processing is needed. The film pack provides details for usage. Kodak DK-50 Developer for developing the diapositive mask is needed. Normal x-ray developers may also be used.

Procedure

A diagrammatic illustration of subtraction technique is shown in Figure 15–1. Basically, the technique consists of producing a diapositive mask (a reversal of the scout radiograph) from the scout radiograph and superimposing the mask over the contrast radiograph, then printing the final subtraction film from this combination.

Scout and Contrast Radiographs

Routine radiographic examination is used to produce the scout film (Fig. 15–2). Contrast radiographs are made after the injection of contrast media while the patient is in exactly the same position (Fig. 15–3). In some angiographic procedures, it may be desirable to use a post-injection radiograph for the scout film, especially if patient movement is produced during the injection manipulation. When negative contrast media such as air are used for retrobulbar or ventricular studies, long clearing time for the media prevents the use of a post-injection radiograph for a scout film. In these cases, it is suggested that a catheter be placed beforehand between the patient and the

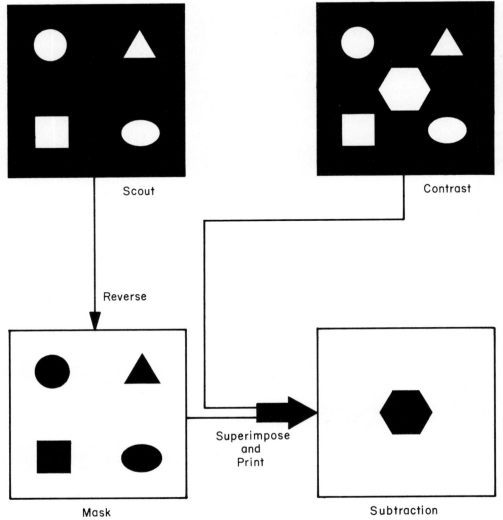

Figure 15–1. Subtraction consists of the production of a diapositive mask from the scout radiograph, the superimposition of the mask over the contrast radiograph, and the production of the subtraction film from the latter combination.

syringe to prevent malpositioning produced by patient manipulation. The preplaced catheter will not interfere with the subtraction film since it represents a radiographic density common to both the scout and contrast radiograph and will be subdued on the subtraction film.

One of the most important considerations in producing good quality subtractions is adequate patient immobilization. Any movement of the body being radiographed between the exposure of the scout and contrast films will drastically mar the results. In veterinary radiography, immobilization must be assured with the use of general anesthesia.

Both scout and contrast radiographs should be of moderate contrast with a density of less than 1.5 units. There should be enough density so that all parts of the radiographs will be exposed. Exposures using a high kilovoltage technique (80 to 100 KV) are important to ensure adequate penetration (Ziedes des Palantes [in press]).

Diapositive Mask

The mask is produced by placing the scout film over the clear glass of the print box. This is then covered with the unexposed mask film[1] with its emulsion facing the scout film (position in the darkroom). The print box or modified cassette is then closed to provide uniform contact of the films.

The mask film is exposed with a 15 watt bulb at a distance of 6 feet for approximately 14 sec. The mask should be developed in a soft developer[2] for approximately five minutes at 20° C (ten Cate et al., 1966). The resultant diapositive mask will possess

reversed densities of the scout radiograph (Fig. 15-4).

The optimum mask should have exactly the same contrast as the scout radiograph. This means that film used to produce the mask should have a long straight density curve corresponding closely to a gamma of one (Wise and Ganson, 1966). Processing the mask in a weak developer will aid in producing this density curve.[3] Incandescent light has been reported to give increased reproducibility of diapositive masks, but several other methods also give satisfactory results (Rice and Barnhardt, 1966).

If the diapositive mask is moderately lighter or darker than the contrast radiograph, only the density of the subtracted

[1]Kodak 4127 Commercial Film for manual processing or Kodak RP/SU X-Omat Subtraction Film for automatic processing.
[2]Kodak DK-50 Developer.

[3]Kodak Dektol Developer diluted 3:1 with water.

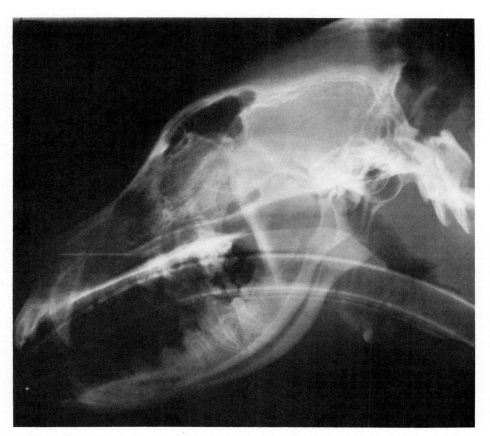

Figure 15–2. Scout film Lateral view of canine skull with radiopaque canula in the infraorbital artery.

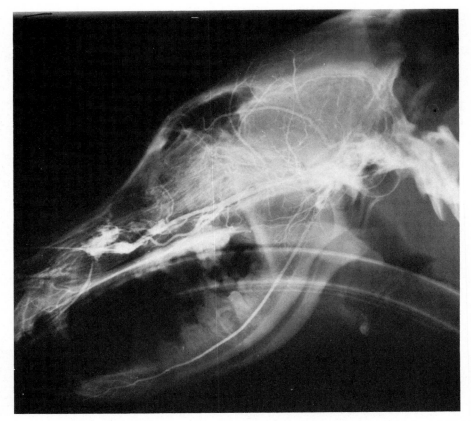

Figure 15–3. Contrast film. Retrograde intraorbital angiogram produced by retrograde injection of 10 cc of 50% Hypaque into the intraorbital artery. Exposure was made immediately after the injection of the contrast medium.

image will be affected. This will minimally affect the masking ability of the diapositive mask. Disproportional densities may greatly impair visualization of the subtracted image, however. The development time of the diapositive mask appears to be a critical factor, and visual control of developing with safelight illumination has been suggested (Levick and Mitchell, 1962). However, it is much better practice to standardize the developing procedure and work with other photographic variables, such as exposure time, rather than alter the developing time.

Because of the difficulty in producing a perfect mask (few films have a density curve over a long enough portion of the curve), a second-order subtraction may be advisable. This is especially important in radiographs that contain large ranges of optical densities. The second-order mask is made by superimposing the scout radiograph and the first-order mask and then exposing them together with an unexposed film to produce the second-order mask. The same materials can be used to make the second-order mask that were used to make the first-order mask; however, exposure should be increased by a factor of approximately three times that of the first-order mask (Oldendorf, 1966). The second-order mask should also be processed in a weak developer.[4] The reverse image of the error of the first-order mask will be represented in the second-order mask. By superimposing both the first and second-order masks over the contrast film, an almost perfect subtraction to the second-order can be obtained.

---

[4]Kodak Dektol Developer diluted 3:1 with water.

Subtraction Film

Place the diapositive mask film next to the glass of the print box. Next, superimpose the contrast radiograph by exactly aligning the common structures. Tape these in place to avoid movement during the placement of the unexposed subtraction film (par speed x-ray film) in the darkroom. The subtracting film is placed adjacent to the felt backing of the print box lid. Superimposition of the mask and the contrast radiograph may be aided by the placement of radiopaque indicators upon the grid before producing the scout and contrast radiographs. The subtraction film is then exposed with a 15 watt bulb at a distance of 6 feet for approximately 30 sec. Development may be accomplished as with routine radiographs.

The resulting subtraction film shows a detailed contrast medium image with a subdued background that represents structures that are common to both the scout and contrast radiographs (Fig. 15–5). In practice, all the background details cannot be cancelled because of the imperfect densitometric diapositive mask (Wise and Ganson, 1966).

A purely photographic technique has the advantage over other methods such as electronic and color subtraction in that it lends itself easily to photographic procedures which may be accomplished at decreased costs. Numerous types of film bases and emulsions may be used advantageously as variables with the photographic technique. Although most radiologists are not photographic experts, the procedures involved in the photographic method are easily learned.

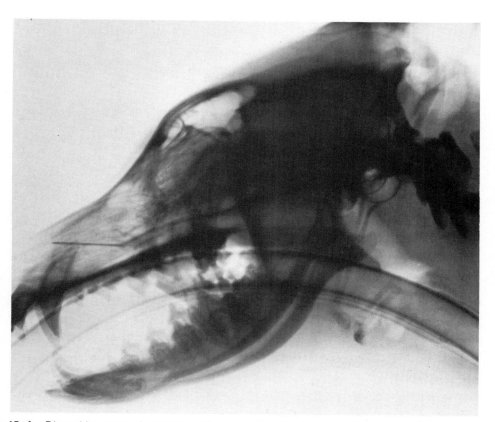

Figure 15–4. Diapositive mask. A reversal of the scout film (Fig. 15–2) produced by exposing Kodak RP/SU X-Omat Subtraction Film to light while in direct contact with the scout film.

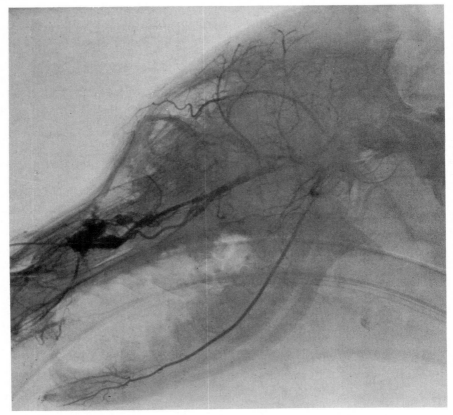

Figure 15–5. Subtraction film. Produced by exposing superimposed contrast film, the diapositive mask and unexposed par speed x-ray film to light. The contrast medium that is not common to the scout and contrast film is enhanced in detail, while common structures such as bone, opaque canula and tracheal tube are subdued as background densities.

REFERENCES

Crittenden, J. J., and Stern, C. A.: Simplified subtraction. Amer. J. Roentgenol., 97:523, 1966.

Hanafee, W., and Stout, P.: Subtraction technique. Radiology, 79:658, 1962.

Holman, C. B.: Evaluation of closed-circuit television techniques in neuroroentgenology. Acta Radiol. (Diagn.) 5:241, 1966.

Levick, R. K., and Mitchell, J.: A simplified method of subtraction and its application of renal arteriography. Brit. J. Radiol., 35:843, 1962.

Oldendorf, W. H.: A modified subtraction technique for extreme enhancement of angiographic detail. Neurology, 15:366, 1966.

Rice, R. P., and Barnhardt, L. E.: A simplified subtraction technique. Amer. J. Roentgenol., 97:529, 1966.

ten Cate, H. W., Jongmans, A., and Ziefes des Palantes, B. G.: Subtraction technique in renal angiography, J. Urol., 95:421, 1966.

Vezina, J. L., and McRae, L. L.: A simple method of subtraction radiography. J. Can. Ass. Radiol., 13:123. 1966.

Wise, R. E.: The value and potential of television in radiologic diagnosis. Surg. Clin. N. Amer., 45:573, 1965.

Wise, R. E., and Ganson, J.: Subtraction of radiographic images by color addition: An inexpensive improved method. Lahey Clin. Found. Bull., 14:131, 1965.

Wise, R. E., and Ganson, J.: Subtraction technique; video and color methods. Radiology, 86:814, 1966.

Ziedes des Palantes, B. G.: Subtraktion: Eine rontgenographische Methode zur separation Abbildung bestimmter Teile des Objekts. Fortschritte Auf dem Gebiete des Rontgenstrahlen, 52:69, 1935.

Ziedes des Palantes, B. G.: Radiographic subtraction. In McLaren, J. W. (Ed.): Modern Trends in Diagnostic Radiology. London, Headley Brothers, Ltd., 1970.

Ziedes des Palantes, B. G.: Subtraction technique. In Newton, T. H. and Potts, D. H. (Eds.): Radiology of the Skull and Brain. Vol. II. St. Louis, C. V. Mosby, 1974.

16

AVIAN RADIOGRAPHIC TECHNIQUE

SAM SILVERMAN

Radiographic examination of the avian patient is a practical procedure applicable to the diagnosis of skeletal, abdominal, and thoracic diseases, some of which are manifested in similar nonspecific clinical signs. When treating avian patients, it is not uncommon to base a diagnosis on specific radiographic changes and nonspecific clinical signs. The inability to rely on clinical pathological tests when treating the avian patient increases the diagnostic and prognostic importance of the radiographic examination (Altman, 1973; Lafeber, 1966, 1968). Over 50 per cent of the avian patients examined at the Veterinary Medical Teaching Hospital at the University of California at Davis are radiographed.

INDICATIONS

Skeletal Conditions

All suspected skeletal diseases or injuries are radiographed in order to obtain the maximum information concerning their extent, chronicity, and possible etiology. The frequency of metabolic bone disease due to dietary imbalance is high. The evaluation of dietary therapy and orthopedic procedures is almost totally dependent on repeated radiographic examinations.

Inflammatory and infectious processes of soft tissue that may extend to skeletal structures such as bumblefoot should also be evaluated radiographically.

Abdominal Diseases

Clinical signs produced by abdominal diseases are often non-organ specific, such as ruffled feathers, general depression, or abdominal distention. The additional information provided by abdominal radiography can supplement physical findings and help to formulate a diagnosis. Identification of altered size, shape, or position of organs (such as hepatomegaly due to fatty infiltration, free abdominal fluid due to peritonitis, and inflammatory processes such as air sacculitis) can be made radiographically.

Respiratory Diseases

Dyspnea is one of the most common clinical signs detected on physical examination of the avian patient. Its etiology often cannot be defined with physical diagnostic techniques, but radiographic examination will usually indicate the site and sometimes the nature of the pathologic condition, and help to differentiate inflammatory, neoplastic, and traumatic etiology. The following are some of the radiographically detectable conditions which may cause dyspnea: tracheitis, tracheal collapse, infraorbital

429

sinusitis, pneumonia, pulmonary hemorrhage, pulmonary gout, air sacculitis, air sac mites, and compression of air sacs and/or lungs by abdominal mass lesions or fluid.

CONTRAINDICATIONS

Radiographic examination of the avian patient is contraindicated when the physical and psychological stresses produced in positioning and restraining the patient are judged to be in excess of what the patient can tolerate. In these cases, radiography is frequently postponed until the patient's general condition is improved by supportive therapy.

ANATOMY

Normal avian abdominal and thoracic structures are easily delineated radiographi-cally—often more completely than is possible in the mammalian species. This phenomenon is due primarily to the presence of the intra-abdominal and intrathoracic gas-filled air sacs, which reproduce the equivalent of a negative contrast study. Figures 16–1 and 16–2 illustrate the normal avian radiographic anatomy (Petrak, 1969).

Alteration in the size, shape, or position of abdominal and thoracic structures can result in the opacification of the air sacs, or in the displacement of other organs. The ventriculus (usually easily identifiable by its radiodense contents) can be displaced characteristically in a number of abdominal diseases. Hepatomegaly displaces the ventriculus caudally and dorsally; caudal abdominal masses displace the ventriculus cranially; and dorsal abdominal masses (e.g., renal tumors) produce ventral displacement of the ventriculus.

Pneumatization and the cortical thickness of the long bones is species-dependent. In-

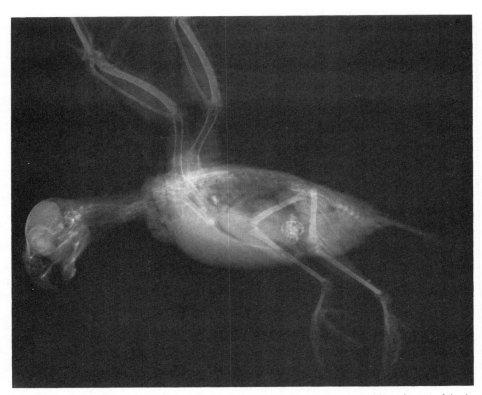

Figure 16–1. Lateral projection of a normal cockatoo. Note that the medullary cavities of most of the long bones show mottled radiodensities that are commonly seen in female birds during egg production.

(Illustration continued on the opposite page.)

creased endosteal and intramedullary bone densities are often noted in egg-producing females. This is a normal finding but can be quite bizarre in appearance.

MATERIALS

X-Ray Machine

The small size of the patient and the rapid respiratory movements necessitate that x-ray exposure times of $\frac{1}{60}$ sec or less be used. Increased radiographic detail can be obtained from an x-ray unit possessing a small focal spot (0.3 mm). If possible, the collimator aluminum equivalent filter should be removed, in order to utilize lower KV X rays.

X-Ray Film and Cassette

Non-screen medical film (Kodak NS 5 4T, Eastman Kodak Co.) or screen film (Cronex 6, E. I. DuPont De Nemours and Co.) with ultra detail intensifying screens (Radelin Ultra Detail Aluminized Maximum Radiation Screens, United States Radium Corporation) may be used. The choice of film depends largely on the detail required in the radiograph and the nature of the examination. The increased detail obtained from nonscreen film must be balanced against the additional exposure required for this film. The longer exposure time required for the nonscreen film often produces radiographs that are less diagnostic than screen film when patient motion is a problem (as in the case of dyspneic patients).

Restraint Apparatus

Positioning the patient on a clear, acrylic material board, utilizing masking tape for restraint, is the method of choice for avian radiography. The masking tape is easy to work with, relatively atraumatic to the patient, and radiolucent compared to other

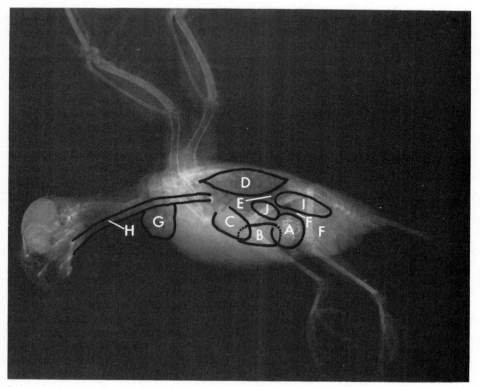

Figure 16–1. *Continued.* Lateral projection of a normal cockatoo. *A,* Ventriculus; *B,* liver; *C,* heart; *D,* lungs; *E,* air sacs; *F,* small intestines; *G,* crop; *H,* trachea; *I,* kidney; *J,* proventriculus.

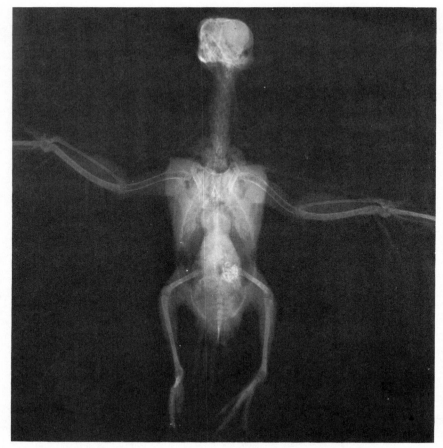

Figure 16–2. Ventrodorsal projection of a normal cockatoo (same patient as in Figure 16–1).

(Illustration continued on the opposite page.)

types of adhesive tape. The acrylic sheet provides a movable restraint surface, which allows the examiner to change film for multiple exposures without having to reposition the patient on a new cassette or film envelope (Figs. 16–3 and 16–4). The acrylic board should not be more than 1/4 inch thick so that the attenuation of the lower KV X rays is minimized.

TECHNIQUE

Anesthesia

Ketamine hydrochloride (Ketamine Hydrocholoride, Vetalar 100 mg/ml, Parke Davis & Co.) administered intramuscularly at a dosage of 10 to 30 mg/lb of body weight, is used routinely when radiographing fractious or excited avian patients. This technique has proven successful in over 200 avian patients, with no adverse reactions attributed to the anesthetic technique. Full recovery usually occurs in 30 to 45 minutes after administration of the anesthesia, thus allowing adequate time to perform the radiographic examination.

Positioning

Abdominal and Thoracic Studies. The entire body cavity of the avian patient is usually radiographed simultaneously, which allows evaluation of abdominal, thoracic,

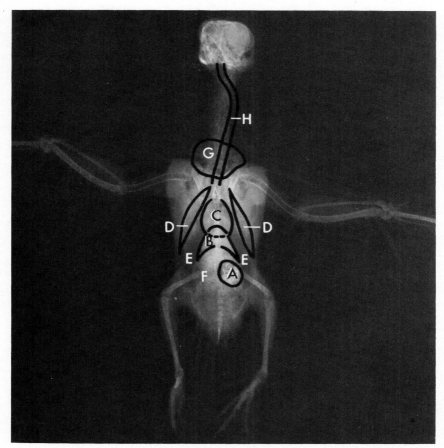

Figure 16–2. *Continued. A,* Ventriculus; *B,* liver; *C,* heart; *D,* lungs; *E,* air sacs, *F,* small intestines; *G,* crop; *H,* trachea.

and a portion of the skeletal structures on a single study.

Patients manifesting marked dyspnea should not be positioned in such a way that the respiratory excursions of their abdominal and thoracic cavities are compromised. Oxygen therapy and the maintenance of body temperature with heat lamps may be used to support the patient during the radiographic examination. On completion of the examination, the patient should be placed in an incubator where temperature, humidity, and oxygen can be regulated.

Lateral body radiographs are produced with the dependent side marked with an appropriate right or left marker, and the dependent extremities positioned cranial to the contralateral extremity (Fig. 16–3). Full extension of the wings and legs will preclude their superimposition on the abdominal or thoracic structures. This projection will also provide a lateral radiograph of the wings or legs. The x-ray beam is centered over the middle of the body.

Ventrodorsal body radiographs require full and symmetrical extension and abduction of the limbs to preclude their superimposition on other organs of interest (Fig. 16–4). The x-ray beam is centered on the midline, slightly cranial to the caudal tip of the sternum. Anteroposterior projections of the legs will be obtained on the ventrodorsal body projections.

Extremity Examinations. Anteroposterior projections of the wings are best obtained with manual positioning of the patient. The

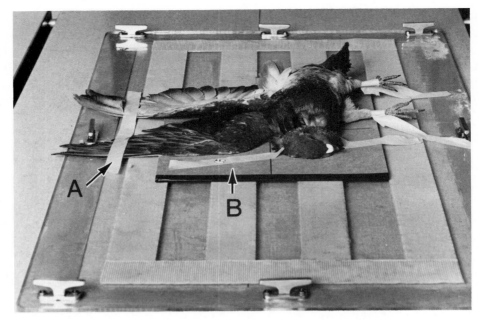

Figure 16–3. Positioning technique for lateral radiograph of an unanesthetized pigeon. The patient is restrained with masking tape (*A*) and is in direct contact with a nonscreen x-ray cassette (*B*). The method shown in Figure 16–4 may also be used if desired.

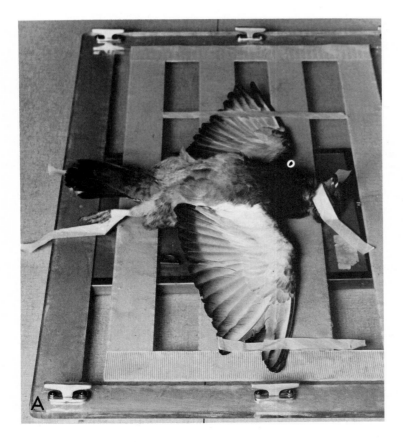

Figure 16–4. Positioning technique for ventrodorsal body radiograph of an unanesthetized pigeon. The bird is attached to a plastic sheet (*A*) with masking tape. The x-ray cassette is placed under the plastic sheet. This method allows for repeated exposures with a minimum of patient movement. The patient may be taped directly to the cassette.

TABLE 16–1

AVIAN RADIOGRAPHIC TECHNIQUES

Subject	Film Type	F.F.D. (Inches)	ma	sec	KV
Canary	NS 54 T	30	100	1/60	70
Parakeet	NS 54 T	27	100	1/60	72
Parrot	NS 54 T	21	100	1/60	72
Red Tail Hawk	Cronex 6*	40	100	1/60	65
Pigeon	Cronex 6*	40	100	1/60	60
Macaw	Cronex 6*	40	100	1/60	72

*Cronex 6 used with ultra-detail cassettes.

remainder of the extremity examination can be obtained with positioning techniques described for abdominal and thoracic radiography. The x-ray beam should be appropriately centered on the area of interest.

Exposure

Exposure factors for some representative avian species are given in Table 16–1. These techniques may require slight modification for use with other x-ray units. Minimization of exposure time and utilization of a small focal spot are desired. Although decreasing the focal film distance from the standard 40 inches will produce some geometric distortion of the image (primarily magnification), it will still produce quality diagnostic radiographs because the patient-film distance is small for most avian species (see Chap. 2).

Radiographic Interpretation

Basic radiographic changes in the avian species are not dissimilar to those detected in the mammalian species. Familiarization with avian anatomy and establishment of a "normal" file of radiographs, arranged according to species, will enhance interpretative ability.

REFERENCES

Altman, R. J.: Cage Birds: Radiography. Vet. Clin. N. Amer., 3:165–173, 1973.

Lafeber, T. J.: Bird clinic cage bird practice today. Animal Hospital, 2:48–55, 1966.

Lafeber, T. J.: Radiography in the caged bird clinic. Animal Hospital, 4:41–48, 1968.

Petrak, M. L.: Diseases of Caged and Aviary Birds. Philadelphia, Lea & Febiger, 1969.

GLOSSARY

Angiocardiography—A contrast study of the cardiovascular system.

Angiography—A contrast study of the arteries.

Anode—The positive terminal of an x-ray tube that contains the target.

Anterior—Situated in front of or in the forward part of, or affecting the forward part of an organ; toward the front part of the body. Used to denote the front surface of a limb.

Anteroposterior (AP) View—A radiograph produced by passing an x-ray beam from the anterior surface to the posterior surface of a limb.

Arthrography—A contrast study of a joint.

Autotransformer—A transformer with insulated primary and secondary windings on one core.

Brachycephalic—Short-headed (such as in breeds like the Bulldog).

Bremsstrahlung X-ray Radiation—X rays that are irradiated from a target atom as a result of electron-target atom attraction which changes the electron direction and decreases velocity, resulting in an energy loss that is irradiated as a continuous spectrum of X rays, depending on the magnitude of direction change that occurs (see Fig. 1–5).

Bucky Diaphragm—The Potter-Bucky diaphragm (named after Dr. Hollis E. Potter, inventor of the movable grid, and Dr. Gustave Bucky, inventor of the grid)—usually shortened to "Bucky" in common usage. This device moves the grid at right angles to the grid strips during exposure so that the white line images of the lead strips are blurred and thereby made indistinguishable.

Cassettes—Light-tight metal cases that are designed to support a pair of intensifying screens and a sheet of x-ray film and to apply moderate pressure to insure good screen-film contact. The front of the cassette is made of plastic or low-atomic-number metal, such as magnesium, and the back of the cassette is a hinged metal lid (see Fig. 2–18).

Cathode—The negative terminal of an x-ray tube that contains a heated, electron-emitting surface.

Caudal—Denoting a position more toward the tail than some specific point of reference.

Characteristic X-ray Radiation—X rays that are irradiated from a target as a result of inner (K or L shell) orbital electron removal by an accelerated electron interaction. Outer orbital electrons then fill the vacated orbits in sequence, and the difference in their binding energies is irradiated. The term "characteristic" is derived from the fact that these radiations are characteristic for a given target atom, since the differences in orbital electron-binding energies are unique (see Fig. 1–5).

Cholecystography — A contrast study of the gallbladder and bile ducts.

Cineradiography — A motion picture filming of the output of image intensification fluoroscopy.

Collisional Interactions — Two types of collisional interactions may occur when a target is bombarded by electrons of the energy range used in medical radiography. Both types result in heat loss. (1) An incoming electron may excite an outer orbital electron of a target atom by passing in near proximity to its orbit, thus transferring energy. This allows the orbital electron to increase its distance from the nucleus. When the excited orbital electron returns to its original orbit, energy is irradiated as heat (see Fig. 1–1*A*). (2) If an incoming electron possesses sufficient energy to remove an outer electron from a target atom, the atom is ionized. The ejected electron and the incoming electron may undergo further interactions with target atoms. The total energy is eventually dissipated as heat (see Fig. 1–1*B*).

Compton Absorption — That mode of electromagnetic energy absorption that is independent of the number of electrons per gram of absorbing material. This mode of x-ray absorption becomes increasingly important in the upper range of x-ray energies used in medical radiography (see Fig. 2–9).

Cone — A cylindrical device that is placed on the output window of the x-ray tube housing for purposes of restricting the size of the primary x-ray beam (see Fig. 2–13).

Contralateral — Situated on or pertaining to the opposite side.

Cranial — Denoting a position more toward the head than some specific point of reference.

Dacryocystorhinography — A contrast study of the nasolacrimal duct.

Developer Solution — A solution of reducing agents that continues the process initiated by the photon interaction that formed the latent image. Electrons made available from the reducing agents allow an increased number of reduced silver atoms (metallic silver) to form, which appear as black foci on the finished radiograph.

Diaphragm — A variable sized rectangular device that is placed on the output window of the x-ray tube housing for purposes of restricting the size of the primary x-ray beam (see Fig. 2–13).

Diaphysis — The shaft of a long bone.

Dolichocephalic — Long-headed (such as in breeds like Collies).

Dorsal — Pertaining to the back or denoting a position more toward the back surface.

Dorsoventral (DV) View — A radiograph produced by passing an x-ray beam from the dorsal to the ventral surface of the skull, neck, trunk or tail.

Epiphysis — The ends of a long bone. Separated from the metaphysis by the physis during the growth of an animal.

Esophagram — A contrast study of the esophagus.

Filter — A thin sheet of aluminum that is placed over the output window of an x-ray tube for the purpose of removing the less energetic, less penetrating X rays from the primary x-ray beam.

Fixer Solution — Fixer solution removes the unexposed (unreduced) silver salts from the x-ray film emulsion after the development process. Sodium or ammonium thiosulfate is the principal chemical used in fixer solutions. These chemicals "clear" the film and leave only black metallic silver atoms in the emulsion. Fixer solutions also contain a hardener (usually salts of aluminum) to prevent excessive swelling and softening of the emulsion during washing and to reduce the drying time.

Fluoroscope—A fluoroscope is a device used to record an x-ray image on a fluorescent screen instead of film.

Focal-Film Distance (FFD)—The distance from the x-ray source (tube target) and the x-ray film surface.

Focal Spot—The area on the surface of the tungsten target that is bombarded by electrons during x-ray production (see Fig. 1–8).

Focused Grid—A grid is composed of strips that are placed parallel to the primary x-ray beam and at increasing angles to the grid surface near the periphery of the grid (see Fig. 2–16). This design allows the primary beam to expose the periphery of the film with nearly the same intensity as the central ray.

Grid—A series of thin, linear strips of alternating radiodense and radiolucent materials, which are encased in a rectangular wafer (see Fig. 2–14) used to reduce scatter radiation.

Grid Efficiency—Grid efficiency is governed by the grid ratio. Grids with greater ratios remove scatter radiation more efficiently.

Grid Ratio—The ratio of the height of the strips to the distance between the radiodense strips.

"Heel Effect"—Unequal distribution of the x-ray beam intensity emitted from the x-ray tube. With a target angle of 20 degrees to the central x-ray beam, the distribution of beam intensity decreases rapidly toward the anode due to absorption of the x-ray beam by target and anode material (see Fig. 1–6).

Image Amplifiers—Electronic devices that are used to amplify a fluoroscopic image. The devices consist of a fluorescent screen which is bonded to a light-sensitive photocathode which produces low energy photoelectrons that are accelerated toward a small fluorescent anode (output viewing screen) (see Fig. 2–21). The net result of photoelectron acceleration and image concentration is image intensification.

Intensifying Screens—Sheets of luminescent chemicals applied to a supporting base, which fluoresce when irradiated and emit foci of light in areas in which X rays have penetrated a patient, thereby exposing the x-ray film that is placed in close contact to the screens.

Ipsilateral—Situated on or pertaining to the same side.

Kilovolts (KV)—1000 volts. KV as applied to radiographic technique indicates the voltage applied across an x-ray tube (from cathode to anode).

Latent Image—When the sensitive speck (silver sulfide incorporated within the silver halide crystals of x-ray film) acquires a negative charge from a liberated outer orbital electron of a silver halide atom during x-ray exposure, the positive silver ion is attracted to the sensitive speck where it is reduced to a silver atom. This process is repeated several times, the number depending upon the number of X rays interacting on a given area of film. Silver halide crystals, in which the sensitive specks have acquired silver atoms during x-ray exposure, are invisible and constitute the latent image.

Metaphysis—A zone of spongy bone located between the physis and diaphysis of long bones.

Milliampere (ma)—1/1000 ampere. Ma as applied to radiographic technique indicates the milliamperes of current flow from cathode to anode in an x-ray tube during the production of a radiograph.

Milliampere-seconds (mas)—The product of the value of milliamperes of current flow across the x-ray tube and the number of seconds the current is allowed to flow. It is thus a measure of the relative number of total X rays generated during an exposure.

Myelography—A contrast study of the subarachnoid space of the spinal cord.

Oligocephalic—Normal-sized head (such as in breeds like the Beagle).

Parallel Grid—A grid composed of strips that are placed perpendicular to the grid surface (see Fig. 2–15).

Photoelectric Absorption—The mode of electromagnetic energy absorption that depends on the number of electrons per gram of absorbing material. This mode of absorption is very important in the energy range used in medical radiography and accounts for the differential absorption of X rays by the various tissues of the body (see Fig. 2–9).

Physis—The cartilaginous growth plate that is located between the metaphysis and epiphysis of growing long bones.

Plantar Surface—That part of the rear limb that is in contact with the surface when standing.

Posterior—Situated behind or toward the rear. Used to denote the rear surface of a limb.

Posteroanterior (PA) View—A radiograph produced by passing an x-ray beam from the posterior surface to the anterior surface.

Pneumoventriculography—An air contrast study of the ventricular system of the brain.

Pronate—To turn a limb inward so that the volar or plantar surface faces downward and the dorsum upward.

Prone—Lying with the ventrum downward.

Radiographic Contrast—Differences in the densities of the various subjects on a finished radiograph. These differences are a function of both film contrast and subject contrast.

Radiographic Density—The degree of blackness possessed by a finished radiograph. Density is a quantitative measure.

Radiographic Detail—The degree of sharpness of the individual shadows on a finished radiograph. Detail is essentially a visual quality.

Radiographic Fog—A general or local deposition of silver on a finished radiograph produced by extraneous radiation or chemical reaction. Fog decreases radiographic detail by imparting a grey appearance to the light areas of a finished radiograph.

Radiative Interactions—If an incoming electron possesses sufficient energy to remove an inner (K or L shell) orbital electron from a target atom, radiative interaction occurs. The ejected electron is replaced by an outer orbital electron and the difference in binding energies is irradiated as characteristic x-ray radiation (see Fig. 1–4A). If an incoming electron approaches the nucleus of a target atom and is attracted toward the positive nucleus, the incoming electron changes direction and loses velocity and the lost energy is irradiated as "bremsstrahlung" x-ray radiation (see Fig. 1–4B).

Reciprocating Bucky—A movable grid driven by a solenoid that works against a spring tension on the opposite end of a slide mechanism. This mechanism oscillates continuously without manual loading.

Recipromatic Bucky—A movable grid that is driven by an electric motor.

Roentgen—A quantity of X or gamma radiation such that the associated corpuscular emission per 0.001293 gm of air (1 cc of dry air at 0° C and 760 mm of Hg barometric pressure) produces, in the air, ions carrying one electrostatic unit of electrical charge of either positive or negative sign.

Roentgen Equivalent Man (rem)—A dose of any ionizing radiation absorbed per gram of living matter such that the relative biological effectiveness (rbe) is the same as 1 rad (radiation absorbed dose) of 200 to 250 KV X rays. For diagnostic x-ray exposure the rem, rad and roentgen of exposure are equal.

Rostral—Denoting a position more near the tip of the nose than some specific point of reference.

Sagittal—Situated in the direction of the ventrodorsal plane or a section parallel to the long axis of the body.

Scale of Contrast—A description of the relative densities on a finished radiograph. A radiograph with an increased scale of contrast possesses more shades of grey and a radiograph with a short scale of contrast possesses a more nearly black and white image.

Scatter Radiation—That radiation that has interacted with the patient's tissues and is scattered multidirectionally. This radiation is reduced in energy compared to the primary x-ray beam.

Sialography—A contrast study of the salivary ducts and glandular ductules.

Spot Film—A radiograph produced during a fluoroscopic examination by a device that places an x-ray cassette in the fluoroscopic beam.

Subtraction Radiography—A photographic technique used to subtract or subdue radiographic densities common to a pair of radiographs produced of the same region and preserve and enhance visualization of densities not common to the two radiographs (see Chapter 15). Common medical usage is found during contrast studies of the brain or other organs where radiographs are produced before and after contrast medium introduction.

Supinate—To turn a limb so that the volar or plantar surface faces upward; also to rotate a limb outward.

Supine—Lying on the back or on the dorsum with the dorsum turned downward.

Target—An area on the surface of an x-ray tube anode that contains a focal spot.

Tomography—A technique of producing radiographs of selected thin planes or layers of the living patient (see Chapter 14).

Urethrogram—A contrast study of the urethra.

Urinary Cystography—A contrast study of the urinary bladder.

Urogram—A contrast study of the kidneys and ureters.

Ventral—Pertaining to the belly or denoting a position more toward the belly surface.

Ventrodorsal (VD) View—A radiograph produced by passing an x-ray beam from the ventral to the dorsal surface of the skull, neck, trunk or tail.

Videoradiography—The display of the output of image intensification fluoroscopy on a television screen. This image may also be recorded on magnetic video tape.

Volar Surface—That surface of the forelimb that is in contact with the surface when standing.

X-ray Film—A photographic film formed by layering a silver halide-containing emulsion on each side of a supporting polyester sheet (see Fig. 2–7).

X Rays—Electromagnetic radiations of wavelengths less than 100 Å produced by the interaction of an electron beam with a material such as tungsten.

INDEX

Page numbers in *italics* refer to illustrations; (t) indicates tables.